Advances in Ophthalmology

Advances in Ophthalmology

Edited by **Ray George**

hayle
medical

New York

Published by Hayle Medical,
30 West, 37th Street, Suite 612,
New York, NY 10018, USA
www.haylemedical.com

Advances in Ophthalmology
Edited by Ray George

International Standard Book Number: 978-1-63241-030-6 (Hardback)

Printed in the United States of America.

Contents

Permissions

List of Contributors

Preface

This book has been a concerted effort by a group of academicians, researchers and scientists, who have contributed their research works for the realization of the book. This book has materialized in the wake of emerging advancements and innovations in this field. Therefore, the need of the hour was to compile all the required researches and disseminate the knowledge to a broad spectrum of people comprising of students, researchers and specialists of the field.

Ophthalmology is advancing at a fast pace. This book deals with diverse features of ophthalmology - the medical discipline of analysis and management of eye diseases. It is separated into a variety of clinical sub-areas of expertise, such as cornea, cataract, glaucoma, uveitis, retina, neuro-ophthalmology, pediatric ophthalmology, oncology, pathology, and oculoplastics. This book presents innovative improvements and forthcoming viewpoints in ophthalmology. It discusses basic concepts regarding ophthalmology. It also elucidates topics related to cornea and ocular surface, refraction and refractive correction, and glaucoma. It intends to provide some fruitful information for experts and students involved in this field.

At the end of the preface, I would like to thank the authors for their brilliant chapters and the publisher for guiding us all-through the making of the book till its final stage. Also, I would like to thank my family for providing the support and encouragement throughout my academic career and research projects.

Editor

Part 1

Basic Concepts in Ophthalmology

Lasers in Ophthalmology

Magdalena Zdybel, Barbara Pilawa and Anna Krzeszewska-Zaręba
Medical University of Silesia in Katowice
Poland

1. Introduction

Lasers emit electromagnetic waves of characteristic properties and energies (Gilmour, 2002; Krzeszewska & Zdybel, 2010; Podbielska et al., 2004; Sieroń et al., 1994; Ziętek, 2009). These specific features are used in the modern ophthalmology (Dick et al., 2010; Evans & Abrahamse, 2009; Gilmour, 2002; Schmidt-Erfurth, 2010; Seitz & Langenbucher, 2000; Soong & Malta, 2009). In this work we described theoretic problems of lasers as the quantum systems, the propagation of laser radiation, the lasers parameters and ranges of them. The historical data about laser apparatus and their applications are cited. The biophysical effects caused by laser radiation in biological structures during therapy are mentioned.

The applications of lasers in ophthalmology are widely taking to account. We described widely the two laser applications in ophthalmology which are connected with paramagnetic species and singlet oxygen. We chose these subjects, because of our experimental experience in spectroscopic studies of paramagnetic centers (Beberok et al., 2010; Buszman et al., 2003, 2005a, 2005b, 2006; Chodurek et al., 2003; Domagała et al., 2008; Latocha et al., 2004, 2005, 2006; Matuszczyk et al., 2004; Najder-Kozdrowska et al., 2009, 2010; Pilawa et al., 2002, 2003a, 2003b, 2005a, 2008c; Zdybel et al., 2009, 2010) and singlet oxygen O_2 with zero spin (Bartłomiejczyk et al., 2008; Latocha et al., 2008; Pilawa et al., 2005b, 2006, 2008a, 2008b). In this work the view of the information in scientific papers is done.

2. Lasers as the quantum systems – Basic theory

2.1 Energy levels

The quantum theory describes the energy levels of atoms and molecules (Glinkowski & Pokora, 1993; Sieroń et al., 1994; Ziętek, 2009). Electrons may move only between these levels, and these transitions are accompanied by emission or absorption of energy by the optical system. The emitted or the absorbed energies reveal the values related to the distances between the energy levels. The system will not absorb the energy, when the energy is lower or higher than the value of the energetic band between the levels. Energy levels of the optical active medium play an important role in laser irradiation. The energy levels of the materials used in laser construction determine the energy necessary to their excitation and the energy of emitted electromagnetic waves is dependent on these levels. The energy (E) of the electromagnetic waves produced by lasers is presented according to the formulas (Bartosz, 2006; Hatfield, 1976; Hewitt, 2001; Jaroszyk, 2008; Ziętek, 2009):

$$E = hv \qquad (1)$$

$$E = hc/\lambda \qquad (2)$$

where h is the Planck constant (h = 6,626 x 10^{-34} Js), c is the speed of the waves (c = 299 792 458 m/s), v is the frequency of electromagnetic waves in Hertz, λ is the wavelength in meters. The frequency and wavelength determine the color of laser radiation.

The emitted energy is fitted to the biological structures treated by the individual lasers, so the reason of the majority of lasers used in ophthalmology is understandable. Summing up, the lasers produce electromagnetic waves with the given energy correspond to the energy levels of their optical systems, and it interact on the specific tissues or cells.

2.2 Optical pumping

Condition of absolute emission of radiation by laser is the previous excitation of its active optical system e.g. molecules formed in this system (Glinkowski & Pokora, 1993; Sieroń et al., 1994; Ziętek, 2009). This excitation is called the optical pumping. Excitation of molecules in laser may be done by electromagnetic waves emitted by lamps, by heating or by energy of electrical field (Podbielska et al., 2004; Sieroń et al., 1994).

2.3 Inversion of electron location on the energy levels

As the result of the optical pumping of the quantum molecular system, higher amount of electrons are located on the levels of the higher energy than those of the lower energy (Glinkowski & Pokora, 1993; Podbielska et al., 2004; Sieroń et al., 1994; Ziętek, 2009). The continuous propagation of energy to the system of electrons in molecules causes that the electrons upon absorption of this energy moves to the higher energy levels. Afterwards they return to the lower energy states via relaxation processes. The time of electron-lattice relaxation processes depends on the molecular structure of the optical system in lasers. Electron-lattice relaxation is the transition of the electrons from the excited energy levels to the ground energy levels via magnetic interactions with diamagnetic lattice molecules (Stankowski & Hilczer, 2005; Wertz & Bolton, 1986). The long time of interactions of electrons with the lattice causes the mentioned above inversion. The pumped electrons stay on the higher energetic level and the former irradiation of the molecular system in laser do not pump electrons to the higher levels, because of their absence in the lower energy levels (Ziętek, 2009). The inversion of electrons location on levels is useful to the former effective stimulation emission of radiation in laser apparatus (Glinkowski & Pokora, 1993).

2.4 Stimulated emission of radiation

The name of the **LASER** apparatus comes from the roles of its work as the "Light Amplification of Stimulated Emission of Radiation" (Maiman, 1960). Two types of emission of electromagnetic waves, the spontaneous and stimulated emissions, are known (Bartosz, 2006; Hatfield, 1976; Hewitt, 2001; Jaroszyk, 2008; Krzeszewska & Zdybel, 2010; Morrish, 1970; Sieroń et al., 1994). Spontaneous emission is the ordinary effect of energy loosening by the excited electrons at the non defined moment. Spontaneous emission is the result of the principle that the optimal state of the system is the state with the lowest energy (Glinkowski & Pokora, 1993; Jóźwiak & Bartosz, 2008; Sieroń et al., 1994; Ziętek, 2009). The stimulated emission is the most important effect to produce laser irradiation. The scheme of stimulated emission of radiation is shown in Figure 1, which was prepared according to the definition of this effect presented in (Sieroń et al., 1994). The stimulated emission of radiation is the controlled effect of energy loosening by the electrons. Before the proper effect of stimulated emission the electron is excited, for example by pumped photons, to the higher energy level. After this the stimulated photon is emitted to the system and at this moment two photons of the same energy are emitted. The energy of the individual emitted photon is equal to the difference between energy of the excited and ground state energy levels. The amplification of the energy of radiation is the effect of emission of these two photons after absorption of one exciting photon by electron. The radiation comes from stimulated emission consist of photons of the same energy so of the same frequency. It means that laser produce monochromatic electromagnetic waves. Monochromatic electromagnetic waves are the same frequency waves (Ziętek, 2009).

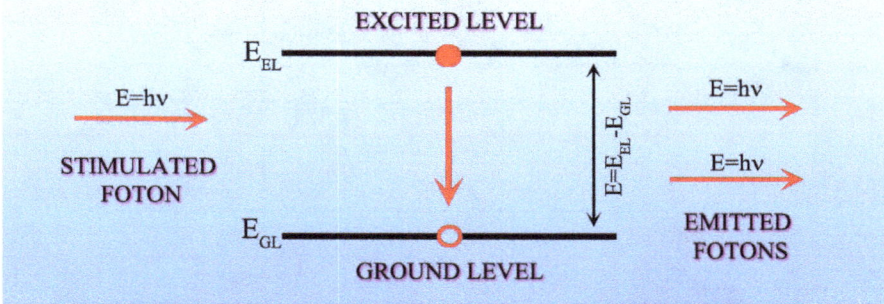

Fig. 1. The scheme of the stimulated emission of radiation prepared according to its definition in (Sieroń et al., 1994).

The exemplary way of the electrons between the three energy levels during laser action is described in work of Sieroń et al. (Sieroń et al., 1994). The main energy levels of electrons are the ground, non-stabile excited, and the quasi-stabile levels, respectively. Electrons are pumped by photons to the non-stabile level with the highest energy in this quantum system. Energy of the pumped photons is equal difference between energy of the non-stabile level and the ground level. Afterwards the electrons without radiation come to the quasi-stabile energy level located lower than the non-stabile level. During the optical pumping there is an increase in number of electrons on quasi-stabile level. At the moment dependent on the type of laser the effect of inversion of distribution of electrons in the energy levels occurs. The higher number of electrons stays on the quasi-stabile level than on the ground level with the lowest energy. The pumping is stopped then and the stimulating photons are sent to the electrons system. At the same time, at the moment of interactions of electrons with stimulated photons the stimulated emission appears. All the electrons located on the quasi-stabile energy level come to the ground energy level. The photons connected with the transition and the stimulated photons are irradiated. The emitted electromagnetic waves have properties of laser radiation, which are described in the next part of this chapter.

3. The properties of laser radiation

Laser radiation as electromagnetic waves differs from the light emitted by the ordinary lamp (Hewitt, 2001). The white light emitted from bulb is superposition of electromagnetic waves with frequencies and wavelengths corresponding to the background colors: red, orange, yellow, green, blue, and violet. The frequencies of the waves increase in the previously given order, and the wavelengths decreases in this manner. The summing of these electromagnetic waves of different colors gives the effect of white light. The component waves in the white light are not coherent. Coherent waves are the waves with the same phase shift (Ziętek, 2009). The component electromagnetic waves in the beam of white light are shown in Figure 2a constructed according to (Hewitt, 2001).

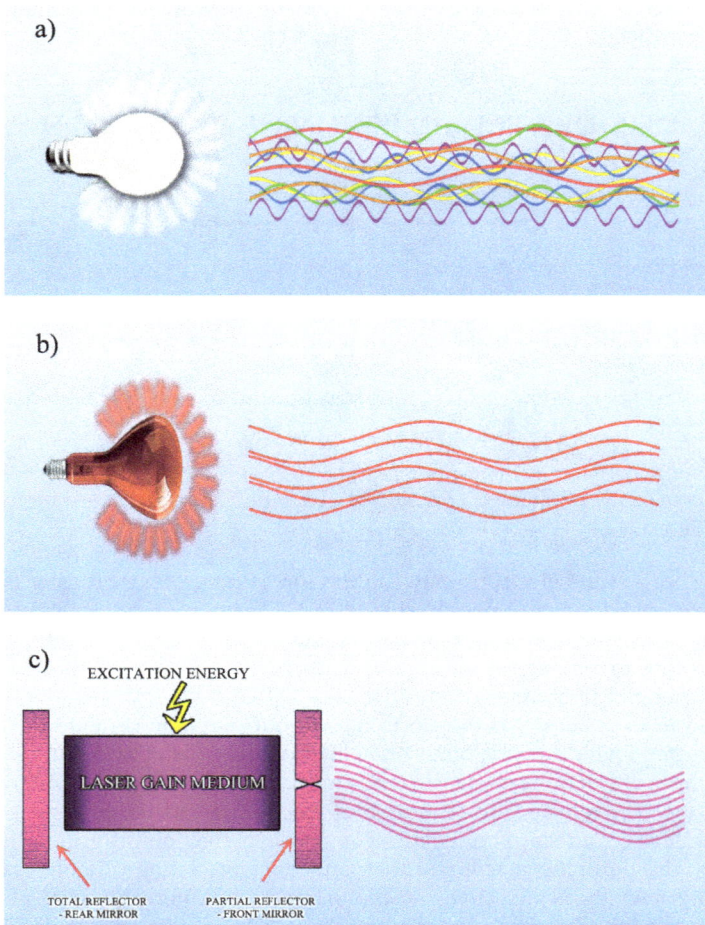

Fig. 2. The electromagnetic waves emitted by: the ordinary lamp produced the white light (a), the source of the monochromatic light (b), and laser (c). The scheme is prepared according to (Hewitt, 2001).

The monochromatic light from the lamp consists of electromagnetic waves of the same frequencies and the same wavelengths (Hewitt, 2001). The waves are not coherent. The electromagnetic waves in the beam of monochromatic light reveal different phases. The monochromatic and incoherent waves are presented in Figure 2b, which was prepared according to (Hewitt, 2001). The fine examples of monochromatic light are the red waves emitted by SOLLUX lamp (Hewitt, 2001).

Lasers produce monochromatic electromagnetic waves (Glinkowski & Pokora, 1993; Hewitt, 2001; Sieroń et al., 1994; Ziętek, 2009). The properties of laser radiation distinguish it from the ordinary white or monochromatic light (Figure 2c) (Hewitt, 2001). The laser waves are monochromatic and coherent. Contrary to white light, laser radiation is monochromatic and in the same phase.

Laser radiation differs from electromagnetic waves sending by the therapeutic BIOPTRON lamps (Straburzyńska-Lupa & Straburzyński, 2004). The BIOPTRON lamp produces electromagnetic waves of the same frequency, but they are incoherent (Figure 3) (Straburzyńska-Lupa & Straburzyński, 2004). The maxima and minima of energy appear on the area of the tissue exposed to coherent laser irradiation. The homogeneous distribution of energy on irradiated area is characteristic for BIOPTRON light.

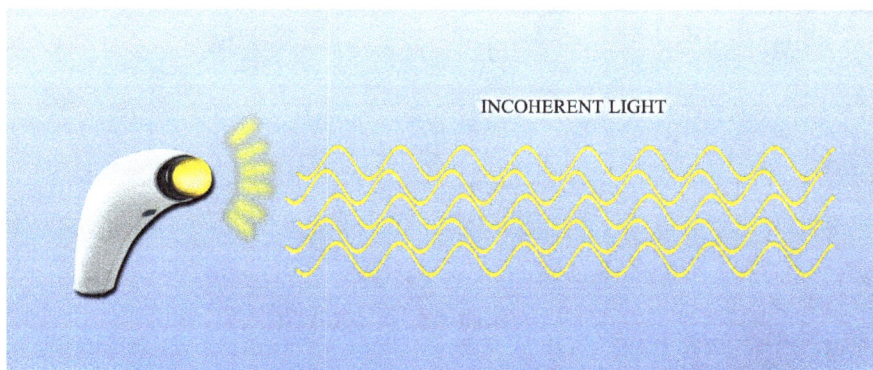

INCOHERENT LIGHT

Fig. 3. The electromagnetic waves emitted by BIOPTRON lamps. Prepared according to (Straburzyńska-Lupa & Straburzyński, 2004).

Laser electromagnetic waves in the environment propagate as perpendicular electric and magnetic fields (Hewitt, 2001). The ranges of wavelength of electromagnetic waves emitted by lasers are showed on figure 4. The values of the wavelengths are cited from (Gilmour, 2002; Ziętek, 2009). The biophysical and biological effects on tissues depend on the energy and the wavelengths of electromagnetic waves (Gilmour, 2002; Jaroszyk, 2008).

There are three basic effects of lasers on biological tissues: photochemical (photoablation and photoradiation), thermal (photocoagulation and photovaporation), and ionizing (photodisruption) (L'Esperance, 1983; Podbielska et al., 2004). The photochemical effects are the result of absorption of energy of laser radiation by molecules in tissues without their destruction. During photoablation the absorption of laser energy causes the increase of temperature of the tissues. Practically the photoablation is caused by the short laser pulses of high energy. Photoradiation is the effect which appears after the transition of the excited by laser molecules in tissues to the ground or the lower energy levels with accompanied radiation of electromagnetic waves. These electromagnetic waves may be responsible for biostimulation effects and tissue temperature rise. Thermal effects interact mainly by the increase of temperature of the tissues after laser irradiation. Photocoagulation causes the increase of temperature in tissues up to 80-90°C via absorption of the laser energy.

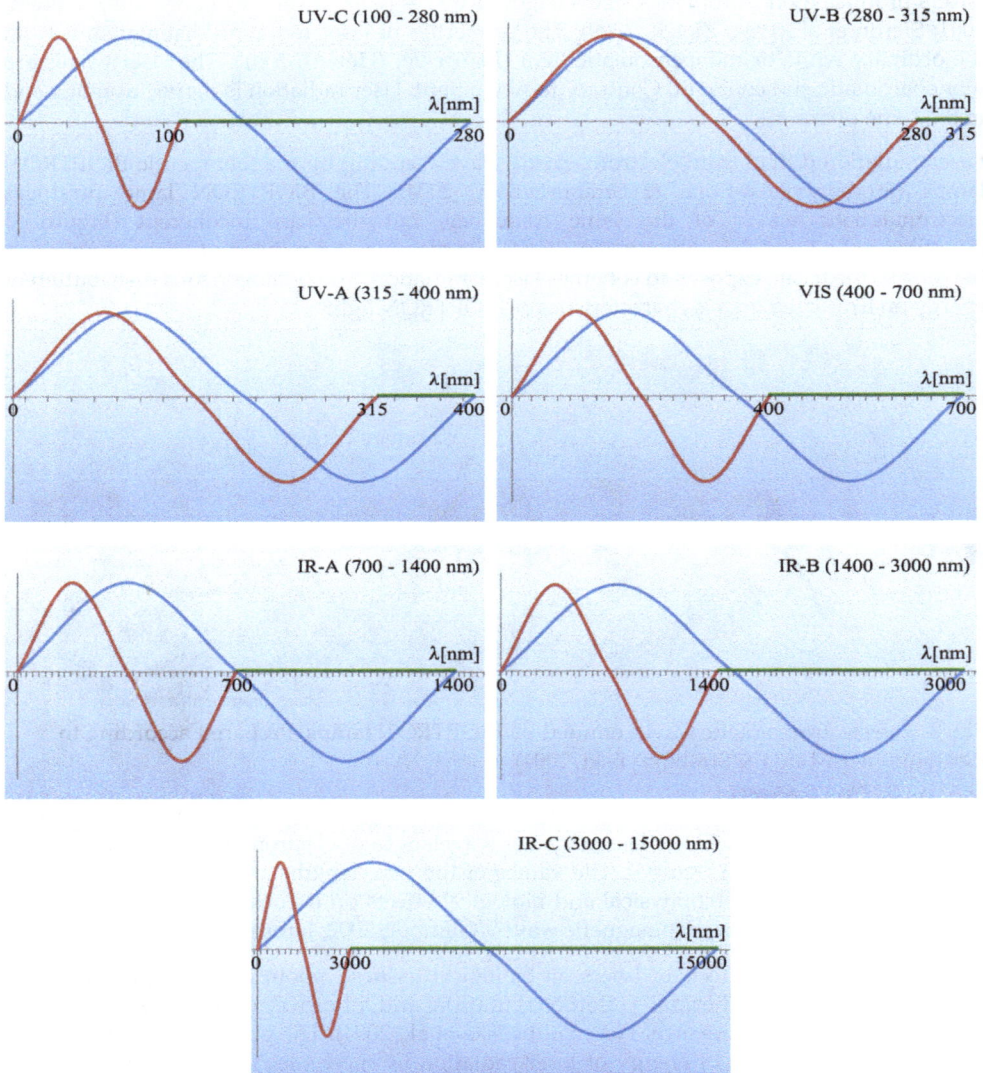

Fig. 4. The ranges of length of electromagnetic waves emitted by lasers. The values of the wavelengths (λ) are cited from (Gilmour, 2002; Ziętek, 2009).

The photocoagulation closes blood and lymphatic vessels, and causes of the necrosis of tissues. Photocoagulation denatures proteins and inactivates enzymes. The laser irradiation of high energy which causes the increase of temperature of the tissues up to 100-300°C is called as the photovaporation. The using of lasers with the high energy of pulse lead to photodisruption effects via ionization in tissues. The ionization is accompanied by the formation of shock waves. The photodisruption effects play an important role in the microsurgery of the front part of the eye.

UV-C and UV-B waves cause increase of pigmentation, burns and photokeratitis (Ziętek, 2009). UV-A waves cause burns, photosensitizing reactions, intensification of dark pigment production, and cataract (Ziętek, 2009). The visible light may destruct retina, lead to burn, and photosensitizing reaction. IR-A and IR-B waves may be responsible for burns and the others thermal destruction of epithelium and cataract. IR-B and IR-C waves may destruct cornea (Ziętek, 2009).

4. History of lasers application in ophthalmology

The history of lasers is connected with the basic theory of quantum radiation presented by Albert Einstein in 1916 (Wróblewski, 2006). This theory defines and characterizes spontaneous and stimulated emission of radiation by atoms. The method of optical pumping of atoms was discovered by Alfred Kastler and Jean Brossel in 1949 (Wróblewski, 2006) and in 1966 Kastler received the Nobel Prize. The inversion of electron localization on energy levels and the effect of stimulated emission of radiation were practically discovered by Edward Purcell and Robert Pound in 1950 (Wróblewski, 2006). In 1960 Theodore Harold Maiman constructed the ruby laser ($Al_2O_3:Cr^{3+}$) emitting light of 694 nm, which is still used in ophthalmology (Seitz & Langenbucher, 2000; Wróblewski, 2006; Ziętek, 2009). In Poland the first ruby laser was constructed by Zbigniew Puziewicz group from Military University of Technology in 1963 (Podbielska et al., 2004). The following types of lasers: helium-neon (He-Ne) (1150 nm), semiconducting, carbon dioxide (CO_2) (10600 nm), argon (476.5 nm, 488.0 nm, 514.5 nm), hydrogen (H_2) (102.5-123.9 nm), excimer (172 nm), and gallium nitride (GaN) (365 nm), were built in 1961, 1962, 1963, 1964, 1970, 1974, 1991, respectively (Ziętek, 2009). The krypton (647.1 nm, 568.2 nm, 530.8 nm) and neodymium: yttrium-aluminum-garnet (Nd:YAG) (1064 nm) lasers were introduced to clinical applications in 1972 and 1980, respectively (L'Esperance, 1983).

The ruby (694 nm) laser is used in the therapy of the following ocular structural defects: retinal tears, peripheral pigmentary degeneration and lattice degeneration of the retina (L'Esperance, 1983). Argon laser is used in the structural defects of the retina and choroid (L'Esperance, 1983). Krypton (647.1 nm) laser is mainly used in outer retinal structural diseases (L'Esperance, 1983). Krypton red laser photocoagulation is exemplary performed in retinal hemorrhagic diseases, retinal edematous diseases, pigment epithelial abnormalities (L'Esperance, 1983). Carbon dioxide laser is applied in operations with the high blood loss (L'Esperance, 1983).

In 1940 light was used in ophthalmology to coagulation of the retina by Gerd Meyer-Schwickerath (Seitz & Langenbucher, 2000). In Poland the first ruby (694 nm) laser coagulator to ophthalmology was constructed in 1965 (Podbielska et al., 2004). In 1961 Campbell applied confocal laser system to retinal coagulation. In 1971 argon laser was by the first used in eye surgery (Seitz & Langenbucher, 2000). In 1977 Nd:YAG (1064 nm) laser was used to microexplosion by Franz Fankhauser and Daniele Aron-Rosa. The history of lasers in ophthalmology is broadly described in the paper of Berthold Seitz (Seitz & Langenbucher, 2000).

5. Types of lasers using in ophthalmology

The group of lasers used in ophthalmology produces coherent electromagnetic radiation of different wavelengths (Dick et al., 2010; Evans & Abrahamse, 2009; Gilmour, 2002; Schmidt-Erfurth, 2010; Seitz & Langenbucher, 2000; Sieroń et al., 1994; Soong & Malta, 2009). Optical systems of ophthalmologic lasers are: CO_2, excimer, argon, tunable dye, Nd:YAG (Gilmour, 2002). Optical systems of excimer lasers contain molecules of dimmers of noble gases as argon fluoride (ArF), krypton fluoride (KrF) and xenon fluoride (XeF) (Ziętek, 2009).

The therapeutic effects as photocoagulation, photoablation, ablation via plasma, interact on eye structures. Photocoagulation is performed by the following lasers: blue-green (488-514 nm) and green (514 nm), argon, krypton red (647 nm), diode infrared (810 nm), Nd:YAG infrared (1064 nm) (Gilmour, 2002). Photoablation is carried on by lasers: excimer ultraviolet (193 nm), holmium: yttrium-aluminum-garnet (Ho:YAG) infrared (2060 nm), erbium: yttrium-aluminum-garnet (Er:YAG) infrared (2940 nm), and CO_2 infrared (10,600 nm). Ablation by plasma is done by pulsed infrared neodymium: yttrium lithium fluoride Nd:YLF (1053 nm) laser (Gilmour, 2002).

6. Parameters of lasers radiation using in ophthalmology

The power of laser is the energy emitted by laser during one second (L'Esperance, 1983; Sieroń et al., 1994). The lasers of low (4-5 mW), medium (6-500 mW), and high (above 500 mW) powers are used in medicine (Sieroń et al., 1994). The examples of lasers of low, medium and high powers are ruby, Nd:YAG, semiconducting (Podbielska et al., 2004; Ziętek, 2009). The lasers of low powers are called the soft lasers, and lasers which emit electromagnetic wave of high power are called hard lasers. The classification of lasers correspond to their irradiated power are shown in Figure 5 (Glinkowski & Pokora, 1993; Sieroń et al., 1994).

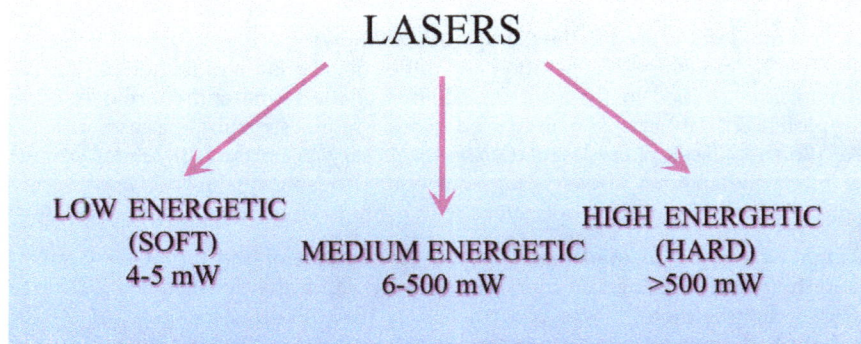

Fig. 5. Classification of lasers corresponds to power of radiation. The values of electromagnetic powers are sited from (Glinkowski & Pokora, 1993; Sieroń et al., 1994).

The biophysical effects in biological systems under laser irradiation are described by Sieroń et al. (Podbielska et al., 2004; Sieroń et al., 1994). Photochemical, thermal and acoustic effects appear during laser radiation propagation in biological samples. Photochemical reactions mainly exist in melanin biopolymers, enzymes, photosensitizers, and hemoglobin, which strongly absorb its energy. Thermal effects take place not only in the irradiated units, but they are also observed in the neighboring structures, because of thermal conductivity of the tissues. The lasers of the highest power cause heating, strong electric field, microplasma formation, increase of pressure, and as the result acoustic effects appear in the tissues.

The soft lasers with the low energy emitted to tissues during one second are used to biostimulation effects (Podbielska et al., 2004; Sieroń et al., 1994). The soft ruby lasers with low energy may be used to biostimulation (Podbielska et al., 2004). The light initiates and increases biochemical reactions. Lasers of medium power are applied in photodynamic therapy. Hard lasers are used to destruction of tissues mainly via thermal effects (Sieroń et al., 1994). Non-thermal effect of photo-destruction occurs in the irradiated structures, when the laser of high power interacts with biological system during the very short time (Podbielska et al., 2004; Sieroń et al., 1994). Free radicals may be produced by lasers of the three mentioned above ranges of power.

The power dose, time, methods, and pulse frequency should be taken to account during planning the laser therapy (Podbielska et al., 2004; Sieroń et al., 1994; Ziętek, 2009). The power, density of power, and density of energy should be correlated to the application of laser. Density of laser power I [W/m^2] is the power related to one square meter of the irradiated area. Density of laser energy H [J/m^2] is the power related to one square meter of the irradiated area (Podbielska et al., 2004; Sieroń et al., 1994; Ziętek, 2009).

7. Application of lasers in ophthalmology

The large amount of laser applications in ophthalmology is known. In that kind of medicine the excimer, argon, krypton, Er:YAG, Nd:YAG and semiconductor lasers are usually used (Dick et al., 2010; Evans & Abrahamse, 2009; Gilmour, 2002; Schmidt-Erfurth, 2010; Seitz & Langenbucher, 2000; Soong & Malta, 2009). The use of lasers in ophthalmology comes down to coagulate, cut and leads to photoablation. Laser radiation can reach the eyeball and focus on the retina and other locations within the eye without surgical intervention. The most common disease which are treated with laser light are glaucoma, cataract, retinal detachment, diabetic retinopathy (Fankhauser & Kwasniewska, 2003; Gilmour, 2002).

Glaucoma is an eye disease in which the optic nerve suffers damage (Chung & Guan, 2006; Eckert, 2010; Herdener & Pache, 2007; Hoffmann & Schulze, 2009; Juzych et al., 2004; Kanamori et al., 2006; Keicher & Stoffelns, 2010; Ngoi et al., 2005; Preußner et al., 2010; Schlote et al., 2008; Wilmsmeyer et al., 2006). It causes permanently decay of vision and if it is untreated it progresses to complete blindness. Glaucoma is often associated with increased pressure of the eye fluid (Gilmour, 2002). The cases in which there is constantly raise of intraocular pressure without any associated optic nerve damage are called ocular hypertension. In that case there is no glaucoma damage. The cases in which there is normal or low ocular pressure with typical for glaucoma visual field are called normal or low tension glaucoma. However, raised intraocular pressure is still the most significant risk factor for glaucoma progression. The permanent damage of the optic nerve and blindness are the effects of untreated glaucoma (Chung & Guan, 2006; Eckert, 2010; Herdener & Pache,

2007; Hoffmann & Schulze, 2009). There are two main categories of glaucoma - open or closed angle. First of them progresses much slower than the other and in this case patient can have any notice of vision lose. In the closed angle glaucoma, the symptoms of disease can appear rapidly (Chung & Guan, 2006). Gradual loss of vision occurs with open angle and chronic angle-closure glaucoma and with acute angle-closure glaucoma. That is why that kind of disorder it is recognized when the disease is quite advanced. In glaucoma once lost visual field cannot be recovered. There is about two percent chance of glaucoma progression in people with a family history of this eye disease. Both laser surgeries and conventional surgeries are performed to treat glaucoma. Selective laser trabeculoplasty (SLT) is one of the newest, efficient methods for the treatment of open angle glaucoma, pseudoexfoliative glaucoma and pigmentary glaucoma. In that kind of treatment Q switch Nd:YAG laser with a wavelength of 532 nm is usually used (Eckert, 2010; Gilmour, 2002). This laser affects on the cells of the trabecular meshwork but it does not cause any destruction or coagulation. The second method of laser treatment in glaucoma is argon laser trabeculoplasty (ALT). That method is focused on drainage correction of fluid from the eye. As a result the intraocular pressure is lower (Wilmsmeyer et al., 2006). In open angle glaucoma the drainage site of the eye does not function normally. In that disorder the iris is encircled by the trabecular meshwork of an eye. The increase of pressure is the result of difficult in drainage. In ALT therapy an argon laser beam is directed at the trabecular meshwork. As the effect the trabecular meshwork drain fluid more effectively (Eckert, 2010; Wilmsmeyer et al., 2006). Nd:YAG and argon lasers are used in iridotomy (L'Esperance, 1983). Argon lasers may be used in iridoplasty (L'Esperance, 1983).

Laser therapy is used in cataract too (Baratz et al., 2001; Çinal et al., 2007; Gilbert, 2011; Hille et al., 2001; Kanellopoulos & Group, 2001; Mahdavi, 2011; Shammas & Shammas, 2007; Verge´s & Llevat, 2003). The cataract is a disease that develops in the crystalline lens of an eye. It can block the passage of light and causes problems from slight to complete opacity. In age-related cataract the power of the lens may be increased, causing near-sightedness called myopia. The opacification of the lens may also reduce the perception of blue colors. Cataract typically progresses slowly and causes vision loss (Gilmour, 2002). That kind of disease potentially induces blinding if it is untreated. Cataract usually affects both eyes, but in most cases one eye is affected earlier than the other. A senile cataract which occurs in the elderly is characterized by an initial opacity and subsequent edema of the lens. One of the most popular cataract treatments nowadays is laser surgery, which uses light to dissolving cataract. The most popular method of cataract surgery is phacoemulsification. In that kind of treatment nucleus is cracking or chopping into smaller pieces. This fragmentation makes emulsification easier. Emulsification of the lens using the Er:YAG laser is very effective for performing small incision cataract surgery in eyes with soft and medium nuclei. The small ablation zones which are created during treatment can help prevent damage to surrounding ocular structures. The Er:YAG technique causes low ablation energy and does not result in thermal injury (Duran & Zato, 2001). Another method involves the removal of almost the entire natural lens while the elastic lens capsule is left intact to allow implantation of an intraocular lens. It is called conventional extracapsular cataract extraction (ECCE). That kind of treatment may be indicated for patients with very hard cataracts or other situations in which phacoemulsification is problematic. Increasingly to remove the pupillary membranes developed after ECCE is used Nd:YAG laser (Kozobolis et al., 1997). Intracapsular cataract extraction (ICCE) is rarely performed kind of cataract surgery, because of high rate of complications. It involves the removal of the lens and the surrounding lens capsule in one piece. After lens removal, an artificial plastic lens - implant is placed (Gilbert, 2011; Kanellopoulos & Group, 2001).

Lasers are also used in medical operations in the field of refractive eye surgery (Gilmour, 2002; Glinkowski & Pokora, 1993; Kim et al., 2011). The main aim of that kind of treatment is to achieve the correct relationship between the length of the eyeball and the power of its optical centers. This is possible by modifying the other shell knobs and intraocular tissues. Refractive surgery can eliminate the necessary of use the contact lenses or glass (Krzeszewska & Zdybel, 2010).

At the beginning of the development of refractive eye surgery procedures used CO_2 lasers (Glinkowski & Pokora, 1993; Kim et al., 2011). However, because of emerging adverse effects they were abandoned. Currently pulsed excimer laser emitting a beam with a wavelength of 193 nm is used during surgeries. The pulses from the beam which is transmitted last from 10 ns to 20 ns. This laser radiation penetrates the cornea to a depth of 1 μm leading to photoablation of the tissue (Krzeszewska & Zdybel, 2010). This is the most common refractive method nowadays. Excimer laser ablation is done under a partial-thickness lamellar corneal flap. While refractive surgery is becoming more affordable and safe, it may not be recommended for everybody. Patients that have medical conditions such as glaucoma, diabetes uncontrolled cardiovascular disease, autoimmune disease, pregnant women or people with certain eye disease are not good candidates for refractive surgery (Kim et al., 2011). Although the risk of complications is decreasing compared to the early days of refractive surgery, there is still a small chance for serious problems. It may appear vision problems such as double-vision, ghosting, halos, starbursts and dry-eye syndrome. Refractive surgery is used in myopia, hyperopia and astigmatism treatment (Gilmour, 2002; Seitz & Langenbucher, 2000).

Myopia is an eyes disease with a refractive defect (Gilmour, 2002). In that kind of disorder while accommodation relaxes, the collimated light produces image focus in front of retina. In other words it is a condition of the eye where the light that comes in does not directly focus on the retina. Because of that the image that one sees is out of focus when looking at a distant object but comes into focus when looking at a close object (Seitz & Langenbucher, 2000).

Hyperopia is a vision defect caused by an imperfection of an eye causing difficulty focusing on near objects and in extreme cases causing a sufferer to be unable to focus on objects at any distance. In that kind of disease power of the cornea and lens is insufficient and the image appears blurred (Gilmour, 2002).

Astigmatism is the visual defect, which is the result of an inability of the cornea to properly focus an image onto the retina. As the effect the image is blurred (Seitz & Langenbucher, 2000).

Laser subephithelial keratomileusis (LASEK) and laser in-situ keratomileusis (LASIK) processes are very common in laser surgery (Gilbert, 2011; Hille et al., 2001; Kanellopoulos & Group, 2001; Verge's & Llevat, 2003). In LASEK which is the laser epithelial keratomileusis, the cornea's surface layer is treated with alcohol and peeled back to reshape the layer underneath. LASIK prevents most problems of postoperative pain, slow rehabilitation and corneal haze (Kanellopoulos & Group, 2001; Shammas & Shammas, 2007).

Lasers are also very useful tools in the management of malignant and benign intraocular lesions, nowadays. One of the most popular methods for small melanomas treatment is transpupillary thermotherepy (TTT) using 810 nm infrared laser. That kind of treatment can be used in medium and large melanomas as combination therapy with other treatment modalities (Gilmour, 2002).

The important application of lasers in the modern ophthalmology is their use in photodynamic therapy (PDT) (Podbielska et al., 2004). Photodynamic therapy was recently used to treat wet age-related macular degeneration (AMD). That kind of therapy was used for monitory of cases in AMD (Gilmour, 2002; Nakata et al., 2011). Now PDT is used in polypoidal choroidal vasculopathy (Akaza et al., 2007; Nakata et al., 2011; Podbielska et al., 2004). In PDT lasers with the medium range of electromagnetic radiation power are used (Podbielska et al., 2004). The molecules of photosensitizers and their excitation by laser play the most important role in this method. Laser radiation of the proper energy excites the photosensitizer molecules, which come to the next excited energy level, and after it comes to the lower energy level via sending the energy to the eye structures. The scheme of the processes in photodynamic therapy is presented in Figure 6. This scheme was prepared according to the work (Podbielska et al., 2004).

These optical processes form reactive free radicals and oxygen molecules O_2 in the singlet state in eye (Fig. 6) (Podbielska et al., 2004). Free radicals and oxygen molecules damage the pathologically changed structures in eye. Free radicals are the paramagnetic molecules containing unpaired electrons and the short lifetime characterize them, because of free radicals interactions with both dia- and paramagnetic molecules in tissues. Mainly the reactive oxygen species are formed upon laser irradiation during photodynamic therapy, especially hydroxyl radicals (OH) and superoxide radical anion (O_2·) (Podbielska et al., 2004). Single oxygen molecules are diamagnetic, but this oxygen form is higher reactive than paramagnetic oxygen molecules in the ground state, because of the most molecules in the environment are diamagnetic, so the reactions between the similar units go easier (Bartosz, 2006; Podbielska et al., 2004).

Free radicals and singlet oxygen in the physiology are not expected, but their formation in the pathological state of organism during photodynamic therapy is the most important effect (Bartosz, 2006; Jóźwiak & Bartosz, 2008; Podbielska et al., 2004). Free radicals and singlet oxygen damage the pathologically changed tissue. The condition of laser irradiation should be fitted to the conditions of the highest formation of free radicals and singlet oxygen.

Free radicals ($S = 1/2$) may be directly detected by electron paramagnetic resonance (EPR) spectroscopy (Eaton et al., 1998; Jóźwiak & Bartosz, 2008; Kęcki, 1999; Kirmse & Stach, 1994; Morrish, 1970; Stankowski & Hilczer, 2005; Symons, 1987; Wertz & Bolton, 1986). Electron paramagnetic resonance effect is characteristic for unpaired electrons located in magnetic field of magnetic induction B (Stankowski & Hilczer, 2005; Symons, 1987; Wertz & Bolton, 1986). The electromagnet and the cavity of EPR spectrometer is presented in Figure 7. The Zeeman splitting of energy levels occurs in magnetic field. The spin magnetic moments orientations - parallel and anti-parallel to magnetic field are responsible for Zeeman Effect. Zeeman Effect is the effect of splitting of energy levels of unpaired electrons in the magnetic field as the result of parallel or non parallel electron magnetic moments orientations in this field (Stankowski & Hilczer, 2005; Wertz & Bolton, 1986). The quantization of magnetic moments of unpaired electrons with spin S in magnetic field results from the $2S + 1$ (S, S-1, ..., -S) possible values of magnetic spin quantum number M_S. Energy of these states is given by the following formula (Stankowski & Hilczer, 2005; Wertz & Bolton, 1986):

$$E(M_S) = g\ \mu_B\ B\ M_S \tag{3}$$

where: E – energy, M_S – magnetic spin number, g – spectroscopic factor, μ_B – Bohr magneton, B – induction of magnetic field.

PHOTODYNAMIC THERAPY

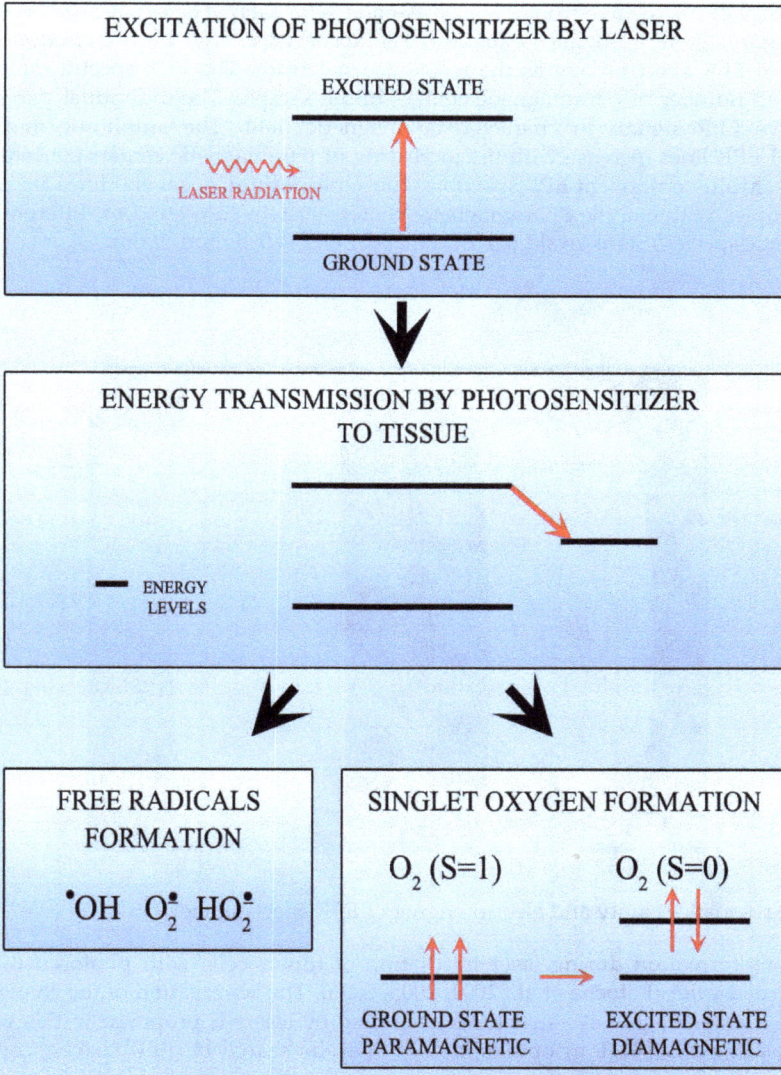

Fig. 6. Photodynamic therapy processes. Prepared according to (Podbielska et al., 2004).

Unpaired electrons are excited to the higher energy levels in magnetic field by microwaves (Stankowski & Hilczer, 2005; Symons, 1987; Wertz & Bolton, 1986). The energy of microwaves (hv) must be fitted to the distances between energy levels (ΔE) of unpaired electrons (Stankowski & Hilczer, 2005; Wertz & Bolton, 1986):

$$hv = \Delta E = g\, \mu_B\, B \tag{4}$$

where v is the frequency of microwaves.

The frequency of microwave from the basic X-band is 9.3 GHz. The equation (4) is called the electron paramagnetic resonance equation. The absorbed energy by unpaired electrons is presented in EPR spectroscopy as the resonance spectrum. The EPR spectra inform about the type and number of paramagnetic centers in the sample. The individual paramagnetic centers give EPR signals in characteristic magnetic field. The amplitude and integral intensity of EPR lines increase with the increasing of paramagnetic centers concentration in the sample. Multi-component EPR spectra as the superposition of several lines are measured for the samples with complex paramagnetic centers system consisting of different types of paramagnetic species (Stankowski & Hilczer, 2005; Wertz & Bolton, 1986).

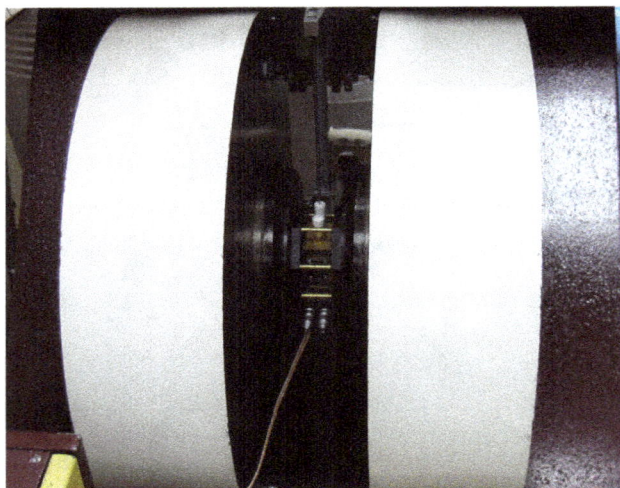

Fig. 7. The resonance cavity and electromagnet of EPR spectrometer.

Free radicals formation during laser irradiation of tumor cells with photosensitizers was studied by us earlier (Latocha et al., 2004, 2005, 2006). The observation of the changes of the amount of free radicals in eye structures irradiated by lasers is proposed in this work. The optimal conditions of PDT in ophthalmology may be search by EPR spectroscopy as the conditions with the highest free radical formation. Similar application was discussed by us for PDT of different tumor cells (Latocha et al., 2004, 2005, 2006).

The optimal conditions of photodynamic therapy are also accompanied by the highest formation of singlet oxygen. Singled oxygen as the diamagnetic molecule may be measured by EPR spectroscopy only by the use of oximetric probes. Oximetric probe is the paramagnetic sample which EPR spectrum strongly changes under changes of the concentration of singlet oxygen in its environment. Our previous results indicates that coal multi-ring aromatic samples may be used as the oximetric probes (Bartłomiejczyk et al., 2008; Latocha et al., 2008; Pilawa et al., 2005b, 2006, 2008a, 2008b). The coal oximetric probes were synthesized by Helena Wachowska group from Institute of Chemistry of Adam Mickiewicz University in Poznań (Poland). Scheme of the idea of application of EPR method and coal oximetric probe is shown in Figure 8. Coal paramagnetic probe contains chemical structures with unpaired electrons with the high probability of interactions with oxygen molecule O_2. Before laser irradiation paramagnetic molecules in the ground triplet state with spin of 1 mainly exist in the environment of the oximetric probe. Paramagnetic oxygen quenches EPR lines of coal probe. After laser irradiation the amount of paramagnetic oxygen molecules decreases, so the amplitudes of the EPR lines of coal probe increase. Under laser irradiation the paramagnetic oxygen molecules become diamagnetic, so the increase of the EPR line of coal probe is proportional to the singlet oxygen formation (Bartłomiejczyk et al., 2008; Latocha et al., 2008; Pilawa et al., 2005b, 2006, 2008a, 2008b). Such methods may be proposed in ophthalmology.

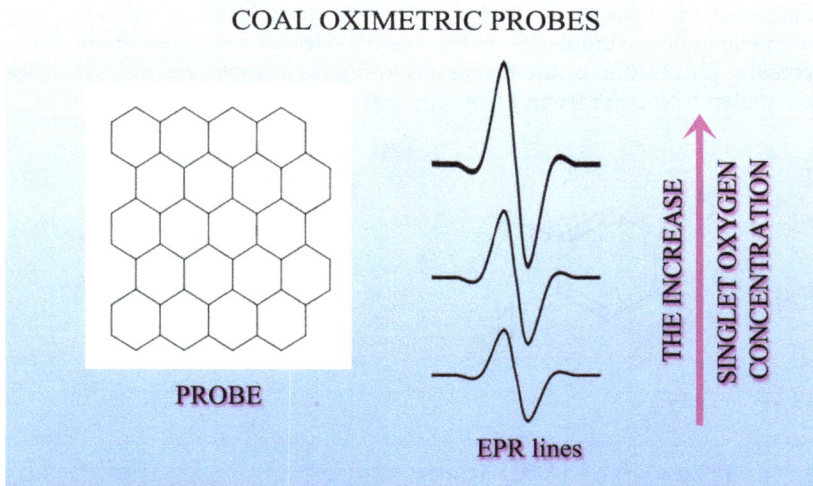

Fig. 8. Potential coal oximetric probe and the changes of its EPR line with increasing of singlet oxygen concentration in the environment.

Lasers in ophthalmology is used to the damage the eye structures via conducting of the energy from melanin biopolymer to them (Gilmour, 2002). Mainly eumelanins with the chemical structure presented in Figure 9 exist in eye (Bilińska et al., 2002; Pasenkiewicz-Gierula, 1990; Sarna, 1981; Zdybel, 2008).

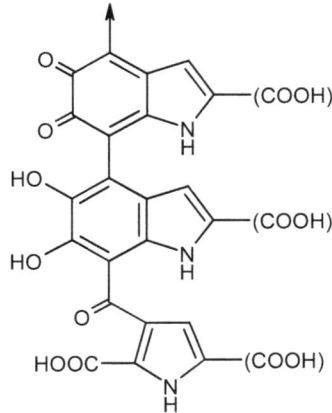

Fig. 9. The chemical structure of eumelanin polymer (Wakamatsu & Ito, 2002).

Melanins are the paramagnetic polymers with o-semiquinone free radicals with spin of 1/2 and biradicals with spin of 1 incorporated in their structure (Kozdrowska, 2006; Najder-Kozdrowska et al., 2009, 2010; Pilawa et al., 2004; Sarna, 1981; Zdybel, 2008). o-Semiquinone free radicals structure is presented in Figure 10 (Kozdrowska, 2006; Pasenkiewicz-Gierula, 1990; Sarna, 1981). Our earlier EPR studies of human retinal pigment epithelium melanosomes from young and old donors pointed out that the amount of free radicals depend on the age and method of irradiation (Bilińska et al., 2002). It seems that free radical reactions in melanin of eye influences on therapeutic effect of laser irradiation. This problem is the interesting proposition of the future electron paramagnetic resonance studies of free radicals and melanin biopolymer and laser application in ophthalmology.

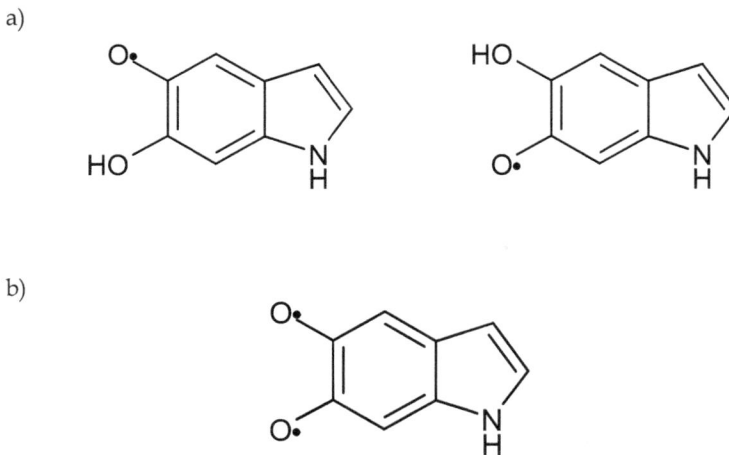

Fig. 10. o-Semiquinone free radicals (a) (Pasenkiewicz-Gierula, 1990; Sarna, 1981) and biradicals (b) (Kozdrowska, 2006) existing in melanin.

The second types of paramagnetic centers – biradicals in melanin were discovered in the last years (Kozdrowska, 2006; Najder-Kozdrowska et al., 2009, 2010; Pilawa et al., 2004; Zdybel, 2008). It is possible that biradicals of melanin could play the role in interactions of laser radiation with eye structures.

The free radicals and biradicals may be differentiated and detected by electron paramagnetic resonance spectroscopy (Kozdrowska, 2006; Najder-Kozdrowska et al., 2009, 2010; Pilawa et al., 2004; Zdybel, 2008). Integral intensities of EPR lines of free radicals and biradicals change differently with the increasing of the measuring temperature (Fig. 11) (Hatfield, 1976). Such dependences were obtained for melanin paramagnetic centers differ in spins (S: 1/2 and 1) (Hatfield, 1976; Kozdrowska, 2006; Najder-Kozdrowska et al., 2009, 2010; Pilawa et al., 2004; Zdybel, 2008).

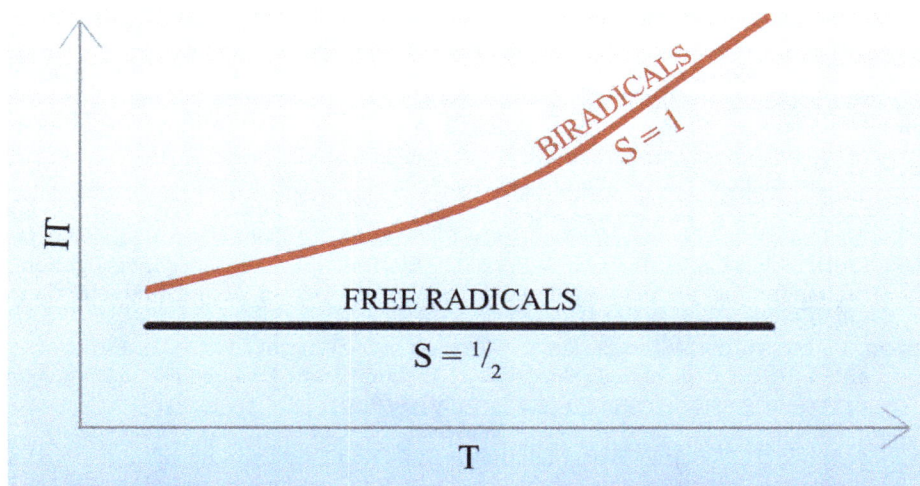

Fig. 11. Changes of integral intensity of EPR lines of free radicals (S = 1/2) and biradicals (S = 1) with the measuring temperature according to functions in (Hatfield, 1976).

The following theoretical functions for free radicals and biradicals in melanin were used (Hatfield, 1976; Kozdrowska, 2006; Zdybel, 2008):

$$IT = C \quad \text{for } S = \tfrac{1}{2} \tag{5}$$

$$IT = D/(3 + \exp(J/kT)) \quad \text{for } S = 1 \tag{6}$$

where: I – integral intensity of EPR lines, T – temperature, S – spin, k – Boltzmann constant, C, D, J – coefficients in the equations.

The electron paramagnetic resonance spectroscopy could be very useful in modern ophthalmology. EPR is the physical method of examination of paramagnetic species which does not damage the sample. The conditions of the laser therapy may be spectroscopically found and the reactions in the eye structures may be tested.

8. Acknowledgements

The EPR studies of paramagnetic centers in Department of Biophysics in 2011 are financially supported by Medical University of Silesia in Katowice, Poland; grant number KNW-1-086/P/1/0.

9. References

Akaza, E.; Yuzawa, M.; Matsumoto, Y.; Kashiwakura, S.; Fujita, K. & Mori R. (2007). Role of photodynamic therapy in polypoidal choroidal vasculopathy. *Japanese Journal of Ophthalmology*, Vol. 51, pp. 270-277

Baratz, K.H.; Cook, B.E. & Hodge D.O. (2001). Probability of Nd:YAG laser capsulotomy after cataract surgery in Olmsted County, Minnesota. *American Journal of Ophthalmology*. Vol.131, No.2, pp. 161-166, ISSN 0002-9394

Bartłomiejczyk, S.; Pilawa, B.; Krzesińska, M.; Pusz, S.; Zachariasz, J. & Wałach, W. (2008). Comparative EPR analysis of oxygen interactions with plants carbonized at different temperatures. *Engineering of Biomaterials*, Vol.73, pp. 1-3

Bartosz G. (2006). *Druga twarz tlenu. Wolne rodniki w przyrodzie*, Wydawnictwo Naukowe PWN, ISBN 978-83-01-13847-9, Warszawa

Beberok, A.; Buszman, E.; Zdybel, M.; Pilawa, B. & Wrześniok, D. (2010). EPR examination of free radical properties of DOPA-melanin complexes with ciprofloxacin, lomefloxacin, norfloxacin and sparfloxacin. *Chemical Physics Letters*, Vol.497, No.1-3, pp. 115-122

Bilińska, B.; Pilawa, B.; Zawada, Z.; Wylęgała, E.; Wilczok, T.; Dontsov, A.E.; Sakina, M.A.; Ostrovsky, M.A. & Ilyasova, V.B. (2002). Electron spin resonance investigations of human retinal pigment epithelium melanosomes from young and old donors. *Spectrochimica Acta A*,Vol.58, pp. 2257-2264

Buszman, E.; Pilawa, B.; Witoszyńska, T.; Latocha, M. & Wilczok, T. (2003). Effect of Zn^{2+} and Cu^{2+} on free radical properties of melanin from *Cladosporium cladosporioides*. *Applied Magnetic Resonance*, Vol.24, pp. 401-407

Buszman, E.; Pilawa, B.; Zdybel, M.; Wilczyński, S.; Gondzik, A.; Witoszyńska, T. & Wilczok, T. (2006). EPR examination of Zn^{2+} and Cu^{2+} binding by pigmented soil fungi *Cladosporium cladosporioides*. *Science of The Total Environment*, Vol.363, No.1-3, pp. 195-205

Buszman, E.; Pilawa, B.; Zdybel, M.; Wrześniok, D.; Grzegorczyk, A. & Wilczok, T. (2005a). EPR examination of Zn^{2+} and Cu^{2+} effect on free radicals in DOPA-melanin-netilmicin complexes. *Chemical Physics Letters*, Vol.403, No.1-3, pp. 22-28

Buszman, E.; Pilawa, B.; Zdybel, M.; Wrześniok, D.; Grzegorczyk, A. & Wilczok, T. (2005b). Paramagnetic center in DOPA-melanin-dihydrostreptomycin complexes. *Acta Physica Polonica A*, Vol.108, No.2, pp. 353-356

Chodurek, E.; Pilawa, B.; Dzierżęga-Lęcznar, A.; Kurkiewicz, S.; Świątkowska, L. & Wilczok, T. (2003). Effect of Cu^{2+} and Zn^{2+} ions on DOPA-melanin structure as analyzed by pyrclysis-gas chromatography-mass spectrometry and EPR spectroscopy. *Journal of Analytical and Applied Pyrolysis*, Vol.70, No.1, pp. 43-54

Chung, R.S.H. & Guan, A.E.K. (2006). Unusual visual disturbance following laser peripheral iridotomy for intermittent angle closure glaucoma. *Graefe's Archive for Clinical and Experimental Ophthalmology*, Vol.244, (October 2005), pp. 532–533

Çinal, A.; Demirok, A.; Yasar, T.; Yazicioglu, A.; Yener, H.I. & Kilic, A. (2007). Nd:YAG laser posterior capsulotomy after pediatric and adult cataract surgery. *Annals of Ophthalmology*, Vol.39, No.4, pp. 321-326, ISSN 1558-9951

Dick, H.B.; Elling, M. & Willert, A. (2010). Femtosecond laser in ophthalmology – A short overview of current Applications. *Medical Laser Application*, Vol.25, pp. 258–261

Domagała, W.; Pilawa, B. & Lapkowski, M. (2008). Quantitative in-situ EPR spectroelectrochemical stuidies of doping processes in poly(3,4-alkylenedioxythiophene)s: Part 1: PEDOT. *Electrochimica Acta*, Vol.53, No.13, pp. 4580-4590

Durán, S. & Zato, M. (2001). Erbium:YAG laser emulsification of the cataractous lens. *Journal of Cataract & Refractive Surgery*, Vol.27, pp. 1025-1032

Eaton, G.R.; Eaton, S.S. & Salikhov, K.M. (1998). *Foundations of modern EPR*, World Scientific, Singapore, New Jersey, London, Hong Kong

Eckert, S. (2010). Lasertrabekuloplastik in der Glaukomtherapie. *Der Ophthalmologe*, Vol.107, (December 2009), pp. 5–7

Evans, D.H. & Abrahamse, H. (2009). A review of laboratory-based methods to investigate second messengers in low-level laser therapy (LLLT). *Medical Laser Application*, Vol.24, pp. 201–215

Fankhauser, F. & Kwasniewska, S. (2003). *Lasers in Ophthalmology - Basic, Diagnostic and Surgical Aspects: A Review*, Kugler Publications, ISBN 90-6299-189-0, The Hague, The Netherlands

Gilbert, W.R. (2011). Advances in cataract surgery: A review for the non-ophthalmic physician. *Northeast Florida Medicine*, Vol.62, No.2, pp. 15-19

Gilmour, M.A. (2002). Lasers in ophthalmology. *The Veterinary Clinics Small Animal Practice*, Vol.32, pp. 649–672

Glinkowski, W. & Pokora, L. (1993). *Lasery w terapii,* Laser Instruments – Centrum Techniki Laserowej, Warszawa

Hatfield, W.E. (1976). Properties of magnetically condensed compounds, In: *Theory and applications of molecular paramagnetism*, Boudreaux E.A., pp. 357-369, John Wiley & Sons, New York, London, Sydney

Herdener, S. & Pache, M. (2007). Minimal-invasive Glaukomchirurgie: Excimer-Laser-Trabekulotomie. *Der Ophthalmologe,* Vol.104, (August 2007), pp. 730–732

Hewitt, P.G. (2001). *Fizyka wokół nas*, Wydawnictwo Naukowe PWN, ISBN 978-83-01-14718-1, Warszawa

Hille, K.; Hans, J.; Manderscheid, T.; Spang, S. & Ruprecht, K.W. (2001). Laser-flare bei kombinierter Katarakt- und Glaukomichirurgie. *Der Ophthalmologe*, Vol.98, pp. 47–53

Hoffmann, E.M. & Schulze, A. (2009). Glaukomdiagnostik mittels Scanning-Laser-Polarimetrie. *Der Ophthalmologe*, Vol.106, (August 2009), pp. 696–701

Jaroszyk, F. (2008). *Biofizyka*, PZWL, ISBN 978-83-20-03676-3, Warszawa

Jóźwiak, Z. & Bartosz, G. (2008). *Biofizyka. Wybrane zagadnienia wraz z ćwiczeniami.* Wydawnictwo Naukowe PWN, ISBN 978-83-01-14461-6, Warszawa

Juzych, M.S.; Chopra, V.; Banitt, M.R.; Hughes, B.A.; Kim, C.; Goulas, M.T. & Shin, D.H. (2004). Comparison of long-term outcomes of selective laser trabeculoplasty versus argon laser trabeculoplasty in Open-Angle Glaucoma. *American Academy of Ophthalmology*, Vol.111, No.10, (October 2004), pp. 1853-1859, ISSN 0161-6420

Kanamori, A.; Nagai-Kusuhara, A.; Escaño, M.F.T.; Maeda, H.; Nakamura, M. & Negi, A. (2006). Comparison of confocal scanning laser ophthalmoscopy, scanning laser polarimetry and optical coherence tomography to discriminate ocular hypertension and glaucoma at an early stage. *Graefe's Archive for Clinical and Experimental Ophthalmology*, Vol.244, (July 2005), pp. 58–68

Kanellopoulos, A.J. & Group, P.I. (2001). Laser cataract surgery. A prospective clinical evaluation of 1000 consecutive laser cataract procedures using the dodick photolysis Nd:YAG system. *Ophthalmology*, Vol.108, (April 2001), pp. 649–655, ISSN 0161-6420

Kęcki, Z. (1999). *Podstawy spektroskopii molekularnej*, Państwowe Wydawnictwo Naukowe, Warszawa

Keicher, A.S. & Stoffelns, B.M. (2010). Argon laser suture lysis following glaucoma filtering surgery – A short introduction to the procedure. *Medical Laser Application*, Vol.25, pp. 209–213

Kim, P.; Sutton, G.L. & Rootman D.S. (2011). Applications of the femtosecond laser in corneal refractive burgery. *Current Opinion in Ophthalmology*, Vol.22, pp. 238–244

Kirmse, R. & Stach, J. (1994). *Spektroskopia EPR. Zastosowania w chemii.* Uniwersytet Jagielloński, Kraków

Kozdrowska, L. (2006). *Właściwości centrów paramagnetycznych kompleksów DOPA-melaniny z kanamycyną i jonami miedzi(II),* Rozprawa doktorska. Uniwersytet Zielonogórski, Zielona Góra

Kozobolis, V.P.; Pallikaris, I.G.; Tsambarlakis, I.G. & Vlachonikolis, I.G. (1997). Nd:YAG laser removal of pupillary membranes developed after ECCE with PC-IOL implantation. *Acta Ophthalmologica Scandinavica*, Vol.75, No.6, pp. 711-715

Krzeszewska, A. & Zdybel, M. (2010). Lasers and their application in medicine and pharmacy. *Scientific Review in Pharmacy*, Vol.6, pp. 24-31

Latocha, M., Pilawa, B., Zdybel, M. & Wilczok, T. (2005). Effect of laser radiation on free radicals in human cancer G361 cells. *Acta Physica Polonica A*, Vol.108, No.2, pp. 409-412

Latocha, M.; Pilawa, B.; Kuśmierz, D.; Zielińska, A. & Nawrocka, D. (2006). Changes in free radicals system of *Imr-90* and *C-32* cells during photodynamic therapy. *Polish Journal of Environmental Studies*, Vol.15, No.4A, pp. 154-156

Latocha, M.; Pilawa, B.; Pietrzak, R.; Nowicki, P. & Wachowska, H. (2008). Conditions of photodynamic therapy of tumor cells examined by carbonized coal and EPR spectroscopy. *Engineering of Biomaterials*, Vol.73, pp. 4-6

Latocha, M.; Pilawa, E.; Chodurek, E.; Buszman, E. & Wilczok, T. (2004). Paramagnetic center in tumor cells. *Applied Magnetic Resonance*, Vol.26, pp. 339-344

L'Esperance, F.A. (1983). *Ophthalmic lasers. Photocoagulation, photoradiation, and surgery,* The C. V. Mosby Company, ISBN 0-8016-2823-7, St. Louis, Toronto, London

Mahdavi, S. (2011). Laser cataract surgery: the next new thing in ophthalmology. *Cataract & Refractive Surgery Today*, Vol.12, (March 2011), pp. 83-87

Maiman, T. (1960). Stimulated optical radiation in ruby. *Nature*, Vol.187, pp. 493-494

Matuszczyk, M.; Buszman, E.; Pilawa, B.; Witoszyńska, T. & Wilczok, T. (2004). Cd^{2+} effect on free radicals in *Cladosporium cladosporioides*-melanin tested by EPR spectroscopy. *Chemical Physics Letters*, Vol.394, No.4-6, pp. 366-371

Morrish, A.H. (1970). *Fizyczne podstawy magnetyzmu*, Państwowe Wydawnictwo Naukowe, Warszawa

Najder-Kozdrowska, L.; Pilawa, B.; Buszman, E.; Więckowski, A.B.; Świątkowska, L.; Wrześniok, D. & Wojtowicz, W. (2010). Triplet states in DOPA-melanin and in its complexes with kanamycin and copper Cu(II) ions. *Acta Physica Polonica A*, Vol.118, No.4, pp. 613-618

Najder-Kozdrowska, L.; Pilawa, B.; Więckowski, A.B.; Buszman, E. & Wrześniok, D. (2009). Influence of copper(II) ions on radicals in DOPA-melanin. *Applied Magnetic Resonance*, Vol.36, No.1, pp. 81-88

Nakata, I.; Yamashiro, K.; Yamada, R.; Gotoh, N.; Nakanishi, H,; Hayashi, H.; Tsujikawa, A.; Otani, A.; Ooto, S.; Tamura, H.; Saito, M.; Saito, K.; Iida, T.; Oishi, A.; Kurimoto, Y.; Matsuda, F. & Yoshimura N. (2011). Genetic variants in pigment epithelium-derived factor influence response of polypoidal choroidal vasculopathy to photodynamic therapy. *American Academy of Ophthalmology*, Vol.118, No.7, pp. 1408-1415

Ngoi, B.K.A.; Hou, D.X.; Koh L.H.K. & Hoh, S.T. (2005). Femtosecond laser for glaucoma treatment: a study on ablation energy in pig iris. *Lasers in Medical Science*, Vol.19, (January 2005), pp. 218–222

Pasenkiewicz-Gierula M. (1990). *Badanie struktury i dynamiki paramagnetycznych układów molekularnych o spinie s = 1/2 metodą elektronowego rezonansu paramagnetycznego (ERP)*, Rozprawa habilitacyjna. Uniwersytet Jagielloński, Kraków

Pilawa, B.; Bartłomiejczyk, S.; Krzesińska, M.; Pusz, S.; Zachariasz, J. & Wałach, W. (2008a). Influence of oxygen O_2 on microwave saturation of EPR lines of plants carbonized at 650^0C and potential application in medicine. *Engineering of Biomaterials*, Vol.73, pp. 7-9

Pilawa, B.; Buszman, E.; Gondzik, A.; Wilczyński, S.; Zdybel, M., Witoszyńska, T. & Wilczok, T. (2005a). Effect of pH on paramagnetic centers in *Cladosporium cladosporioides*. *Acta Physica Polonica A*, Vol.108, No.1, pp. 147-150

Pilawa, B.; Buszman, E.; Wrześniok, D.; Latocha, M. & Wilczok, T. (2002). Application of EPR spectroscopy to examination of gentamicin and kanamycin binding to DOPA-melanin. *Applied Magnetic Resonance*, Vol.23, pp. 181-192

Pilawa, B.; Chodurek, E. & Wilczok, T. (2003a). Types of paramagnetic centres in Cu^{2+} complexes with model neuromelanins. *Applied Magnetic Resonance*, Vol.24, pp. 417-422

Pilawa, B.; Latocha, M.; Buszman, E. & Wilczok, T. (2003b). Effect of oxygen on spin-spin and spin-lattice relaxation in DOPA-melanin. Complexes with chloroquine and metal ions. *Applied Magnetic Resonance*, Vol.25, pp. 105-111

Pilawa, B.; Latocha, M.; Kościelniak, M.; Pietrzak, R. & Wachowska, H. (2006). Oxygen effects in tumor cells during photodynamic therapy. *Polish Journal of Environmental Studies*, Vol.15, No.4A, pp. 160-162

Pilawa, B.; Latocha, M.; Krzyminiewski, R.; Kruczyński, Z.; Buszman, E. & Wilczok, T. (2004). Effect of temperature on melanin EPR spectra. *Physica Medica*, Vol.1, pp. 96-98

Pilawa, B.; Latocha, M.; Ramos, P; Kościelniak, M.; Pietrzak, R. & Wachowska, H. (2008b). New paramagnetic probes and singlet oxygen formation in cells. *Current Topics in Biophysics*, Vol.31, pp. 10-15

Pilawa, B.; Pietrzak, R.; Wachowska, H. & Babeł, K. (2005b). EPR studies of carbonized cellulose – oxygen interactions. *Acta Physica Polonica A*, Vol.108, No.2, pp. 151-154

Pilawa, B.; Zdybel, M.; Latocha, M.; Krzyminiewski, R. & Kruczyński, Z. (2008c). Analysis of lineshape of black *Drosophila melanogaster* EPR spectra. *Current Topics in Biophysics*, Vol.31, pp. 5-9

Podbielska, H.; Sieroń, A. & Stręk, W. (2004). *Diagnostyka i terapia fotodynamiczna*, Wydawnictwo Medyczne Urban & Partner, ISBN: 83-87944-79-3, Wrocław

Preußner, P.R.; Ngounou, F. & Kouogan, G. (2010). Controlled cyclophotocoagulation with the 940 nm laser for primary open angle glaucoma in African eyes. *Graefe's Archive for Clinical and Experimental Ophthalmology*, Vol.248, (May 2010), pp. 1473–1479

Sarna T. (1981). Badanie struktury i właściwości centrów aktywnych melanin. *Zagadnienia Biofizyki Współczesnej*, Vol.6, pp. 201-219

Schlote, T.; Grüb, M. & Kynigopoulos, M. (2008). Long-term results after transscleral diode laser cyclophotocoagulation in refractory posttraumatic glaucoma and glaucoma in aphakia. *Graefe's Archive for Clinical and Experimental Ophthalmology*, Vol.246, (October 2007), pp. 405–410

Schmidt-Erfurth, U. (2010). Current concepts in the management of diabetic macular edema. *Johns Hopkins Advanced Studies in Ophthalmology*, Vol.7, No.2, (December 2010), pp. 52–59

Seitz, B. & Langenbucher, A. (2000). Lasers in ophthalmology. *The Lancet Perspectives*, Vol.356, (December 2000), pp. S26-S28

Shammas, H.J. & Shammas, M.C. (2007). No-history method of intraocular lens power calculation for cataract surgery after myopic laser in situ keratomileusis. *Journal of Cataract & Refractive Surgery*, Vol.33, pp. 31–36

Sieroń, A.; Cieślar, G. & Adamek M. (1994). *Magnetoterapia i laseroterapia. Podstawy teoretyczne. Oddziaływania biologiczne. Zastosowania kliniczne*, Śląska Akademia Medyczna, Katowice

Soong, H.K. & Malta, J.B. (2009). Perspective femtosecond lasers in ophthalmology. *American Journal of Ophthalmology*, Vol.147, No.2, pp. 189-197

Stankowski, J. & Hilczer, W. (2005). *Wstęp do spektroskopii rezonansów magnetycznych*, Wydawnictwo Naukowe PWN, Warszawa

Straburzyńska-Lupa, A. & Straburzyński, G. (2004). *Fizjoterapia*, Wydawnictwo Lekarskie PZWL, ISBN 83-200-2904-X, Warszawa

Symons, M. (1987). *Spektroskopia EPR w chemii i biochemii*, Państwowe Wydawnictwo Naukowe, Warszawa

Verge's, C. & Llevat, E. (2003). Laser cataract surgery: Technique and clinical results. *Journal of Cataract & Refractive Surgery*, Vol.29, pp. 1339–1345

Wakamatsu, K. & Ito, S. (2002). Advanced chemical methods in melanin determination. *Pigment Cell Research*, Vol.15, No.3, pp. 174-183

Wertz, J.E. & Bolton, J.R. (1986). *Electron Spin Resonance Theory and Practical Applications*, Springer Verlag, ISBN 0-412-01161-1, New York, London

Wilmsmeyer, S.; Philippin, H. & Funk, J. (2006). Excimer laser trabeculotomy: a new, minimally invasive procedure for patients with glaucoma. *Graefe's Archive for Clinical and Experimental Ophthalmology*, Vol.244, (October 2006), pp. 670–676

Wróblewski, A.K. (2007). *Historia fizyki*, Wydawnictwo Naukowe PWN, ISBN 83-01-14635-1, Warszawa

Zdybel, M. (2008). *Złożony układ centrów paramagnetycznych kompleksów DOPA-melaniny z netilmicyną, jonami cynku(II) i miedzi(II)*, Rozprawa doktorska. Śląski Uniwersytet Medyczna, Katowice

Zdybel, M.; Pilawa, B.; Buszman, E. & Witoszyńska, T. & Cieśla, H. (2010). EPR studies of *Cladosporium cladosporioides* mecelium with flucytosine. *Current Topics in Biophysics*, Vol.3, pp. 271-275

Zdybel, M.; Pilawa, B.; Buszman, E. & Wrześniok, D. (2009). Zastosowanie spektroskopii EPR do badania melanin oraz kompleksów melanin z jonami metali i substancjami leczniczymi. *Farmaceutyczny Przegląd Naukowy*, Vol.6, No.6, pp. 42-46

Ziętek, B. (2009). *Lasery*, Wydawnictwo Naukowe Uniwersytetu Mikołaja Kopernika, ISBN 978-83-231-2345-3, Toruń

Transient Receptor Potential (TRP) Channels in the Eye

Zan Pan[1], José E. Capó-Aponte[2,3] and Peter S. Reinach[3]
[1]Margaret Dyson Vision Institute,
Weill Cornell Medical College, New York, NY,
[2]Visual Sciences Branch,
U.S. Army Aeromedical Research Laboratory, Fort Rucker, AL,
[3]Department of Biological Science, State University of New York,
College of Optometry, New York, NY,
USA

1. Introduction

The first member of transient receptor potential (TRP) channel superfamily was discovered in photoreceptors of *Drosophila* over 30 years ago.[1] Since then this protein superfamily has been extensively characterized based on exponential increases in the number of publications related to TRP channels. With 28 TRP homologous genes identified in mammals, TRP channels have been detected in both neural and non-neural tissues.

In humans, 27 different TRP genes are classified into two groups and six different subfamilies based on their amino acid homology and phenotypes associated with mutant genes. The genes of TRP channel in Group 1 and Group 2 are only distantly related. The Group 1 of TRP genes are comprised of TRPC (canonical), TRPM (melastatin), TRPV (vanilloid) channel subfamilies, with TRPA (ankyrin) being more recently assigned to this group.[2] Such categorization is based on their resemblance to the amino acid sequence of the *Drosophila* TRP channel. The nomenclature of TRP channel genes in Group 2 is based on the human phenotypes generated by the mutation of the founding genes of each subfamily, including polycystic kinase disease (PKD) and mucolipidosis type IV (MCOLN, mucolipin). Their encoded proteins have also been referred to as TRPP (polycystin) and TRPML (mucolipin), respectively (Figure 1).

The TRP superfamily is evolutionarily conserved from nematodes to mammals.[3] The common features of TRP channels are six putative transmembrane spanning domains and a cation-permeable pore formed by a short hydrophobic region between transmembrane domains 5 and 6. They are configured as homo- or hetero-tetramers to form non-selective cation channels (Figure 2). Their permeability ratios to Ca^{2+}/Na^+ vary significantly among individual members. TRPV5 and TRPV6 channels exhibit a Ca^{2+}/Na^+ permeability ratio of greater than 100, indicating high Ca^{2+} selectivity.[4] In contrast, TRPM4 and TRPM5 channels are impermeable to Ca^{2+} but are selective for monovalent cations (Na^+, K^+).[5, 6] Such intra-family variability is unique to the TRP channel superfamily whereas most other ion channel families have little difference in ionic permeability within a family.[7]

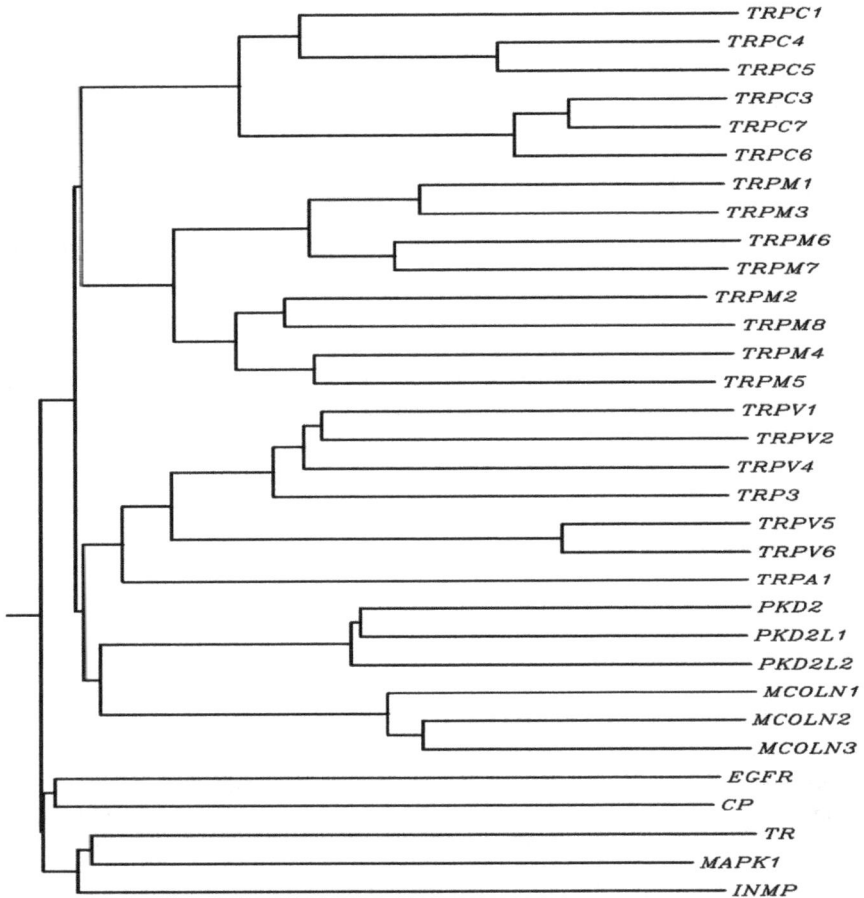

Fig. 1. Human TRP channel superfamily dendrogram. Random proteins bound to the plasma membrane (i.e., EGF receptor, EGFR), endoplasmic reticulum (i.e., calreticulin precursor, CP), mitochondria (thioredoxin reductase, TR), cytosolic protein (i.e., mitogen-activated protein kinase 1, MAPK1) and nuclear membrane (i.e., inner nuclear membrane protein, INMP) are shown to illustrate that PKD and MCOLN are evolutionarily related to TRP channels or are the results of convergent evolution. The dendrogram shows that PKD and MCOLN belong to the TRP channel superfamily, since random genes extend from branches distinct from the TRP channel superfamily.[8]

TRP channel subfamilies in Group 1 share substantial sequence homology in the transmembrane domain 6. What divides each subfamily is differences in their intracellular domains. TRPC, TRPV and TRPA channels contain ankyrin repeats near the intracellular N-terminal domain, whereas the TRPC and TRPM channels subfamilies possess proline-rich 'TRP domain' in the region of the C-terminal near the putative transmembrane segment. TRPM6 and TRPM7 channels have a protein kinase domain in the C-terminal.

The TRPC subfamily consists of seven genes (TRPC1–7) in mammals, but TRPC2 channel is a pseudogene in humans. TRPC channels are widely expressed in multiple systems. TRPC4, TRPC5, TRPC6 and TRPC7 channels are identified in the various ocular tissues of mammals.[9-12] The TRPM channel subfamily comprises eight genes (TRPM 1–8), of which three encode channel-like proteins and five non-channel proteins. TRPM1 channels are expressed in retinas and TRPM8 channels in corneas.[13, 14] The TRPV channels subfamily contains six members (TRPV1–6). TRPV1, TRPV2, TRPV3 and TRPV4 channels are expressed in the cornea whereas TRPV1, TRPV2, TRPV5 and TRPV6 channels are expressed in the retina.[15-20] The TRPA channel subfamily has only one member, TRPA1.

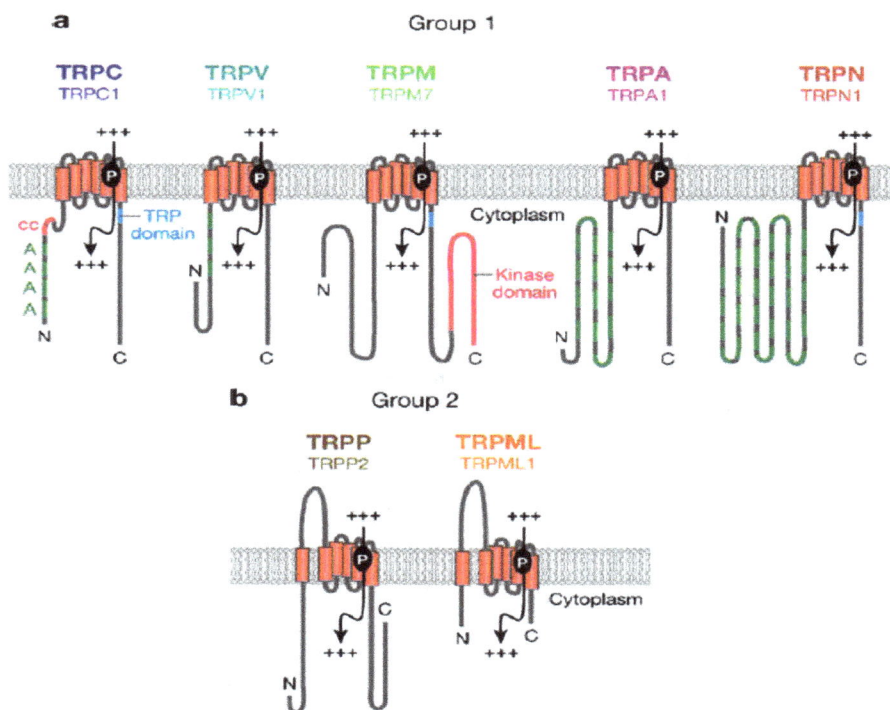

Fig. 2. Domain structure of the TRP channel superfamily. There are five TRP channel subfamilies in Group 1 (TRPN, no mechanoreceptor potential C channels are expressed in mammals) (a) and two TRP channel subfamilies in Group 2 (b). All subfamilies contain a six-transmembrane domain unit with a cation-permeable pore between domains 5 and 6. Four of such units are assembled as a homo- or hetero-tetramer to form a TRP channel. Domain indications: ankyrin repeats (A), coiled-coil domain (cc), protein kinase domain (TRPM6 and TRPM7 channels only), cation-permeable pore (P), transmembrane (TM) domain, cation-permeable (+++), TRP channels domain (TRPC and TRPM channels only), large extracellular loop between transmembrane domains 1 and 2 (TRPP and TRPML channels only). Adapted with permission from Venkatachalam and Montell.[21]

TRPP and TRPML channel subfamilies belong to Group 2. They contain limited sequence homology to TRP channels in Group 1, although such resemblance to classical TRP channels is still larger than those of random genes (e.g., EGFR, INMP) (Figure 1). TRPP channel proteins share 25 percent amino acid sequence homology to TRPC3 and TRPC6 channels over a region including transmembrane domains 4 and 5 and the hydrophobic pore loop between domains 5 and 6. TRPML channel proteins consist of three small proteins compared with other TRP channel proteins. Homology of their amino acid sequence with TRPC channels proteins is restricted to the region spanning transmembrane domains 4 to 6 (amino acids 331 to 521). TRP channels in Group 2 have a unique large extracellular loop between their first and second transmembrane domains. They are named as TRP channels based on the six transmembrane domains that they contain and function as cation-permeable channels.

The activation mechanisms of TRP channels are unique in that there are a diverse host of stimuli that can activate TRP channels and exhibit sharp differences in stimulatory modes even within each TRP channel subfamily. TRP channels were initially recognized as sensory mechanisms to a variety of stimuli, ranging from light, temperature, osmotic pressure, smell, taste, mechanical stress and acidity. There is also increasing awareness of their roles in mediating wound healing, inflammation, apoptosis and excretion. These channels are sensitive to intracellular and extracellular messengers, as well as declines in the calcium content of intracellular calcium stores (ICS).

Their activation following conformation changes modulates Ca^{2+}/Na^+ cell permeability ratios, which is dependent on TRP channel subunit composition. Transient increases in intracellular calcium concentration trigger intracellular activation of mediators including: 1) phospholipase C (PLC) by coupled GTP-binding protein, leading to stimulation of store-operated Ca^{2+} channels; 2) transactivation of EGF tyrosine receptors through MMP-mediated HB-EGF shedding.[4, 10, 16] The physiological significance of TRP channel expression is indicated by the finding that TRP channel mutations are linked to human diseases.[22]

There is compelling evidence that the TRP channel superfamily plays a critical role in ocular homeostasis and pathogenesis. Functional importances of TRP isotypes expressed in different ocular tissues are multi-faceted. Their activation is essential for retaining corneal deturgescence and clarity, mediating aqueous humor outflow through trabecular meshwork and ciliary body as well as inducing light sensation in retina. Mutation of TRP channels is associated with ocular pathological phenotypes either due to loss of its homeostatic role or over-activation of its function. The realization of the importance of TRP channel has prompted much research effort to investigate novel strategies for regulating TRP channels function in a number of ocular diseases.

2. Roles of TRP channels in corneal sensation and wound healing

Continuous renewal of corneal epithelial layer is essential to maintain corneal transparency. The intact epithelium not only offers a smooth and clear optical surface, but also provides corneal barrier function. This property protects the underlying stroma from swelling and pathogenic invasion. Should such protection become compromised by ocular surface diseases, outcomes can range from mild symptoms, such as irritation, photophobia, to severe consequences including corneal opacity, ulceration and even perforation. TRP channel functions have been indicated to associate with maintaining corneal sensation and integrity. Corneas express ample collection of TRP channel isotypes in various mammalians. There are TRPC1, TRPC3, TRPC4, TRPC6 and TRPC7 as well as TRPV1–4 channels in the corneal epithelium, TRPV1-4 in the corneal endothelium, TRPV1, TRPA1, and TRPM8 in the corneal nerves.[10, 15-17, 23, 24, 25-27] These channels are involved in corneal regenerative, protective and sensory mechanisms.

TRPC4 channels protein is localized in plasma membranes of cultured human corneal epithelial cells (HCEC) and mediate epidermal growth factor (EGF)-promoted epithelial proliferation. They are activated by EGF-induced depletion of ICS content in the endoplasmic reticulum. This depletion occurs as a consequence of stimulation of PLC activity which results in increases in inositol 1,4,5-trisphosphate (IP3) formation. This response leads to declines in ICS content and activation of TRPC4 store operated channel (SOC) function. Its activation induces intracellular Ca^{2+} influx leading to stimulation of downstream signalling cascades. They include the mitogen activated protein kinase (MAPK) cascade composed of ERK, JNK and p38 casettes as well as protein kinase A (PKA), protein kinase C (PKC), JAK/STAT and PI3-K/AKT/GSK-3. All of their activations contribute to the control of increases in cell survival and proliferation elicited by EGF. The importance of TRPC4 channels activation to mediate EGF-induced mitogenic responses is indicated by the finding that knockdown of its gene expression in HCEC eliminated the mitogenic response to EGF.[10]

TRPV1 channel expression was first identified on the ophthalmic branch of the trigeminal nerve. More recently, the functional expression of this channel was also identified in the corneal epithelial and endothelial layers. A hallmark of its activity is that the vanilloid compounds (such as capsaicin isolated from hot chilli pepper), hyperosmolarity, acidity (pH below 6) and high temperatures (above 43°C) stimulate TRPV1 channels. In the mouse corneal epithelium, severe chemical injury to corneal epithelium induces TRPV1 channel activation leading to dysregulated inflammation, scarring and loss of corneal transparency. On the other hand, its activation stimulates in HCEC proliferation and migration through EGF receptor (EGFR) transactivation.[28] The involvement of TRPV1 channel activation in inducing these diverse responses is indicated by the finding that in homozygous TRPV1 knockout mice the wound healing response to an alkali burn does not result in losses of corneal transparency. Similarly, TRPV1 channel activation in some types of dry eye disease resulting from exposure to hyperosmolar tears may account for chronic inflammation since TRPV1 channels activation caused by exposure to a hyperosmolar challenge induced large increases in a host of proinflammatory cytokines (e.g., IL-6, IL-8, TNFα and IL-1β) and chemoattractants (e.g., MCP-1) in HCEC. On the other hand, pre-exposure to a selective TRPV1 channel antagonist obviated all of these responses, suggesting that TRPV1 channels are potential drug target for the treatment of dry eye syndrome because suppression of its activation may reduce ocular surface inflammation.[16, 23]

In contrast with TRPV1, its cohort, TRPV4 channel reacts to a different spectrum of stresses. Unlike TRPV1, which is thought to only be activated by a hyperosmolar stress, TRPV4 channels may instead be an osmosensor for a hypoosmolar challenge.[17] Such a stress is encountered by the cornea during exposure to fresh water (e.g., swimming, bathing, use of some eye drops). This hypotonic exposure results initially in corneal epithelial swelling due to obligatory water influx in order to reach equilibration between the cell interior and surface tears. However, excessive swelling can lead to cell lysis. To counter the initial swelling, corneal epithelial cells mediate regulatory volume decrease (RVD) behavior by stimulating volume-sensitive potassium and chloride channels as well as potassium-chloride co-transporter (KCC) activity to restore isotonic cell volume through osmotically coupled net fluid efflux.

TRPV1–4 channel isoforms also serve as thermosensors over defined temperature ranges in the corneal epithelium. In addition, TRPV3 channel activation, either by temperatures above 33°C or by its selective agonist, carvacrol, not only contributes to thermosensation, but also accelerates epithelial wound recovery by enhancing cell survival, proliferation and migration.[15, 29] TRPV1–3 and TRPC4 channels are also expressed in corneal endothelial cells.[9, 30] TRPV1–3 channels are sensitive to temperatures from 25 to 40°C, similar to their epithelial counterparts.

TRP channels play an important role in mediating corneal sensations. The cornea has the highest sensory nerve density of any tissue in the body. The corneal sensory nerves originate from the ophthalmic branch of the trigeminal ganglion and are responsible for eliciting nociception to thermal, chemical and mechanical stimuli.[31] TRPV1 channels colocalize with substance P (SP) and calcitonin-gene-related peptide (CGRP) in the ophthalmic branch of the trigeminal nerve indicating their role in eliciting nociceptive perception. This realization makes TRPV1 channel tenable as a potential drug target for treating neurotrophic keratopathy.[31, 32] Additionally, the TRPM8 channel contributes to corneal cold sensation and basal tear secretion required to maintain corneal surface hydration.[14, 33]

Taken together, these studies on the corneal epithelial, endothelial cells and corneal nerves indicate that functional expression of TRP channels are essential for maintaining corneal transparency and eliciting adaptive responses to stresses. This indicates the importance of further studies on TRP channel regulation since such insight may lead to novel strategies for treating corneal diseases and better management of ocular surface inflammatory pain.

3. Roles of TRP channels in glaucoma

Some members of the TRPC and TRPV channel subfamilies are expressed in trabecular meshwork, ciliary muscle and retinal ganglion cells.[34, 35] Their roles have been associated with regulating intraocular pressure through modulation of aqueous humor flows and ganglion cell survival. The trabecular meshwork contains contractile elements whose tension modulation changes fluid drainage rate from the anterior chamber into the Canal of Schlemm. The contractile state of trabecular meshwork is governed by tension imparted from the ciliary muscle and possibly trabecular meshwork itself.[35, 36] The trabecular meshwork and the ciliary muscle act as functional antagonists. Such opposition is evident since ciliary muscle contraction leads to relaxation of the trabecular meshwork with subsequent increases in fluid outflow whereas trabecular meshwork contraction has the opposite effect.[35] Malfunction of trabecular meshwork and ciliary muscle contractility often leads to ocular hypertension and glaucoma.[37] Their contractile states are modulated by changes in intracellular Ca^{2+} concentration and Ca^{2+} channel activity. Specifically, increases in cytoplasmic Ca^{2+} resulting from the stimulation of TRP channels enhance contractility. Other types of Ca^{2+} channels that regulate intracellular Ca^{2+} concentration include L-type voltage-gated Ca^{2+} channels, receptor operated Ca^{2+} channels and store-operated calcium entry (SOCE) pathways. In bovine trabecular meshwork cells, TRPC1 and TRPC4 channels are implicated in the formation of heteromeric SOCE channels which contribute to rises in cytoplasmic Ca^{2+} store and therefore trabecular meshwork contractility during exposure to bradykinin or endothelin-1.[4]

Similarly TRPC1, TRPC3, TRPC4 and TRPC6 channels are also present in ciliary muscle cells. The ciliary muscle is densely innervated by parasympathetic nerves that stimulate muscle contraction through acetylcholine-mediated muscarinic receptor stimulation on neighboring muscle cells. Such activation leads to a surge in intracellular Ca^{2+} concentration resulting in membrane voltage depolarization via receptor-operated non-selective cation channels. TRPC1, TRPC3, TRPC4 and TRPV6 channels are considered as potential candidates for such channels as they are co-localized with muscarinic receptor type 3 in ciliary muscle fibres.[38, 39]

Modulation of TRPC channel activity in turn alters aqueous humor outflow and therefore intraocular pressure through changes in trabecular meshwork contractility. The dual localization of TRPC channels on ciliary muscles and trabecular meshwork cells suggests that strategies targeted towards their selective modulation may prove to be advantageous in providing better control of intraocular pressure in patients with ocular hypertension or glaucoma. Such an outcome is possible once there is definitive identification of the TRP channels subtypes on each of these tissues. At this point, it may be possible to maximize fluid outflow rates by selectively decreasing trabecular meshwork resistance through a decrease in its contractile state. Accordingly, additional studies are needed to map the TRP channels subtypes and characterize their mechanisms of regulation in the ciliary muscle and trabecular meshwork.

Chronic intraocular hypertension is a risk factor which in some cases can induce glaucoma due to damage to retinal ganglion cells. Such damage can result from either increased hydrostatic pressure, declines in retrograde neutrophin flow, ischemic or oxidative stress. Irreversible loss of retinal ganglion cells leads to gradual and often insidious vision impairment and possible blindness. Elevated intraocular pressures can activate TRP channels in retinal ganglion cells. TRP channel sensitivity to hydrostatic pressure has been described in the bladder, lungs and skin.[40-42] Sappington et al. showed *in vitro* that exposure of retinal ganglion cells to elevated hydrostatic pressure induced transient rises of intracellular Ca^{2+} accumulation due to TRPV1 channel activation. This effect promoted apoptosis of retinal ganglion cells whereas suppression of TRPV1 channel activation protected retinal ganglion cells from pressure-induced death.[34] Recently, similar stresses were identified to stimulate TRPV4 channel and induce apoptosis in retinal ganglion cells.[43] The increased levels of cytoplasmic Ca^{2+} are the underlying mechanism leading to retinal ganglion cells apoptosis.[44] Ca^{2+}-dependent calcineurin and calpain are a phosphatase and a protease, respectively, that trigger apoptosis signalling. Both of them induce cytochrome c release from mitochondria and trigger pro-apoptotic signalling. In contrast, the TRPV1 channel in the retinal microglia appears to have a retinoprotective effect. Retina microglia cells are essential to neuronal homeostasis and provide innate immunity for retina to defend against pathogenic infiltration. Exposure of microglia to chronic stress is associated with various neurodegenerative diseases, including retinal dystrophies. TRPV1 channel activation in the cultured retinal microglia cells by hydrostatic pressure induces increases in IL-6 and TNF-α release through transient rises in intracellular Ca^{2+} levels. Rises in IL-6 suppress pro-apoptotic signalling pathways and cell death.[45] Therefore, provided strategies can be devised to selectively induce increases in microglial TRPV1 channels expression, TRPV1 channels may be a potential drug target in managing pressure-induced retinal ganglion cell loss in glaucoma.

4. Possible roles of TRP channels in cataract development

Maintenance of intracellular Ca^{2+} levels is imperative to crystalline lens clarity.[46] Lenses with cortical cataracts have intracellular Ca^{2+} levels that are above those in the physiological range.[47] Accordingly, a better understanding of the mechanisms mediating control of lens intracellular Ca^{2+} levels is pertinent for identifying economical and novel drug strategies to preserve lens transparency or slow cataract progression.

As previously described, store-operated calcium entry (SOCE) channels are composed of TRP subunits and are heterogeneously expressed in the lens epithelial cells. Epithelial cells in the lens equatorial region have higher SOCE expression than that in the central anterior region. This difference is attributable to the fact that the size of the intracellular calcium storage is larger in the equatorial than the central anterior epithelial cells.[48] The higher intracellular Ca^{2+} load in the equatorial epithelium is required for its more rapid proliferative rate than other parts of the lens epithelium. However, the equatorial epithelium is more susceptible to damage that can induce cortical cataracts since the development of such cataracts is associated with Ca^{2+} overload in the lens epithelial cells. The identity of the TRP channels isoforms constituting SOCE channels is elusive since drugs that modulate SOCE channels activity have poor selectivity for each of the different TRP subunits in the TRPV and TRPC channel subfamilies. For example, the inhibitory effects of lanthanum are used as a criterion to distinguish between SOCE and TRPC channel involvement in the development of cataract. At lower concentrations (i.e., in the nanomolar range), lanthanum inhibits SOCE channels, whereas at higher concentrations it blocks TRPC-containing channels.[49, 50] However, this approach is problematic because a cut-off between lanthanum concentration ranges having the inhibitory effect on either SOCE or TRPC channel is poorly defined. Another complication is that, in the micromolar range, Ca^{2+} influx is potentiated through TRPC4- and TRPC5-containing pathways. Nevertheless, the current understanding is that SOCE channels are the major pathway for Ca^{2+} influx in the lens. Better insight into the specific involvement of TRP channels dysfunction in cataractogenesis will be clarified once either more selective Ca^{2+} channel modulators become available or genetic approaches are employed to selectively modulate levels of TRP channel isoform expression.

5. Roles of TRP channels in retinopathy

TRP channels are abundantly expressed in the entire retinal layer including the retinal pigment epithelium (RPE), photoreceptors, retinal ganglion cells, Müller cells, and microglia. Initially, TRP channel-mediated phototransduction was identified in *Drosophila* and 13 of the known 28 homologues of the mutant insect channels were next identified in the mammalian retina.[51] For example, the TRPC channels in mammals are most closely related to the *Drosophila* TRP channels. The difference is that in mammals the six TRPC subfamily genes (i.e., trpc 1, 3–7) encode seven proteins (TRPC1–7 channels), since TRPC2 is a pseudogene.

In *Drosophila* retinal photoreceptors, TRPC channels lead to photoexcitation. Light absorption converts rhodopsin to active metarhodopsin, which activates PLC. PLC hydrolyzes phosphatidylinositol 4,5-bisphosphate (PIP$_2$) to IP$_3$ and diacylglycerol (DAG). DAG can be degraded to release polyunsaturated fatty acids and protons. TRPC channel activation occurs as a consequence of phosphoinositide depletion and acidification resulting from PLC-induced PIP$_2$ hydrolysis and proton release associated with IP$_3$ formation.[34] TRPC channel activation by phosphoinositide metabolites suggests that these channels are part of the light-sensing mechanism for *Drosophila,* but their role in humans is still unclear.

TRP channel dysfunction has been implicated in mammalian retinopathy. Mutation of TRPM1 channels in ON bipolar cells has been linked to autosomal-recessive congenital stationary night blindness (CSNB), a heterogeneous group of retinal disorders characterized by non-progressive impaired night vision and variable decreased visual acuity.[52] On the other hand, Wang et al. reported that TRPC6 channel activation has a neuroprotective effect on retinal ischemia-reperfusion (IR) injury in the rat.[53] Following IR, the expression of TRPC6 channels decreases in retinal ganglion cells. Activation of TRPC6 channels before IR reduces retinal ganglion cell losses whereas suppression of TRPC6 channels has an opposite effect. Such protection by TRPC6 channels of retinal ganglion cells is dependent on brain-derived neurotrophic factor (BDNF) signalling.

The RPE layer has essential roles in sustaining normal retinal function. It regulates the hydration and ionic composition of the subretinal space, as well as rod outer segment function. RPE also secretes cytokines that are essential for retinal health. TRPV5 and TRPV6 expressions were identified *in vitro* in the human RPE, implicating that these two most calcium-selective channels of the TRP channel superfamily contribute to the regulation of the subretinal space calcium composition accompanying light/dark transitions.[19] TRPV2 channels were shown in another study to control RPE release of vascular endothelial growth factor (VEGF). Insulin-like growth factor-1 (IGF-1) is a TRPV2 channel activator that selectively induces the intracellular Ca^{2+} transients required for inducing VEGF release. Control of this response is needed to reduce retinal neovascularization, since wet age-related macular degeneration (AMD) is decreased or stabilized by treatment with anti-VEGF antibodies. These results suggest that reducing TRPV2 channels activity may provide another option for managing wet AMD.[54]

6. Summary

TRP channels are involved in ocular sensory and cellular functions. In mammals, TRP channel subunit proteins are encoded by 27 genes and are classified into two groups and six different subfamilies, based on differences in amino acid sequence homology. Group 1 and Group 2 of TRP channels are only remotely related, but share similar cation channel-forming structures of six transmembrane domains. Their cation selectivity and activation mechanisms are very diverse and depend on individual TRP channel. TRP channel activation induces a host of responses to variations in ambient temperature, pressure, osmolarity and pH. In addition, their activation by injury induces inflammation, neovascularization, pain and cell death, as well as wound healing. There is emerging interest in characterizing their roles in inducing ocular surface disease, glaucoma, cataracts and retinopathy. Such efforts could lead to the identification of novel drug targets for improving management of many ocular diseases.

7. References

[1] Minke B. Drosophila mutant with a transducer defect. *Biophys Struct Mech* 1977;3:59-64.
[2] Clapham DE. TRP channels as cellular sensors. *Nature* 2003;426:517-524.
[3] Harteneck C, Plant TD, Schultz G. From worm to man: three subfamilies of TRP channels. *Trends Neurosci* 2000;23:159-166.
[4] Montell C. The TRP superfamily of cation channels. *Sci STKE* 2005;2005:re3.
[5] Launay P, Fleig A, Perraud AL, Scharenberg AM, Penner R, Kinet JP. TRPM4 is a Ca2+-activated nonselective cation channel mediating cell membrane depolarization. *Cell* 2002;109:397-407.
[6] Hofmann T, Chubanov V, Gudermann T, Montell C. TRPM5 is a voltage-modulated and Ca(2+)-activated monovalent selective cation channel. *Curr Biol* 2003;13:1153-1158.
[7] Voets T, Janssens A, Droogmans G, Nilius B. Outer pore architecture of a Ca2+-selective TRP channel. *J Biol Chem* 2004;279:15223-15230.
[8] Pan Z, Yang H, Reinach PS. Transient receptor potential (TRP) gene superfamily encoding cation channels. *Hum Genomics* 2011;5:108-116.
[9] Xie Q, Zhang Y, Cai Sun X, Zhai C, Bonanno JA. Expression and functional evaluation of transient receptor potential channel 4 in bovine corneal endothelial cells. *Exp Eye Res* 2005;81:5-14.
[10] Yang H, Mergler S, Sun X, et al. TRPC4 knockdown suppresses epidermal growth factor-induced store-operated channel activation and growth in human corneal epithelial cells. *J Biol Chem* 2005;280:32230-32237.
[11] Warren EJ, Allen CN, Brown RL, Robinson DW. The light-activated signaling pathway in SCN-projecting rat retinal ganglion cells. *Eur J Neurosci* 2006;23:2477-2487.
[12] Da Silva N, Herron CE, Stevens K, Jollimore CA, Barnes S, Kelly ME. Metabotropic receptor-activated calcium increases and store-operated calcium influx in mouse Muller cells. *Invest Ophthalmol Vis Sci* 2008;49:3065-3073.
[13] Oancea E, Vriens J, Brauchi S, Jun J, Splawski I, Clapham DE. TRPM1 forms ion channels associated with melanin content in melanocytes. *Sci Signal* 2009;2:ra21.
[14] Madrid R, Donovan-Rodriguez T, Meseguer V, Acosta MC, Belmonte C, Viana F. Contribution of TRPM8 channels to cold transduction in primary sensory neurons and peripheral nerve terminals. *J Neurosci* 2006;26:12512-12525.
[15] Mergler S, Garreis F, Sahlmuller M, Reinach PS, Paulsen F, Pleyer U. Thermosensitive transient receptor potential channels (thermo-TRPs) in human corneal epithelial cells. *J Cellular Physiol (in press)* 2010.
[16] Pan Z, Wang Z, Yang H, Zhang F, Reinach PS. TRPV1 Activation is Required for Hypertonicity Stimulated Inflammatory Cytokine Release in Human Corneal Epithelial Cells. *Invest Ophthalmol Vis Sci (in press)* 2010.
[17] Pan Z, Yang H, Mergler S, et al. Dependence of regulatory volume decrease on transient receptor potential vanilloid 4 (TRPV4) expression in human corneal epithelial cells. *Cell Calcium* 2008;44:374-385.
[18] Sappington RM, Calkins DJ. Contribution of TRPV1 to microglia-derived IL-6 and NFkappaB translocation with elevated hydrostatic pressure. *Invest Ophthalmol Vis Sci* 2008;49:3004-3017.
[19] Kennedy BG, Torabi AJ, Kurzawa R, Echtenkamp SF, Mangini NJ. Expression of transient receptor potential vanilloid channels TRPV5 and TRPV6 in retinal pigment epithelium. *Mol Vis* 2010;16:665-675.

[20] Leonelli M, Martins DO, Kihara AH, Britto LR. Ontogenetic expression of the vanilloid receptors TRPV1 and TRPV2 in the rat retina. *Int J Dev Neurosci* 2009;27:709-718.

[21] Venkatachalam K, Montell C. TRP channels. *Annu Rev Biochem* 2007;76:387-417.

[22] Nilius B, Voets T, Peters J. TRP channels in disease. *Sci STKE* 2005;2005:re8.

[23] Zhang F, Yang H, Wang Z, et al. Transient receptor potential vanilloid 1 activation induces inflammatory cytokine release in corneal epithelium through MAPK signaling. *J Cell Physiol* 2007;213:730-739.

[24] Yang H, Sun X, Wang Z, et al. EGF stimulates growth by enhancing capacitative calcium entry in corneal epithelial cells. *J Membr Biol* 2003;194:47-58.

[25] Yamamoto Y, Hatakeyama T, Taniguchi K. Immunohistochemical colocalization of TREK-1, TREK-2 and TRAAK with TRP channels in the trigeminal ganglion cells. *Neurosci Lett* 2009;454:129-133.

[26] Salas MM, Hargreaves KM, Akopian AN. TRPA1-mediated responses in trigeminal sensory neurons: interaction between TRPA1 and TRPV1. *Eur J Neurosci* 2009;29:1568-1578.

[27] Bang S, Kim KY, Yoo S, Kim YG, Hwang SW. Transient receptor potential A1 mediates acetaldehyde-evoked pain sensation. *Eur J Neurosci* 2007;26:2516-2523.

[28] Yang H, Wang Z, Capo-Aponte JE, Zhang F, Pan Z, Reinach PS. Epidermal growth factor receptor transactivation by the cannabinoid receptor (CB1) and transient receptor potential vanilloid 1 (TRPV1) induces differential responses in corneal epithelial cells. *Exp Eye Res* 2010;91:462-471.

[29] Yamada T, Ueda T, Ugawa S, et al. Functional expression of transient receptor potential vanilloid 3 (TRPV3) in corneal epithelial cells: involvement in thermosensation and wound healing. *Exp Eye Res* 2010;90:121-129.

[30] Mergler S, Valtink M, Coulson-Thomas VJ, et al. TRPV channels mediate temperature-sensing in human corneal endothelial cells. *Exp Eye Res* 2010;90:758-770.

[31] Murata Y, Masuko S. Peripheral and central distribution of TRPV1, substance P and CGRP of rat corneal neurons. *Brain Res* 2006;1085:87-94.

[32] Okada Y, Reinach PS, Kitano A, Shirai K, Kao WW, Saika S. Neurotrophic keratopathy; its pathophysiology and treatment. *Histol Histopathol* 2010;25:771-780.

[33] Parra A, Madrid R, Echevarria D, et al. Ocular surface wetness is regulated by TRPM8-dependent cold thermoreceptors of the cornea. *Nat Med* 2010;16:1396-1399.

[34] Sappington RM, Sidorova T, Long DJ, Calkins DJ. TRPV1: contribution to retinal ganglion cell apoptosis and increased intracellular Ca2+ with exposure to hydrostatic pressure. *Invest Ophthalmol Vis Sci* 2009;50:717-728.

[35] Wiederholt M, Thieme H, Stumpff F. The regulation of trabecular meshwork and ciliary muscle contractility. *Prog Retin Eye Res* 2000;19:271-295.

[36] Wiederholt M. Direct involvement of trabecular meshwork in the regulation of aqueous humor outflow. *Curr Opin Ophthalmol* 1998;9:46-49.

[37] Weinreb RN, Khaw PT. Primary open-angle glaucoma. *Lancet* 2004;363:1711-1720.

[38] Salmon MD, Ahluwalia J. Discrimination between receptor- and store-operated Ca(2+) influx in human neutrophils. *Cell Immunol* 2010;265:1-5.

[39] Sugawara R, Takai Y, Miyazu M, Ohinata H, Yoshida A, Takai A. Agonist and antagonist sensitivity of non-selective cation channel currents evoked by muscarinic receptor stimulation in bovine ciliary muscle cells. *Auton Autacoid Pharmacol* 2006;26:285-292.

[40] Goto M, Ikeyama K, Tsutsumi M, Denda S, Denda M. Calcium ion propagation in cultured keratinocytes and other cells in skin in response to hydraulic pressure stimulation. *J Cell Physiol* 2010;224:229-233.

[41] Yin J, Kuebler WM. Mechanotransduction by TRP channels: general concepts and specific role in the vasculature. *Cell Biochem Biophys* 2010;56:1-18.

[42] Birder LA. TRPs in bladder diseases. *Biochim Biophys Acta* 2007;1772:879-884.

[43] Ryskamp DA, Witkovsky P, Barabas P, et al. The polymodal ion channel transient receptor potential vanilloid 4 modulates calcium flux, spiking rate, and apoptosis of mouse retinal ganglion cells. *J Neurosci* 2011;31:7089-7101.

[44] Qu J, Wang D, Grosskreutz CL. Mechanisms of retinal ganglion cell injury and defense in glaucoma. *Exp Eye Res* 2010;91:48-53.

[45] Sappington RM, Chan M, Calkins DJ. Interleukin-6 protects retinal ganglion cells from pressure-induced death. *Invest Ophthalmol Vis Sci* 2006;47:2932-2942.

[46] Duncan G, Williamsa MR, Riacha RA. Calcium, cell signalling and cataract. *Progress in Retinal and Eye Research* 1994;13:623-652.

[47] Duncan G, Bushell AR. Ion analyses of human cataractous lenses. *Exp Eye Res* 1975;20:223-230.

[48] Rhodes JD, Russell SL, Illingworth CD, Duncan G, Wormstone IM. Regional differences in store-operated Ca2+ entry in the epithelium of the intact human lens. *Invest Ophthalmol Vis Sci* 2009;50:4330-4336.

[49] Gwack Y, Srikanth S, Feske S, et al. Biochemical and functional characterization of Orai proteins. *J Biol Chem* 2007;282:16232-16243.

[50] Nilius B, Owsianik G, Voets T, Peters JA. Transient receptor potential cation channels in disease. *Physiol Rev* 2007;87:165-217.

[51] Gudermann T, Mederos y Schnitzler M. Phototransduction: keep an eye out for acid-labile TRPs. *Curr Biol* 2010;20:R149-152.

[52] van Genderen MM, Bijveld MM, Claassen YB, et al. Mutations in TRPM1 are a common cause of complete congenital stationary night blindness. *Am J Hum Genet* 2009;85:730-736.

[53] Wang X, Teng L, Li A, Ge J, Laties AM, Zhang X. TRPC6 channel protects retinal ganglion cells in a rat model of retinal ischemia/reperfusion-induced cell death. *Invest Ophthalmol Vis Sci* 2010;51:5751-5758.

[54] Cordeiro S, Seyler S, Stindl J, Milenkovic VM, Strauss O. Heat-Sensitive Trpv Channels Regulate Vegf-a Secretion in Retinal Pigment Epithelial Cells. *Invest Ophthalmol Vis Sci* 2010;51:6001-6008.

3

Microsurgical Techniques in Ophthalmology – Current Procedures and Future Directions

Pradeep Prasad[1,2], Allen Hu[1,2],
Robert Beardsley[1,2] and Jean-Pierre Hubschman[1,2]
[1]Retina Division, Jules Stein Eye Institute,
[2]Department of Ophthalmology,
David Geffen School of Medicine at University of California, Los Angeles, California,
USA

1. Introduction

Given the small dimensions of the human eye, ocular surgery demands the ability to both visualize and precisely manipulate delicate tissue within a microscopic space. Microsurgical technological advancements have rapidly changed the way in which ophthalmic microsurgery is performed and have provided for greater surgical efficiency and improved functional outcomes.

A thorough understanding of normal ocular anatomy is critical to define pathologic anatomic conditions, to delineate surgical goals, and to develop and utilize surgical tools to optimize patient outcomes. The anatomy of the eye and orbit can be broadly categorized as extraocular structures (including the eyelids, lacrimal gland, canalicular system, conjunctiva, and extraocular muscles) and intraocular structures, located within the globe of the eye. Intraocular structures are further grouped based on their location in the anterior or posterior segments of the eye (figure 1). The anterior segment consists of (from anterior to posterior): the cornea, anterior chamber, iris, and crystalline lens. The crystalline lens is suspended in place by hundreds of zonular fibers, which extend from the ciliary body to a thin capsule surrounding the lens. Contraction of the ciliary body changes the tension of the zonular fibers on the lens, allowing the lens to change its shape and focusing power. The cornea and lens are of particular importance as a majority of ophthalmic surgical interventions are performed on these structures, such as corneal transplantation, refractive corneal surgery, and cataract extraction.

The posterior segment of the eye consists of the vitreous humor (a clear gelatinous substance composed primarily of water, type II collagen, and hyaluronic acid), the neurosensory retina, the retinal pigment epithelium (which promotes the function and viability of the neurosensory retina), and the choroid (a vascular layer interposed between the retinal pigment epithelium and the sclera). The neurosensory retina is a highly organized extension of the central nervous system composed of photoreceptors and multiple layers of interconnected neurons. These neurons ultimately synapse on ganglion cells, whose axons coalesce into the optic nerve. Posterior segment ophthalmic surgery generally involves removal of the vitreous humor to: 1) relieve traction of the vitreous on the retina, 2) remove visually-significant opacities within the vitreous, or 3) to gain access to the retina or sub-retinal space for further surgical manipulation.

The origins of ophthalmic surgery date back as far as the sixth century B.C. when ancient Indian surgeons used curved needle-like instruments to dislodge a cataract, a technique termed "couching". Further contributions by Greek, Middle Eastern and European physicians provided detailed functional knowledge of the eye and intraocular structures.

Development of the surgical microscope further revolutionized ophthalmic microsurgery. Although initially little more that a binocular telescope worn by the surgeon, the modern ophthalmic microscope provides a well-lit binocular stereoscopic view with a high-level optical clarity (figure 2). Foot pedal controls allow the surgeon to adjust magnification (approximately 10-30x), illumination intensity, x-y axis movement and level of focus. Furthermore, both contact and non-contact lens based systems are now employed to provide a wide-angle stereoscopic view of the posterior segment. Indeed, the ophthalmic microscope has enabled precise visualization of both anterior and posterior segment structures making modern ophthalmic microsurgery possible. Two such ophthalmic surgeries, cataract extraction and pars plana vitrectomy, are described below in detail.

1.1 Cataract extraction

1.1.1 Technique overview

Over two million cataract extractions are performed yearly in the United States making it the most common ophthalmic surgery, and among the most frequently performed surgeries in any field. A "cataract" refers to a focal or diffuse opacification of the crystalline lens, a structure that is normally optically clear and measures approximately 10mm wide and 6mm deep. Opacities within the lens limit the normal focusing ability of the lens resulting in blurred vision. Although cataract formation is most commonly an age-related process, cataracts may form at any age due to a number of different etiologies including medications, systemic metabolic disease, and ocular trauma. Although many methods have been developed to remove cataracts, the most common technique employed in modern ophthalmic microsurgery is "phacoemulsification".

Standard phacoemulsification for cataract extraction typically begins with the creation of a 2.2 to 3 mm tunnel or wound in the peripheral cornea to gain access to the anterior chamber. The anterior chamber is stabilized during intraocular manipulation with an ophthalmic viscoelastic device (a clear, removable, gel-like substance composed primarily of water and hyaluronic acid). A circular opening is then created in the anterior face of the lens capsule, termed a "continuous curvilinear capsulorrhexis". With the lens contents now accessible, the tip of a handpiece connected to a phacoemulsification machine is placed within the anterior chamber. This handpiece performs three functions: 1) administration of ultrasonic energy to fracture the lens material into small pieces; 2) aspiration to remove the small lens particles; 3) irrigation of a saline-like solution to maintain the volume of the anterior chamber (Figure 3).

Once the lens material is successfully removed, a clear artificial lens is typically placed within the intact capsule of the lens. Although early intraocular lenses were composed of rigid polymethylmethacrylate (PMMA) requiring enlargement of the corneal wound for intraocular placement, modern intraocular lenses are composed of silicone or acrylic, both of which are biologically inert and can be folded and placed into the eye through a small corneal incision.

2. Principles of phacoemulsification

The fluid dynamics of phacoemulsification require constant fluid irrigation into the anterior chamber to maintain normal depth while lens material is aspirated. Due to the small volume of the anterior chamber, fluid circulation during phacoemulsification is critical to ensure efficient removal of the cataract while preventing complications due to anterior chamber collapse. Indeed, if outflow, or aspiration through the handpiece is allowed to exceed inflow, or irrigation, even for a fraction of a second, anterior chamber instability may result in unintended damage to intraocular tissue.

The formula that governs fluid flow during phacoemulsification surgery is Poiseuille's law:

$$Q = \Delta P \, \pi \, r^4 \, / \, 8 \, \eta L,$$

where Q is flow rate, ΔP is the pressure gradient, r is the radius of instrument tip, η is fluid viscosity, and L is length of the tubing. Given that the viscosity of the fluid and length of the tube are constant, flow is essentially proportional to the change in pressure and radius of the tubing.

In the case of phacoemulsification surgery, ΔP is the pressure gradient between the infusion pressure and the vacuum driving aspiration. The source of fluid inflow is a bottle of balanced salt solution, the height of which can be adjusted relative to the patient's eye to control infusion pressure. Fluid outflow is dependent on the vacuum level generated by the machine. The surgeon can control both the infusion pressure and vacuum or aspiration.

3. Phacoemulsificaiton instruments

The primary tool of phacoemulsification is the handpiece (figure 4). The tip of this tool delivers ultrasonic energy to break up the lens, aspirate fluid and lens material, and provide inflow of fluid to the anterior chamber. The handpiece is connected to a machine that regulates the aspiration pressure, the infusion pressure, and the intensity of the ultrasonic energy delivered by the handpiece. The design of the handpiece tip varies with respect to the angle and size of the lumen. Steeper tip bevels (less angled) provide better cutting ability into dense lens nuclear material whereas flatter tip bevels provide a larger surface area for improved aspiration of large lens fragments.

Modern phacoemulsification machines also employ foot pedal controls with at least three positions that allow the surgeon to control the fluidics of phacoemulsification. The first position typically provides irrigation only, which cools the handpiece and keeps the anterior chamber formed. The second position, in addition to irrigating, engages the aspiration mode at a constant or variable rate, depending on the settings selected by the surgeon. In the third position, ultrasound energy is delivered in addition to irrigation and aspiration. Many other microsurgical instruments are also utilized in conjunction with the phacoemulsification probe to facilitate manipulation of the lens material and to improve the efficiency of cataract extraction.

Ultrasonic power for phacoemulsification is generated by applying a time-varying electric field across a piezoelectric crystal in the phacoemulsification handpiece. The oscillating crystal deforms in response to the electric field, resulting in the conversion of electrical to mechanical energy. Oscillation of the tip occurs at a preset frequency that varies from 27 kHz to 60 kHz. The amplitude of the movement, or stroke length, ranges from 50 µm to 100 µm and is modulated when the phacoemulsification power is changed. As the tip retracts, a vacuum is created resulting in the formation of "cavitation bubbles". When the bubbles implode, they release heat and shock waves that fracture the lens material. Phacoemulsification power can also be modulated by varying the duty cycle; the period of time when the phacoemulsification power is being delivered. Varying the duty cycle allows for efficient administration of phacoemulsification energy to promote fracturing of lens material while minimizing excess heat and energy that may damage the cornea or other intraocular structures.

4. Phacoemulsification systems

While there are a variety of phacoemulsification machine manufacturers and configurations, they all generate the required vacuum and aspiration based on one of two pump types: Venturi and peristaltic.

A peristaltic system (figure 5) utilizes a series of rollers to displace fluid, producing flow in a compressible tube that is wound tightly around a rotating wheel. As the wheel turns, a segment of fluid trapped between two rollers is moved, resulting in more fluid being drawn into the tubing. Therefore, the flow rate is directly proportional to the speed of the rotary mechanism. Significant vacuum is generated only when the tip is occluded. The surgeon sets a desired flow rate and vacuum limit. The flow rate determines how rapidly the vacuum builds up when the handpiece tip is occluded and flow is restricted.

The Venturi pump (figure 6) utilizes the Venturi effect to create vacuum. The Venturi effect refers to the creation of vacuum secondary to the flow of a fluid (typically nitrogen or air in a phacoemulsification machine) over an opening. Thus, a Venturi pump allows a given vacuum level to be generated immediately, without occlusion of the phacoemulsification tip as is required in the peristaltic system. As such, flow cannot be directly modulated and is dependent on the vacuum level generated. The Venturi system provides the surgeon with near instantaneous vacuum levels and potentially higher flow rates.

5. Femtosecond laser technology and the future of phacoemulsification

In the near future, a new application of an existing technology may alter the way in which cataract surgery is performed. The femtosecond laser is a device that emits coherent optical pulses with a wavelength of 800nm and duration on the order of 10^{-15} seconds. It has been used extensively in ophthalmology due to its ability to alter delicate tissue in a precise and predictable way. In addition to its precision, the femtosecond laser can cut tissue with practically no heat development. Clinical trials utilizing the femtosecond laser to perform the incisional steps of cataract surgery, including cornea wound creation, capsulorrhexis creation, and disassembly of the lens are currently ongoing. Future applications of this laser may allow many steps of phacoemulsification to be automated, thus minimizing risk and error while increasing surgical efficiency.

5.1 Vitreoretinal surgery

5.1.1 Basic techniques

Vitreoretinal surgery, in its modern form, is a minimally invasive technique similar to laparoscopic surgery whereby small entry ports or trocars are placed on the surface of the eye to gain surgical access to intraocular structures. A variety of instruments including surgical manipulators, illuminating probes, laser probes, and infusing and aspirating devices can be placed through the trocars for a variety of surgical procedures. The trocars are placed at a safe anatomic entry point, the pars plana, located within a narrow band around the eye 3 to 4 mm posterior to the corneoscleral junction. This space lies just posterior to the highly vascularized ciliary body but anterior to the retina. Placing trocars too far anteriorly or posteriorly can lead to significant complications and surgical failure.

The vitreous body, a clear gelatinous structure located between the crystalline lens and the retina, occupies approximately 80% of the volume of the human eye. It is mainly composed of water (99%), collagen fibrils (type II collagen), and hyaluronic acid. The vitreous gel is integral in the pathogenesis of many posterior segment diseases. For example, in diabetic retinopathy, bleeding into the vitreous cavity can severely reduce visual acuity since dense hemorrhages can become loculated within the vitreous body. In some instances where the hemorrhage does not dissipate on its own, vitrectomy is necessary to remove the vitreous and blood. The vitreous body is adherent to a number of structures in the posterior segment including tight adhesions over the optic disc, the macula, retinal blood vessels and the ora serrata (a band which straddles the anterior retina and the pars plana where the vitreous and retina are anatomically fused and cannot be surgically separated). Thus, vitreous removal must be performed in a precise and controlled fashion to minimize excessive traction of the retina, which may result in complications such as retinal tears and detachment. Although the vitreous plays an important role in ocular development *in utero*, removal of the vitreous in the adult eye has no deleterious effects on the health of the retina. Once vitrectomy is performed, the vitreous cavity is typically replaced by the surgeon with balanced salt solution, which is eventually replaced by the eye with aqueous humor. Therefore, the vitreous body does not reform once it is removed.

5.2 Principles of vitreoretinal surgery

Surgery within the posterior segment of the eye is bound by the same principles as anterior segment surgery: the volume of the eye must be maintained as material is removed. Adding complexity to vitreoretinal surgery is the difficulty in visualization of the posterior segment during intraocular surgical maneuvers. External illumination is generally inadequate to visualize the retina and, despite advances in modern lens systems, the surgeon's view of the retinal periphery can be limited while operating near the posterior pole.

The first pars plana vitrectomy was performed by Robert Machemer in 1970 using a 17-gauge (1.42 mm diameter) one-port system that combined an infusion cannula and vitreous cutter in one handpiece. Since that time, numerous innovations have improved the efficiency and outcomes of this procedure and led to the development of the modern 3-port 20-gauge pars plana vitrectomy. In this procedure, three 20-gauge sclerotomies are created within the pars plana. One sclerotomy is used to anchor a cannula that infuses balanced salt solution into the posterior cavity while the vitrectomy is performed, thus maintaining intraocular pressure. The remaining ports are used for the vitrectomy probe and a light probe to remove the vitreous and illuminate intraocular structures respectively. Following removal of the vitreous, the sclerotomy can be used to introduce other instruments such as intraocular forceps and laser probes to further manipulate and treat the retina (figure 7).

Visualization during pars plana vitrectomy is performed using the operating microscope in conjunction with a contact lens (which can be held by the assistant or sewn onto the eye at the corneoscleral junction) or a non-contact lens viewing system. Direct contact visualization systems allow for greater field of view and enhanced three-dimensional perception. Non-contact lens viewing systems are easier to use and do not require an assistant or additional surgical maneuvers to anchor the lens to the ocular surface, but sacrifice some field of view and three-dimensional perception.

5.3 Vitrectomy instruments

The basic tools of pars plana vitrectomy are a vitreous cutter, illuminating device, laser probe, various tissue manipulators such as micro-forceps for delicate intraocular work, and an infusion cannula to maintain intraocular pressure. The workhorse of pars plana vitrectomy is the vitreous cutter, whose basic function is to remove the vitreous in a controlled fashion. Because the vitreous is a semi-solid structure with adhesions to the retina, simple aspiration of the vitreous results in excess traction on the retina. To minimize such traction, the vitrectomy probe is designed with both an aspiration port and a cutting mechanism to aspirate a small volume of vitreous into the handpiece and to cut and remove it. High cut speeds allow for incremental removal of small amounts of vitreous while minimizing tractional forces of the vitreous on the retina. Lower cut speeds result in removal of larger volumes of vitreous, thereby increasing the rate at which vitreous is removed. Most modern high-speed (600-5000 cuts per minute) vitrectomy probes are pneumatically driven with a side-cutting guillotine port near the tip of the instrument (figure 8).

Most vitrectomy machines are equipped with a built-in light source employing either yellow or white light from a halogen or metal-halide light source. The light probe, a fiberoptic cable encased in a plastic handpiece, is connected to the light source and can function as a separate instrument or, in some cases, can be combined with the infusion cannula to simultaneously illuminate and irrigate the posterior segment. A recent innovation has been the introduction of a xenon light source, which can provide bright illumination through a narrow probe. This has facilitated the performance of smaller gauge surgery and eliminated light wavelengths under 400 nm that can be phototoxic to the retina.

Many surgical instruments have been developed to facilitate surgical procedures on the macula. The macula is located at the center of the posterior pole of the retina and has the highest concentration of photoreceptors. It is responsible for fine central visual acuity needed for such tasks as reading, driving and other activities of daily living. Pars plana vitrectomy may be required to treat a variety of macular diseases including epiretinal membranes, macular holes, vitreo-macular traction, and hemorrhagic age-related macular degeneration. Instruments used to manipulate and treat the macula include a variety of micro-forceps (e.g. end-grasping and pick forceps), scissors, needles and cannulas.

The intraocular laser probe allows for minimally invasive and precise ablation of retinal tissues and is used in a wide variety of surgical procedures. Similar to the light probe, the "endolaser" probe is also a fiber-optic cable encased in a plastic handpiece. The intensity of the laser ablation is controlled by the surgeon by modulating the power and duration of the laser as well as by altering the distance of the probe tip to the retina. Intraocular laser is typically employed for two key purposes: 1) to treat retinal tears by creating a fibrous scar between the retina and the underlying choroid thus preventing fluid in the eye from collecting underneath the retina; and 2) to ablate non-perfused or ischemic retinal tissue (as in diabetic retinopathy and other occlusive retinal vascular diseases) to decrease the pathologic production of growth factors that result in retinal neovascularization, intraocular hemorrhage and retinal edema.

5.4 Vitrectomy systems

Vitrectomy machines, similar to phacoemulsification machines, are complex devices that drive the vitreous probe cutter, provide irrigation at an adjustable level to control intraocular pressure, aspirate and remove intraocular material, and provide a light source for intraocular illumination. Many of these functions are controlled via foot pedal by the surgeon, similar to the previously-described phacoemulsification machine.

Two major types of systems are used to drive the vitrectomy probe cutter: electric guillotine and pneumatic guillotine. The electric guillotine employs an electric drive motor with a sinusoidal transmission, translating the rotary motion of an electric motor shaft to the linear guillotine motion of the cutter tip. The profile of motion of the guillotine remains constant as the cut rate is altered. That is to say, the duty cycle, or ratio of time the cutter port is open or closed, remains constant regardless of the cut rate.

The second type of handpiece, which is pneumatically driven, uses pulses of air or gas to close the cutter tip. The pneumatically-driven guillotine is attached to a diaphragm. When a pulse of air is delivered, the diaphragm and guillotine extend, closing the cutter tip and completing a cut. The guillotine then retracts to its original position either through a spring mechanism or through a "dual drive" system where an additional pulse of air pushes the guillotine back, thus opening the cutter tip. In the spring mechanism, as the cut rate is increased, the duration of open time per cut decreases, while the closed time remains constant (decreasing the duty-cycle). The "dual drive" system allows for improved duty cycle compared with the spring mechanism, but the duty cycle still decreases at high cut rates.

6. Current directions

Recent advances in vitreous surgery have resulted in the development of smaller instruments: the 23- and 25-gauge transconjunctival suture-less vitrectomy systems (figure 9). A standard 20-gauge (0.9 mm diameter) vitrectomy requires removal of the conjunctiva and sutures to close the sclerotomies used to access the posterior segment. 23-gauge (0.6 mm diameter) and 25-gauge (0.5 mm diameter) entry wounds, when constructed properly, are small enough to self-seal and thus can be placed through the conjunctiva and sclera without the need for closing sutures. To allow for easy entry and exit of surgical instruments during vitrectomy and to align the entry holes in the conjunctiva and sclera, a 23- or 25-gauge trocar is placed at the site of the desired sclerotomy. The trocar consists of two components: a polyimide cannula and a polymer hub. The polyimide cannula maintains the transconjunctival and transcleral tunnel through which surgical instruments are passed. The polyimide cannula material provides both strength and flexibility, allowing the cannula wall to be thin while avoiding collapse or buckling. The polymer hub is the part of the trocar visible on the surface of the eye and prevents the trocar from sliding into the vitreous cavity. The hub has a central hole that is continuous with the cannula, allowing for instruments to be inserted into the vitreous cavity.

Many surgeons believe the potential advantages of smaller gauge, suture-less techniques include shortened operative time and faster patient recovery. However, the reduction in port diameter results in reduced flow rates compared with 20-gauge cutters, and therefore, smaller-gauge surgery may require more time to remove the same amount of vitreous or may be inadequate to remove dense or highly organized vitreous. Other concerns with suture-less techniques include the increased risk of post-operative hypotony and infection if the sclerotomies are not constructed properly.

7. The future of ophthalmic surgery – Robot-assisted microsurgery?

With recent innovations in engineering and the demands for increasingly precise and efficient ophthalmic microsurgery, the next major advancement in ophthalmic surgery may be the integration of mechanization and robotics into ophthalmic microsurgical techniques. The potential benefits of robotic surgery in ocular surgery include increased precision, reduction of human error, task automation and the capacity for remote surgery.

Guerrouad and Vidal described one of the first ocular robotic systems in 1989. Named the "Stereotaxical Microtelemanipulator" (SMOS), it provided relatively good range of motion for basic surgical tasks but the technology was too premature at that time to raise tangible interest for further development. In the 1990s, Steve Charles and researchers at Northwestern University demonstrated the use of robotic platforms for ophthalmic surgery with precise position measurement and fine incremental motion but these prototypes were limited by the complexity of its software control and the need for increased robotic responsiveness to human controls.

Presently, the Food and Drug Administration has approved the *da Vinci* Surgical System (Intuitive Surgical, Sunnyvale, CA), which has become the most commonly employed robotic platform in human surgery (figure 10). Although it has been used in the fields of general surgery, urology, gynecology and cardiac surgery, its use in ophthalmic surgery is in its early phases. Preliminary studies have demonstrated good robot arm responsiveness to human controls for external and intraocular surgical tasks. However, the remote center of motion (pivot point) and limited range of motion of the robot arm make intraocular manoeuvrability difficult with excessive distortion of the globe of the eye. Furthermore, while the visualization system of the *da Vinci* system is adequate for extraocular and some anterior segment surgical procedures, posterior segment surgery is hampered by a limited field of view. Finally, the surgical instruments of the *da Vinci* instruments are not well-suited to ophthalmic microsurgery due to their bulkiness. Recent studies have better defined the range of motion required for robot-assisted ophthalmic surgery and further refinements to the robot surgery platform are underway to make this technology a tangible option in the near future.

Ocular robotic surgery poses a myriad of unique challenges and the application of this technology will undoubtedly require many stages of evolution. Further work will be required to continue to integrate traditional surgical techniques with new devices to bring the advantages of robotics to the field of ophthalmology.

8. Conclusion

Ophthalmic microsurgery has rapidly evolved in recent history as advances in medical device technology have led to the development of numerous minimally invasive procedures for the treatment of ocular diseases. The multi-disciplinary integration of technology and knowledge from the fields of biomaterials, optics, lasers, ultrasonics and pneumatics have helped to refine the surgical tools available to ophthalmic surgeons, increasing their efficiency and surgical outcomes. As life expectancy and the prevalence of various systemic diseases continue to rise, so too will the burden of ocular disease. Further advances to better address these demands will undoubtedly lead to novel surgical techniques and devices, expanding the role of ophthalmic surgery to undiscovered heights.

9. References

American Academy of Ophthalmology. Basic and Clinical Science Course: Lens and Cataract. Basic Principles of Ophthalmic Surgery. San Francisco: American Academy of Ophthalmology, 2006.

American Academy of Ophthalmology. Basic and Clinical Science Course: Retina and Vitreous. San Francisco: American Academy of Ophthalmology, 2006.

American Academy of Ophthalmology. Basic and Clinical Science Course: Fundamentals and Principles of Ophthalmology. San Francisco: American Academy of Ophthalmology, 2006.

Apple, DJ. Sims, J. Harold Ridley and the Invention of the Intraocular Lens. Survey of Ophthalmology 1996 Feb; 40(4): 279-292.

Beebe DC . The lens. In PL Kaufman, A Alm, eds., Adler's Physiology of the Eye, 10th ed., pp. 117–158. St. Louis: Mosby, 2003.

Bourla, D. H., J. P. Hubschman, et al. (2008). Feasibility study of intraocular robotic surgery with the da Vinci surgical system. Retina 28(1): 154-8.

Charles S, Das H, Ohm T, et al. Dexterity-enhanced telerobotic microsurgery. Proc IEEE Int Conf Adv Robot 1997;July:5–10

Charles S. Debating the pros and cons of 23-g vs 25-g vitrectomy: the pros of 25-g vitrectomy. Retina Physician 2006; 3: 24–25.

Devgan, U. Phaco Fundamentals for the Beginning Phaco Surgeon. Bausch and Lomb Ophthalmology World Report Series, 2009: 1-54.

Georgescu, D., A. F. Kuo, et al. (2008). A fluidics comparison of Alcon Infiniti, Bausch & Lomb Stellaris, and Advanced Medical Optics Signature phacoemulsification machines. Am J Ophthalmol 145(6): 1014-1017.

Guerrouad, A. and D. Jolly (1989). Automatic analysis of weariness during a micromanipulation task by SMOS. IEEE Conference Proceeding 3: 906-907

Guerrouad, A. and P. Vidal (1989). SMOS: stereotaxical microtelemanipulator for ocular surgery. IEEE Conference Proceeding 3 879-880.

Guerrouad, A. and P. Vidal (1991). Advantage of computer aided teleoperation (CAT) in microsurgery. IEEE Conference Proceeding 1: 910- 914.

Hubschmar, J. P., J. L. Bourges, et al. The Microhand': a new concept of micro-forceps for ocular robotic surgery. Eye 2010 Feb; (24(2): 364-367

Hubschmar, J. P., J. L. Bourges, et al. Effect of Cutting Phases on Flow Rate in 20-, 23-, and 25-Gauge Vitreous Cutters. Retina 2009: Oct; 29(9): 1289-93.

Jensen, P. S., K. W. Grace, et al. (1997). Toward robot-assisted vascular microsurgery in the retina. Graefes Arch Clin Exp Ophthalmol 235(11): 696-701.

Machemer R, Parel JM, Norton EW. Vitrectomy: a pars plana approach: technical improvements and further results. Trans Am Acad Ophthalmol Otolaryngol 1972; 76: 462–466.

Nagy Z, Takacs A, Filkorn T, Sarayba M. Initial clinical evaluation of an intraocular femtosecond laser in cataract surgery. J Refract Surg 2009 Dec;25(12):1053-60.

O'Malley C, Heintz Sr RM. Vitrectomy with an alternative instrument system. Ann Ophthalmol 1975; 7: 585–588: 91–94.

Siebel, Barry. Phacodynamics: Mastering the Tools and Techniques of Phacoemulsification Surgery. New Jersey: Slack Incorporated, 2005.

Son, J., J. L. Bourges, et al. Quantification of intraocular surgery motions with an electromagnetic tracking system. Stud Health Technol Inform 2009; 142: 337-9.

Tsirbas, A., C. Mango, et al. Robotic ocular surgery. Br J Ophthalmol 2007; 91(1): 18-21.

Williams, GA. 25-, 23-, or 20-gauge instrumentation for vitreous surgery? Eye 2008; 22: 1263–1266.

Zabriskie, Norman. The Operating Microscope and Surgical Loupes. American Academy of Ophthalmology. Basic and Clinical Science Course: Basic Principles of Ophthalmic Surgery. Basic Principles of Ophthalmic Surgery. San Francisco: American Academy of Ophthalmology, 2006.

Part 2

Cornea and Ocular Surface

4

Trafficking of Immune Cells in the Cornea and Ocular Surface

Yureeda Qazi,
Aslihan Turhan and Pedram Hamrah
Cornea Service, Massachusetts Eye and Ear Infirmary,
Department of Ophthalmology, Harvard Medical School
USA

1. Introduction

The role of immuno-inflammatory responses in the cornea and ocular surface has continuously been evolving over the past decades and has been becoming the center stage for therapeutic approaches for many diseases. In fact, the relevance of inflammation as a significant component in the pathophysiology of most acute and chronic forms of corneal and ocular surface diseases (e.g., microbial keratitis, allergy, and dry eye syndrome) has become evident. Both local and systemic immunomodulation with anti-inflammatory agents have been used successfully in improving these conditions or bringing these conditions under control. Thus, understanding the cellular and molecular mechanisms by which the ocular surface participates in immuno-inflammatory disorders is crucial for a more rational clinical approach to treating these diseases.

There are several unique anatomical and physiological features of the cornea and ocular surface as compared to other tissues in the body, which translate into specific mechanisms by which they are involved in both inciting and expressing immunity, as well as preventing unnecessary inflammation. There are a very large number of immune and inflammatory disorders that involve the cornea and ocular surface. Control of leukocyte entry and migration within the cornea and ocular surface is thus vital to regulate protective and pathological responses. While local control of pathogens is dependent on the ability of immune cells to access and operate within these sites, too much inflammation can be deleterious and lead to loss of vision. In this chapter, the current knowledge on the coordinated migratory events that regulate leukocyte trafficking in the cornea and ocular surface are discussed. The aim is to first provide an overview of the contribution of resident bone marrow (BM)-derived cells of the cornea and ocular surface. Second, the role of infiltrating leucocytes in some of the innate defense mechanisms will be discussed. Third, we will provide a summary of the mechanisms that dictate immune cell trafficking to the cornea and ocular surface in response to inflammation. Finally, we will discuss trafficking mechanisms of antigen presenting cells from the cornea and ocular surface to draining lymph nodes where the immune responses are initiated.

2. Role of leukocytes in disease

2.1 Overview of resident leukocytes

The cornea and ocular surface have constant and direct contact with the external world. This necessitates a powerful and intrinsic immune surveillance system involved in their natural defense. Resident ocular tissue elements together with circulating bone marrow-derived cells are important components of this system, delicately balancing defense and tolerance under steady sate conditions. The ocular surface consists of three distinct anatomical regions: the cornea, limbus, and the conjunctiva. These regions function both in concert and independently against microbial, immunogenic and traumatic insults.

Antigen presenting cells (APCs) and in particular dendritic cells (DCs) orchestrate the immune response through their capacity to capture, process and subsequently present antigens. APCs serve as the principal immune sentinels to the foreign world. They can be divided into 'professional' and 'nonprofessional' types. While the latter are found among nonlymphoid tissues (e.g., vascular endothelial or some tissue epithelial cells), professional APC are BM-derived, and form an integral part of the immune system. Professional APCs include DCs (including epithelial Langerhans cells; LCs), macrophages, and B cells, although DCs are the most potent APCs. Expression of major histocompatibility class II (MHC-II) antigens on DCs, whose primary function is to distinguish between self and non-self, plays an integral role in antigen recognition and presentation. DCs have a dual function as key regulators of T cell immunity and tolerance induction to both self and foreign antigens. Precursor and progenitor DCs constitutively repopulate normal tissues from the bloodstream, and are recruited in elevated numbers to sites of inflammation. A second type of DC precursors is constituted by peripheral blood monocytes that are recruited during an inflammation.

DCs originate from bone marrow hematopoietic stem cells. (Traver et al., 2000; Wu et al., 2001) DC progenitors are not restricted to the BM and can be found in multiple locations. These progenitors can differentiate into DC upon challenge in peripheral tissues. Fully differentiated DC are found in healthy tissues as immunologically immature cells, being able to sample foreign antigens, but not able activate T cells. Although rare in numbers in the circulation, one fully mature DC is capable to interact with ten thousand T cells per day.(O'Keeffe et al., 2003) DC consist of several distinct populations that can be differentiated by surface and intracellular phenotypic markers, immunological function, and anatomic location. Irrespective of their phenotype and immunological role, DC exert their activity in the eye remote from their place of origin, where they utilize their advanced migratory skills for navigation. Currently, factors leading to the development from precursor DC to differentiated mature DC are still largely unknown. It has been shown that depending on the environmental cues, different forms of DC may be generated.(Naik et al., 2006) Further, while in lymphoid as well as in some non-lymphoid organs,(Kabashima et al., 2005; Merad et al., 2002) DC have been shown to proliferate locally, it is yet unclear whether resident corneal DC have the same proliferative potential, or are alternatively replenished through circulating DC. The diverse functions of DC in immune regulation depend on the diversity of DC subsets and lineages and on the functional plasticity of DCs at their immature stage.

Over the last several decades, the search for corneal APC, largely reliant on their presumed and universal MHC-II expression, had led to the dogma that APC are essentially absent in the central corneal. This absence of corneal APC was assumed to be a critical component of corneal immune privilege. However, this paradigm has now shifted with the demonstration of a diverse population of resident APC over the last years.(Hamrah et al., 2003a; Hamrah et al., 2003b, c) Dendritic cells, the sentinels of the immune system, were recently discovered to reside not only in the peripheral cornea, but also in the centreal cornea (**Fig 1**).(Hamrah et al., 2003c; Hamrah et al., 2002b; Liu et al., 2002) While a large number of DC are MHC class II+ in the periphery, a large population of MHC class II-*negative* immature/precursor DC are present both in the central epithelium and stroma.(Hamrah et al., 2003c; Hamrah et al., 2002b) Immature DC do neither express major histocompatibility complex (MHC)-II nor costimulatory molecules unless they are incited by cytokines. Thus, in contrast to other organs, where terminally differentiated populations of resident DC and/or macrophages outnumber colonizing precursors, large numbers of DCs within the cornea remain in an undifferentiated state.

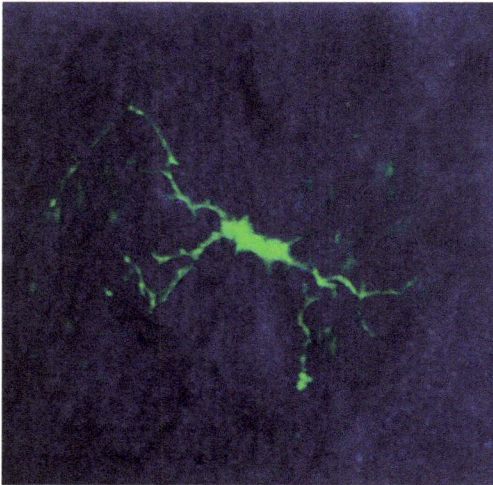

Fig. 1. Dendritic Cell in central corneal epithelium in CD11c-Yellow fluorescent protein (YFP) transgenic mouse

The constitutive presence of these DCs in the cornea focuses now attention on the cornea as a participant in immune and inflammatory responses, rather than the cornea being essentially a collagenous tissue that simply responds to the activity of infiltrating cells. Other immune cells that populate the cornea and ocular surface are T cells, B cells, macrophages, plasma cells, and neutrophils (PMN). Further, macrophages and neutrophils together with natural killer (NK) cells, initially constitute the primary innate immune response, while DCs, T cells and B cells largely play a role in the secondary, adaptive response.(Janeway C, 2004) While the primary innate immune response is non-specific, rapid, and lacks memory, the secondary adaptive immune response is slower, but highly specific. Further, T and B cell responses maintain immunological memory, such that any following encounters with the same antigen will lead to rapid and robust immune responses.

2.2 Microbial keratitis

2.2.1 Herpes simplex virus type-1 (HSV-1)

HSV-1, is a member of the α-herpesviridae family of double-stranded DNA (dsDNA) viruses.(Shukla & Spear, 2001) HSV-1 infections are prevalent both in the developed and developing countries with a higher and earlier onset of seroconversion in population groups of lower socioeconomic status.(Whitley & Roizman, 2001) 60% to 90% of the global adult population is infected with this pathogen, with a remarkably high prevalence of approximately 90% in the United States.(Carr et al., 2001; Whitley & Roizman, 2001) The two main forms of ocular HSV-1 infections are epithelial keratitis, and immune stromal keratitis.(Thomas, J. & Rouse, 1997) In the West, HSV-1 is also the leading cause of blindness secondary to recurrent infection, corneal stromal inflammation (herpes stromal keratitis; HSK), stromal thinning, neovascularisation and scarring.(Dana, M. R. et al., 2000)

The ocular surface, through several means, is able retard host invasion by external pathogens. The tear film which forms the outermost layer of the ocular surface presents the first barrier to viral invasion.(Farris, 1998) Some of the anti-viral factors in the tear film include, but are not limited to, tear film proteins such as lysozyme, immunoglobulin A (IgA), lactate dehydrogenase (LDH), complement proteins, amylase, peroxidase, as well as interferons alpha (IFNα) and beta (IFNβ). (Babu et al., 1995; Chatterjee et al., 1984; Chen et al., 1994) Since herpes viruses rely on replication and dissemination in metabolically active cells (Schang et al., 1998; Schang et al., 2000), the terminally differentiated outer layers of the corneal epithelium act as both a physical and metabolic barrier against viral entry. In the event of a breach in the integrity of the corneal epithelium, the virion attaches to epithelial cells via interaction of its surface glycoproteins with cognate receptors, (Campadelli-Fiume et al., 2007; Shukla et al., 1999; Spear, 2004) leading to either attachment, surfing and fusion of the virion envelope to the host cell plasma membrane, or, via endocytosis of the nucleocapsid into the host cell cytoplasm. Having intercepted the barriers to entry, HSV-1 inhibits its host's programmed cell death, assembles its immune-defying, host-crippling machinery to invade, replicate and infect the cornea, nerves and eventually the trigeminal ganglion where the virus maintains lifelong latency, leading to recurrent infections and potentially irreversible damage to the corneal tissue.(Akhtar & Shukla, 2009; Whitley & Roizman, 2001) Transmission may occur through cell lysis and shedding of viral progeny or cell-to-cell spread of the virion. Once the host corneal epithelial layers are penetrated, HSV replicates in the corneal epithelial cells. Following host infection, the outcome of viral latency or resolution has been shown to be dependent on the initial viral load.(Kintner & Brandt, 1995).

Cytokines are low molecular weight proteins produced by various resident corneal cells such as epithelial cells, stromal cells, and APCs.(Torres & Kijlstra, 2001) They are responsible for recruiting inflammatory and immune cells via cell-to-cell signalling through autocrine, paracrine and endocrine pathways, thus promoting tissue damage.(Balkwill & Burke, 1989) As the disease course changes, expression profiles of cytokines follow suit. During the early phase of HSK, the cornea expresses interleukin (IL)-1α, interferon (IFN)-γ and IL-2, whereas IL-4 is expressed later, indicating that the Th1 T cell response is required for induction of HSK. (Babu et al., 1995; Niemialtowski & Rouse, 1992b) (Heiligenhaus et al., 1999) While IL-2 may be responsible for incurring destructive effects on the stroma, IL-2 knockout mice are more prone to severe HSV infection, which is ameliorated by providing recombinant IL-2 treatment, hence indicating that the Th1 T cell response not only plays a role in tissue destruction, but also plays a protective role against HSV-1 invasion.(Ghiasi et al., 1999) Paradoxically, IFN-γ has also been implicated in the clearance of virus from the cells thus reducing latency, (Bouley et al., 1995; Smith et al., 1994) (Hendricks et al., 1991) yet driving immunopathogenesis as exemplified by the reduction in HSK severity following neutralisation of IFN-γ titres beforehand. (Hendricks et al., 1992b; Niemialtowski & Rouse, 1992a, b) Among the array of cytokines produced, IL-1 is particularly pertinent to corneal melting by induction of LC migration into the cornea thereby priming the tissue for further destruction. In order to combat the effects of IL-1, human corneal epithelium and stroma constitutively express interleukin-1 receptor antagonist (IL-1 RA), which helps maintain corneal immune privilege.(Dana, M. R. et al., 1998; Kennedy et al., 1995) Finally, while proinflammatory cytokines contribute to the augmentation of the immune response, vascular endothelial growth factor (VEGF) secreted by polymorphonuclear (PMN) cells, and local epithelial cells, contributes to corneal neovascularization in HSK.(Lee, S. et al., 2002; Zheng, M. et al., 2001)

Chemokines are specific, small cytokines of 8-10 kDa and can be classified according to their structure and function. Structurally, they fall into four families, the two most important of which are the CXC (alpha) and CC (beta) families. The CC and CXC chemokines are named based on intervening residues between their amino (N)-terminal cysteine amino acids. Hence, the CC family of chemokines have two adjacent cysteine amino acids near the N-terminus without an intervening residue. However, in the CXC family of chemokines, these N-terminal cysteine residues are separated by an amino acid "X", thus their "CXC" salutation. Chemokine receptors (CCR) CCR1, CCR2, CCR5, CXC chemokine receptor (CXCR) CXCR2 and their ligands (CCL/CXCL) have a well-defined role in HSV. Viral replication leads to expression of chemokines such as macrophage inflammatory protein (MIP)-1α/CCL3, KC/CXCL1, MIP-1β/CCL4, MIP-2/CXCL2, monocyte chemotactic protein (MCP)-1/CCL2 and lymphotactin/XCL1. (Thomas, J. et al., 1998) (Wolpe et al., 1989) Of these, MIP-1 α /CCL3 plays the most pivotal role in causing stromal inflammation, possibly by recruiting neutrophils and T cells as seen in experimental studies on murine corneas.(Tumpey et al., 1998; Wolpe et al., 1988) Furthermore, CXCR3 and its ligands, namely, monokine induced by gamma interferon (MIG)/CXCL9, interferon gamma-induced protein 10 (IP-10)/CXCL10 and interferon-inducible T-cell alpha chemoattractant (I-TAC)/CXCL11 may also contribute to the development of a protective, anti-viral immune response seen in the cornea following HSV-1 infection. (Carr et al., 2008; Wuest & Carr, 2008) These chemokines may form potential targets for therapy in HSK.

It is well established that primary infection with HSV-1 incites both a localized innate immune response, and systemic immunity through the adaptive arm of the immune cascade. The localized innate immune response involves PMNs, natural killer (NK) cells, and macrophages, with the adaptive immune response involving DCs and T cells.(Brandt & Salkowski, 1992; Ghiasi et al., 2000; Hendricks & Tumpey, 1990; Meyers-Elliott & Chitjian, 1981; Niemialtowski & Rouse, 1992a; Pepose, 1991; Tullo et al., 1983; Tumpey et al., 1996) Clinically, the collection of these cells is seen as infiltrates in the corneal stroma. Within 48 hours following infection, PMN cells, which constitute the first line of defense, are recruited to the cornea by means of the limbus vasculature, following a multi-step adhesion cascade, including selectins, integrins, and chemokines.(Thomas, J. et al., 1997) A cytokine and chemokine response by recruited PMN cells, including tumor necrosis factor (TNF-α),(Daheshia et al., 1998) then quickly translates into recruitment of other cells to the site of infection. Additionally, toll-like receptors (TLRs) expressed on the corneal epithelium and stroma, recognise pathogens and their activation leads to generation of both an innate and acquired adaptive immune responses. Of particular note are TLRs 3, 4, 7, and 9 which mediate an anti-viral response to corneal epithelial infection with HSV-1 (Redfern & McDermott) Binding of the pathogen to TLRs causes release of cytokines and chemokines which provide alert signals to draw in inflammatory cells such as neutrophils and lymphocytes. TLR activation also induces resident corneal APCs to express MHC-II and costimulatory molecules thus engaging the acquired immune response.(Hamrah & Dana, 2007) The anti-viral immune response of TLR7 has been successfully tested in clinical trials treating HSV following the success of Imiquimod, an FDA-approved TLR7 agonist used in the treatment of infection with the human papilloma virus (HPV).(Miller, R. L. et al., 2008) Despite encouraging results of TLR agonist therapy for HSV, one must exercise caution in their use since excessive TLR stimulation can lead to an unfavourably strong immune response with much damage to bystander cells and tissues of the eye.

Langerhans cells have been found in abundance near the limbus and are recruited to the site of inflammation within a few days in the wake of HSV-1 infection.(Streilein et al., 1979) (Asbell & Kamenar, 1987; Hendricks et al., 1992a) There they process the viral antigens for presentation to naïve T-helper (Th0) cells in draining lymph nodes. These Th0 cells mature into Th1 or Th2 cells depending upon the type of cytokines, prostaglandins and costimulatory molecules released by LCs and cells of the innate immune system.(Torres & Kijlstra, 2001) The extent of stromal damage in HSK is affected by the density of LCs in the cornea.(Asbell & Kamenar, 1987; Hendricks et al., 1992a; Jager et al., 1991; Jager et al., 1992; Miller, J. K. et al., 1993) Virally-induced migration or maturation of LCs in the cornea precedes the development of HSK. Induction of LC migration into the central cornea before HSV-1 infection results in an accelerated and enhanced delayed type hypersensitivity (DTH) response to HSV-1 antigens, and an increased severity of HSK. On the contrary, depletion of DCs reduces the incidence and severity of HSK, suggesting a role for DCs in the induction of a T cell response. These findings have led to the conclusion that HSV-1 infection results in de novo migration of LCs from the limbus, which in turn might play a role in the immunopathology of HSK through presentation of antigens to T cells in the infected cornea. Thus, patients that have a higher density of corneal LCs are likely to get more severe forms of HSK, which highlights the role of LCs as a potential therapeutic target in HSK.

HSK has been studied extensively using mouse models of disease and CD4+ T helper 1 (Th1) cells have been purported to be key mediators in the immunopathogenesis of corneal HSV-1 infection. (Hendricks, 1997; Streilein et al., 1997) In mice depleted of CD4+ cells, HSK development and progression was prevented or retarded, whereas depletion of CD8+ cells either made no difference or made the severity of HSK worse. (Newell et al., 1989a; Newell et al., 1989b) Corticosteroids, which are commonly prescribed in addition to antiviral therapy in HSK, work partially via inhibition of CD4+ T-cell response and are thus effective in controlling inflammatory damage to the eye. Among other local tissue factors, the kind of T-helper response generated is orchestrated by a fine balance between cytokines IL-12 and IFN-α, and IL-4 and IL-10, which mature Th0 cells into Th1 or Th2 respectively. (Torres &

Kijlstra, 2001) The predominant expression of cytokines IL-2 and IFN- α in HSK further corroborates the role of CD4+ Th1 immune response in HSK pathogenesis.(Hendricks et al., 1992b; Niemialtowski & Rouse, 1992b) The role of Th2 cells in HSK is far more controversial and inconclusive. While some groups state that Th2 cells have negligible involvement in HSK, (Niemialtowski & Rouse, 1992a, b) others either ascribe Th2 cells as inducers of HSK, (Foster et al., 1993; Jayaraman et al., 1993) or ascribe their role to convalescent phase of HSK.(Jayaraman et al., 1993) There is however one caveat; the kind of response generated is also driven by the strain of HSV-1. Corneal infections with the reticuloendotheliosis (RE) strain of HSV-1 are predominantly CD4+ driven, whereas the relatively less neuroinvasive (KOS) strain recruits and activates CD8+ T cells. (Hendricks & Tumpey, 1990; Newell et al., 1989a; Russell et al., 1984) T cell mediated delayed type hypersensitivity eventually is critical for the elimination of the virus. After this point circulating memory T and B lymphocytes continuously scan the cornea.

The suggested T-cell mediated immune response in HSK, is supported by the fact that specific HSV epitopes have been shown to mount an immune response by generation of autoreactive T cells. (Zhao et al., 1998) Murine studies of chronic HSK further demonstrated that despite clinical signs of active disease and lesions, 10-15 days post viral inoculation, viral antigens and messenger RNA (mRNA) were undetectable in the corneas of these mice.(Babu et al., 1996) Furthermore, Avery and colleagues performed elegant experiments, demonstrating that transfer of autoreactive CD4+ T cells to into athymic mice infected with HSV-1, results in the development of HSK.(Avery et al., 1995) However, there is ongoing debate regarding the source of antigenic response elicited in HSK. Verjans et al. have shown that T cells harvested and cultured from HSK donor corneas failed to show reactivity against human corneal antigens.(Verjans et al., 2000) Moreover, human studies to date have been inconclusive and it has been hypothesised that a variable clinical spectrum of disease in patients with recurrent HSK may either be due to a heterogeneous immune response to the HSV epitopes, or, to heterogeneity in the expression of corneal autoantigens in the host.(Ellison et al., 2003)

Based on the ability of HSV-1 to circumvent the immune response and maintain latency, along with the complexity of immune players that orchestrate signalling cascades leading to a spectrum of disease seen clinically, it is challenging for clinicians to treat HSK effectively. Attempts towards immunomodulation of HSK have been made, ranging from induction of apoptosis in T cells by amniotic membrane transfer,(Bauer et al., 2009) to suppression of chemotaxis and activation of CD4+T cells by targeting chemokine receptors.(Komatsu et al., 2008; Lee, S. K. et al., 2008). However, with an evolving and deeper understanding of the molecular mediators of HSV-1 infection, new molecular targets may provide platforms for emerging therapies.

2.2.2 Pseudomonas keratitis

One of the most important organisms in the group of bacterial keratitides is the Gram-negative bacterium *Pseudomonas aeruginosa. P. aeruginosa* is an opportunistic pathogen, which like other microbes, requires a breach in the corneal surface for infection.(Hazlett et al., 1978) Such infections are typically seen in individuals who wear contact lenses for extended periods of time, and in nosocomial or tropical settings stemming from the ability of the bacterium to grow in any niche without much nutritional support.(Hazlett, 2004)

Pseudomonal keratitis is highly invasive and can lead to corneal perforation within 24-48 hours post-infection.(Jones, 1973) Pseudomonal infections of the cornea are marked by inflammation and necrosis; there is a suppurative stromal infiltrate, coagulative necrosis, epithelial edema, a mucopurulent exudate, and in some cases a paracentral corneal ring infiltrate that can be seen in addition to a hypopyon.(Hazlett, 2004) One of the main host factors that is the culprit for a stromal meltdown is the massive recruitment of neutrophils, which release lysosomal enzymes and oxidative compounds, digesting collagen of the stromal extracellular matrix. (Carubelli et al., 1990; Nicas & Iglewski, 1985; Trinkaus-Randall et al., 1991; Van Horn et al., 1978; Weiss, 1989) IL-6, one of the cytokines expressed within 24 hours of *P.aeruginosa* invasion, may be involved in recruitment of PMNs to the site of inflammation by upregulating the expression intercellular adhesion molecule-1 (ICAM-1), a key molecule involved in migration of neutrophils.(Cole et al., 1999; Youker et al., 1992) Integrin-mediated neutrophil migration is a critical phenomenon that occurs not only within the proteoglycan matrix, but also among stromal keratocytes which express adhesion molecules.(Burns et al., 2005)

The rapid spread of infection in the early stages of disease has been attributed in part to a delayed response from the responsible TLRs, TLR-2, -4 and -5, which are expressed at a later stage in the disease thus leading to a delay in activation of both the innate and adaptive arms of the immune response. (Jin et al.) Using a murine model of pseudomonal keratitis, Sun and colleagues demonstrated that *P.aeruginosa* activates expression of TLR-4/5 on resident corneal bone marrow-derived macrophages, inducing transcription of chemokines and cytokines such as KC/CXCL1, as well as IL-1α and IL-1β. Subsequent recruitment of neutrophils into the corneal stroma leads to destruction of *P.aeruginosa*. The produced IL-1 has a positive feedback effect by activating the IL-1 receptor in macrophages and other cells of the cornea, thus ensuring a sustained response against the bacteria.(Sun et al.) While a sustained immune response favours reducing bacterial load, it is also associated with bystander local tissue damage from dysregulation of cytokines and chemokines as seen by elevated expression of TNF- α , MIP-2/CXCL2, IL-1α but low levels of IL-10.(Zhou et al.) It is evident that the role of a prompt and efficient immune response is critical in curtailing the spread and severity of pseudomonal keratitis, and eventually in preventing loss of vision. However, the caveat to a robust immune response remains the collateral damage incurred to surrounding cells and tissues.

From a therapeutic standpoint, TLRs make interesting molecular targets. Particularly, TLR-9 is one of the first in its class to be expressed when the cornea is invaded by *P. aeruginosa*. Huang and colleagues used RNA interference (RNAi) to knockdown TLR-9 in mice which resulted in decreased corneal opacity, fewer corneal perforations, with decreases in PMNs, inductors of the Th1 pathway IFN-γ and IL-12, and mediators of chemotaxis IL-1 β and MIP-2/CXCL2, but higher bacterial titers than controls.(Huang et al., 2005) Further, when mice were either depleted of CD4+ T cells or received IFN- γ neutralising antibodies prior to inoculation, they were spared corneal perforation and had a reduced DTH response, corroborating the role of a CD4+ T-cell mediated immunopathogenesis of this disease.(Kwon & Hazlett, 1997) Cytokines released by CD4+ T cell and LC result in infiltration of higher numbers of PMN, eventually leading to increased corneal.(Hazlett et al., 2001; Hazlett et al., 2002) While some propose that in order to minimise this collateral damage to ocular tissues, therapies should consider directing the immune response from

CD4+/Th1 mediated towards a Th2 pathway, (Kijlstra, 1994) others are of the opinion that it is the balance between pro-and anti-inflammatory mediators that is of greater significance in pseudomonal keratitis. (Hazlett, 2004) (O'Callaghan et al., 1996)

2.2.3 Fungal keratitis

Fungal keratitis is a vision-threatening infection and has seen a recent continual rise in incidence, with a spike during 2005-2006, following *Fusarium* contamination of a commercial contact lens solution. The three most common risk factors for fungal keratitis are contact lens use, trauma and penetrating keratoplasty. (Yildiz et al.) (Iyer et al., 2006) Filamentous fungi form the majority of causative organisms with *Fusarium* (41%), *Candida* (14%), *Aspergillus* (12%) and *Curvularia* (12%) being among the top contenders.(Iyer et al., 2006; Jurkunas et al., 2009) Fungal infections of the cornea, if not treated immediately and managed appropriately, can rapidly lead to corneal ulceration, perforation, corneal neovascularisation, loss of vision and possibly, loss of the eye. (Yuan & Wilhelmus, 2009) (Thomas, P. A. & Geraldine, 2007) It is thus imperative to understand the molecular underpinnings of fungal keratitis, especially the involvement of immune players, for a more thorough understanding towards devising novel and efficacious treatment modalities.

Contact lens wear can compromise the integrity of the corneal epithelium, making it susceptible to fungal invasion. It is known that contact lens wear can induce a subclinical host immune response with recruitment of LCs into the cornea. (Sankaridurg et al., 2000) TLRs on APCs, such as LCs or macrophages, recognize fungi, thereby activating the innate and adaptive immune response to clear the infection.(Barton & Medzhitov, 2003; Johnson et al., 2005) Hu et al. demonstrated the importance of macrophages through depletion of these cells, showing the contribution of macrophages in two different fungal infection models 5 and 7 days following infection. In this study development of more severe keratomycosis in mice depleted of macrophages points the contribution of macrophages in limiting fungal disease. (Hu et al., 2009) *In vitro* studies have shown that inactivated hyphae of *Fusarium solani* upregulate gene expression of TLRs-2, 3, 4 and 6, along with protein expression of TLRs 2 and 4 with resultant increases in cytokine expression of IL-6 and IL-8. The importance of TLR-4 in modulating the host defense mechanisms to fungi, especially *Fusarium* keratitis, has been demonstrated by several groups. In an experimental model of infectious keratitis, it was observed that resolution of *Fusarium* keratitis involved activation of both the innate immune response along with the adaptive arm through TLR-4.(Sun et al.) In another murine study, inoculation in knockout models of TLR-4, lead to impaired host anti-fungal defense mechanisms, decreased production of CXCL1 with subsequent decreased recruitment of neutrophils into the cornea, as well as uncontrolled fungal growth and eventually corneal perforation (Tarabishy et al., 2008) On the contrary, hydrocortisone treatment *in vitro* leads to a TLR-mediated increase in resistance to *Fusarium solani* with a concomitant increase in IL-6 expression by human corneal endothelial cells (HCEC).(Jin et al., 2007)

Similarly, in humans, fungal keratitis secondary to *Aspergillus* and *Candida* species also rely on human corneal TLRs 2 and 4 for hosting an immune response.(Mambula et al., 2002; Netea et al., 2002; Netea et al., 2003) TLRs 2 and 4 recognise fungal zymosan and mannan, leading to an expected increase in the production of IL-6 and IL-1β when challenged with *Aspergillus*, which is diminished by knocking down these innate receptors, confirming the putative role of TLRs 2 and 4 in Aspergillus keratitis.(Guo & Wu, 2009) In a recent study from the same group investigated the effect of targeting TLR2 by a small interfering RNA (siRNA) construct applied subconjunctively and topically to the cornea, showed that suppressing TLR2 expression in the cornea results in a decrease in neutrophil infiltration, allowing the cornea to preserve its morphological integrity. Suppressing TLR2 expression also caused a decrease in TNF-α, IL-1β, IL-6, IL-12, monocyte chemoattractant protein (MCP-1)/CCL2 and macrophage inflammatory protein (MIP-2)/CXCL2 expression. Immunomodulation by targeting TLR2 might be a treatment approach in fungal keratitis to avoid damage to the cornea by an immune response.(Guo et al.) *Aspergillus fumigatus* also induces IL-10 expression, and taken together, these cytokines attract and direct PMNs into the cornea, inciting innate immunity.(Redfern & McDermott) Thus, in addition to anti-fungal therapy, modulating fungus-specific TLR responses and controlling the host's immune response to the patient's advantage, is an exciting avenue to explore in the field of molecular anti-fungal therapy towards quicker resolution of infection with minimal residual damage.

2.2.4 *Acanthamoeba* keratitis

Acanthamoeba keratitis (AK) is a resilient, vision-threatening infection of the cornea. *Acanthamoeba* is an ubiquitous protozoa, which is exceptionally difficult to treat. Infection with *Acanthamoeba* either resolves spontaneously, or, as often seen, results in progressive infection and eventual corneal melting, suggesting a role of the immune system in its pathophysiology. Corneal transplantation is indicated in cases of severe infection, however, reinfection can commonly occur due to the presence of *Acanthamoeba* cysts within the host graft bed. Reinfection and recrudescence indicates the absence of memory against this parasite, and hence a poor activation of the adaptive arm of the immune response. *Acanthamoeba species* exist freely in the environment and on certain mucosal surfaces of healthy individuals.(Alizadeh et al. 1996; Niederkorn et al. 1999) Two of the most critical risk factors for AK include contact lens use and corneal trauma.(Niederkorn et al. 1999) Trophozoites attach to the surface of the contact lens which are then introduced to the ocular surface. Integrity of the host immune machinery predicts the severity of infection and incidence of disease as patients with AK have lower tear levels of IgA against *Acanthamoeba* antigens as compared to healthy controls, implicating the role of mucosa-mediated immunity in AK. (Alizadeh et al. 2001) The unique resilience of the double-layered cellulose wall of *Acanthamoeba* cysts, which are resistant to extreme temperatures, UV and gamma irradiation, underlies the challenges of treating AK. Systemic immunization to *Acanthamoeba* antigens does not confer immunity unlike mucosa-induced immunity.

Once the trophozoites invade the corneal epithelium through dislodgement of the epithelial cells caused by contact-lens induced microabrasions, there is a TLR-4-mediated immune response in corneal epithelial cells with release of cytokines IL-8 and TNF-α as shown in rats (Ren and Wu 2011). The innate immune response is activated with recruitment of neutrophils and macrophages. Macrophages are believed to be pivotal to the resolution of AK. They have a chemotactic response to the pathogen, and bear an inherent ability to kill the trophozoites *in vivo*. This phenomenon can be demonstrated by the depletion of macrophages in Clodronate treated animals which develop severe, chronic AK. (Stewart et al. 1992; van Klink et al. 1996) Although cysts are more difficult to eradicate, macrophages forming the first line of defence in AK may also attack *Acanthamoeba* cysts by direct phagocytosis as seen *in vitro* (Hurt et al. 2003). Like macrophages, neutrophils also form the first-line defence against both *Acanthamoeba* cysts and trophozoites, but demonstrate a more robust and efficient response. They are found in large numbers in corneas with AK, where they clear the protozoan using myeloperoxidase-dependent killing. Neutrophils are important both in the prevention and resolution of AK.(Hurt et al. 2003; Clarke et al. 2005).

The most convincing and potent response from the adaptive arm of the immune system is the secretion of IgA antibody. IgA antibody promotes neutrophil-mediated killing of trophozoites hence preventing adhesion of the trophozoites to the corneal epithelium. Furthermore, it shuts down the corneal melt-down plant of the trophozoites by inhibiting mannose-induced cytopathic protein 133 (MIP-133)-induced digestion of the corneal epithelium and stroma. The role of corticosteroids in the treatment of AK remains controversial. This issue arises from the contrary effects of dexamethasone on the eye; on the one hand they help in the resolution of AK-associated ocular inflammation, but on the other hand, they induce excystment of dormant cysts leading to recrudescence. Thus, targeting MIP-133 offers an attractive target in the therapy of AK. Earlier detection of disease by visualization of cysts in the cornea using *in vivo* confocal microscopy (IVCM) may offer an advantage in the management of AK.(Kumar et al. 2010) Through a more sensitive approach in the detection and consequent treatment of AK, the prognosis may be improved leading to fewer cases of corneal melting and associated complications.

2.3 Corneal transplantation

Corneal transplantation is the most common form of solid tissue transplantation with approximately 45,000 cases being performed annually in the United States alone.(CCTS, 1992; Niederkorn, 1999; Streilein, 1999) Unlike other solid tissue transplants, corneal allotransplants enjoy immune privilege, and neither require standard human leukocyte antigen (HLA) matching, nor permanent systemic immunosuppression. First time recipients of corneal allografts enjoy a 2-year graft survival rate of greater than 90% if the recipient corneal bed is avascular and free of inflammation.(Niederkorn, 1990) Corneal immune privilege is attributed to: (a) an avascular corneal bed which prevents recruitment of immune cells and leukocytes to the graft site, thus preventing recognition of non-self HLA antigens; (b) lack of lymphatic vessels, which eliminates transport and presentation of non-self HLA antigens and egress of APCs to T cells in draining lymph nodes, thus decreasing sensitisation (c) paucity of mature MHC-II+/HLA-DR+ resident corneal dendritic cells, including LC, thus decreasing direct presentation of unmatched HLA antigens to T cells; (d) constitutive expression of Fas ligand (CD95; FasL), which programs cell death of activated Fas+ T cells; (e) local ocular production of immunomodulatory neuropeptides and factors in aqueous humour such as transforming growth factor beta (TGF)-β_2 and alpha-melanocyte stimulating hormone (α -MSH), which inhibits alloantigen-driven T cell activation and DTH.(Dana, M. R. et al., 2000; Dua & Azuara-Blanco, 1999; Griffith et al., 1995; Jager et al., 1995; Niederkorn, 1990; Niederkorn et al., 1989; Streilein, 1993, 1995; Stuart et al., 1997; Thiel et al., 2009)

Neovascularization of the corneal graft greatly increases the rate of rejection.(Alldredge & Krachmer, 1981; Maguire et al., 1994) As per guidelines of the Collaborative Corneal Transplantation Studies, the recipient cornea is considered "high-risk" if there is stromal vascularisation in two or more quadrants preoperatively.(1992) The other factors which lead to graft rejection include growth of lymphatic vessels into the cornea, thereby establishing drainage to the cervical lymph nodes;(Hamrah et al., 2002a) migration of LCs into the cornea; maturation of resident LCs and DCs of the cornea, which can then serve as APCs;(Dekaris et al., 1999; Hamrah & Dana, 2007; Hamrah et al., 2002b; Liu et al., 2002) increased expression of cytokines IL-1 and TNF- α , which lead to recruitment of neutrophils, suppression of anterior chamber-associated immune deviation (ACAID), maturation of corneal APCs, upregulation of vascular adhesion molecules, and recruitment of leukocytes.(Dana, M. R. & Streilein, 1996; Dana, R., 2007; Hamrah et al., 2007; Pepose et al., 1985; Streilein et al., 1996; Yamagami et al., 1999; Zhu, S. et al., 1999; Zhu, S. N. & Dana, 1999)

The process of corneal transplant rejection includes an induction phase, called the "afferent" arm, and an expression phase, called the "efferent" arm. In the afferent arm, the host becomes sensitized to the donor antigens by APCs (e.g., MHC class II-positive DC, LC, macrophages, etc.) that present antigens to T cells in draining lymph nodes. This sensitization process involves two different pathways. The *direct* pathway, which involves *donor* APCs that sensitize the host *directly* when T cells recognize the donor class II MHC, thus generating direct alloreactive T cells, and the *indirect* pathway, which involves *host* APCs that migrate to the graft, take up donor antigens, process it, migrate to draining lymph nodes, and then present their antigens to T cells. Host sensitization to donor antigens of corneal grafts occurs through both pathways of sensitization, especially in high-risk corneal grafting. Further, the critical role of draining cervical lymph nodes in the process of allosensitization has been clearly demonstrated by recent studies. Upon arrival in the lymph nodes, APCs upregulate surface expression of co-stimulatory molecules, secrete cytokines, leading to activation of T cells. The subsequent efferent phase is then responsible for the actual rejection of the graft. This phase consists of the proliferation of alloreactive T cells in lymphoid organs, migration of these cells to the cornea, and the development of "memory" that can assist the alloimmune response in case of repeated exposure to the same antigens. Both CD8+ cytotoxic T lymphocyte (CTL) and CD4+ T helper (Th) cells have been implicated in the rejection process. Th1 cells uniquely secrete IL-2, IFN-γ, and lymphotoxin, and have the purpose of eradicating offending pathogens by promoting inflammation. Th2 cells secrete IL-4 and IL-10, suppress Th1 cells, and promote B cell differentiation, leading to the production of antibodies. CD4+ Th1 cells are the primary mediators of the efferent arm and act directly as effector cells and not as helper cells in corneal graft rejection. IL-2, secreted by these cells, stimulates the activation and proliferation of other T and B cells, whereas IFN-γ activates macrophages and induces expression of class II antigens in the donor tissue. The role of CD8+ T cells in the rejection of allogeneic corneal grafts remains controversial. While CD8+ T cells can contribute to graft rejection, corneal grafts can still be rejected in their absence, hence making CD8+ T cells sufficient but not necessary for graft rejection.

A major factor directing the recruitment of T cells and other leukocytes into grafts are chemokines. Surgical trauma induces release of early cytokines such as TNF-α and IL-1 by corneal epithelial cells. These cytokines in turn stimulate the production of early neutrophil- and macrophage-attractant chemokines, including MIP-2/CXCL2, MCP-1/CCL2, regulated upon activation normal T-cell expressed and secreted protein (RANTES)/CCL5, MIP-1α/CCL3, MIP-1β/CCL4 and eotaxin/CCL11, especially after high-risk corneal transplantation.(Flynn et al., 2008; Yamagami et al., 2005; Yamagami et al., 2000; Yamagami et al., 1999) While early chemokines direct non-antigen-specific leukocytes to the graft, late chemokines as stated above produced by the graft and infiltrating leukocytes recruit alloantigen-primed T cells into the graft. In addition, recipients of high-risk transplants express very high levels of the IP-10/CXCL10 chemokine. Chemokines function together with other molecular mediators including integrins and adhesion molecules to direct the immune response toward the graft. Therapeutic endeavours seek to inhibit either or both arms of the immune response to prolong graft survival. Regulatory T cells (Foxp3$^+$T$_{regs}$) have been shown to promote graft survival by inhibiting alloimmunity in draining lymph nodes as opposed to altering to the effector arm of the immune response.(Chauhan et al., 2009; Cunnusamy et al.; Tang & Bluestone, 2008) Measures devised to enhance graft survival should essentially revolve around three main goals: (a) to prevent induction of alloimmune response, (b) to inhibit or deplete immune effector cells, and, (c) to induce tolerance to specific alloantigens.(Niederkorn, 2002)

2.4 Dry Eye Disease

Dry eye disease (DED) is one of the most common diagnoses made in ophthalmic practice. DED affects millions of people around the world. It is more prevalent in women than men and is of inflammatory etiology.(Calonge et al.; 2007b) In epidemiologic studies conducted by Schaumberg and colleagues, they found a prevalence of 5.7% in women aged 50 years or younger, and 9.8% in women aged 75 years or above.(Schaumberg et al., 2003) Patients usually present with ocular irritation and in severe cases, there may be accompanying ocular pain, punctate keratopathy and filamentary keratitis.(Pflugfelder, 1998) The definition of DED has been modified over the years to integrate evolving concepts of the involvement of tear film hyperosmolarity, inflammation of the ocular surface, and the effects of DED on vision. In 2007, the International Dry Eye Workshop (DEWS) defined DED as: "a multifactorial disease of the tears and ocular surface that results in symptoms of discomfort, visual disturbance, and tear film instability with potential damage to the ocular surface. It is accompanied by increased osmolarity of the tear film and inflammation of the ocular surface."(DEWS, 2007a)

Clinically, DED can be categorised into (a) aqueous deficient and, (b) evaporative dry eye. (Lemp, 1995) Aqueous deficient DED consists of disorders that affect the lacrimal functional unit (LFU). The term "lacrimal functional unit" was coined in 1998 by Stern and group, comprising the ocular surface, lacrimal glands, associated innervation, and neuroendocrine factors.(Stern et al., 1998; Stern et al., 2004) The clinical diagnosis of DED is made using a combination of examination techniques, including Schirmer's test, tear film osmolarity, and fluorescein tear break-up time (fTBUT). A reading of less than 15mm on the Schirmer's strip in conjunction with elevated tear film osmolarity (>315 mOsm) is indicative of decreased tear production, hence, suggestive of aqueous-deficient DED. When fTBUT is less than 10 seconds, there is increased suspicion of evaporative DED. Diseases that lead to aqueous deficient dry eye disease include Sjögren's syndrome and non-Sjögren's autoimmune conditions. Whereas, evaporative dry eye is due to diseases that affect the production, quality and distribution of the tear film lipid layer, namely, meibomian gland dysfunction (MGD) and chronic blepharitis.(Barabino & Dana, 2007; Calonge et al.) It has been demonstrated that regardless of the etiology of dry eye, inflammation of the ocular surface and homing of immune cells to the target tissue, are hallmarks of DED. These immuno-inflammatory processes are culprits of corneal and conjunctival damage leading to the presenting symptoms.(Barabino & Dana, 2007; Dana, M. R. & Hamrah, 2002)

Recent evidence suggests a role for chemokines in the pathogenesis of dry eye syndromes. Increased RNA levels of IL-8, which is chemotactic for neutrophils, are found in the conjunctival epithelium of Sjogren's syndrome patients compared to controls. Furthermore, increased levels of select chemokines in the lacrimal glands of nonobese diabetic (NOD) mice, an animal model of Sjogren's syndrome, have been detected. NOD mice are a murine model for type-1 insulin-dependent diabetes with an autoimmune component. They represent a murine model of Sjogren's syndrome based on the similar histopathological picture of sialoadenitis. These mice have lymphocytic infiltration of not just the pancreas but also the submandibular and lacrimal glands. Both RANTES/CCL5 and IP-10/CXCL10 gene transcripts are detected in lacrimal glands at 8 weeks of age increased markedly during the course of active disease, concomitant with induction of their receptors CCR1, CCR5 and CXCR3. The examination of lacrimal glands indicated that lymphocytes in the inflammatory infiltrates are responsible for the production of these chemokines. Moreover, anti-RANTES treatment significantly reduced inflammation in the lacrimal glands of these mice. Further, patients with DED have a significant increase in the number of ocular surface cells that express CCR5, the receptor for RANTES/CCL5 and MIP-1β/CCL4. These data suggest that a better understanding of the role of chemokines and chemokine receptors in DES could open new doors for development of molecular strategies for immune modulation in this common disorder.

Numerous studies have demonstrated the enhanced expression of pro-inflammatory cytokines (e.g., IL-1, IL-6, IL-8, TNF-α) mRNA and protein by the ocular surface epithelium or tear film. The increase of these proinflammatory cytokines can lead to epithelial cell proliferation, keratinization, and angiogenesis, and thereby could link ocular surface disease with a number of lid margin disorders, such as rosacea, characterized by inflammation. In addition, IL-1 may lead to upregulation of matrix proteases, including collagenases, and thereby exacerbate stromal pathology as well as alter the paracrine effect of other cytokines on resident DCs, macrophages, fibroblasts, and epithelial cells by altering the matrix milieu in which these cytokines bind their respective receptors. Corneal epithelial cells respond to stress signals by producing cytokine mediators of inflammation such as TNF- α , IL-1β, IL- 8 and MMPs.(Li et al., 2006; Luo et al., 2004) Subsequently, maturing resident and recruited DC carry antigen to the draining lymph nodes to present and activate T cells. T cell-mediated responses have recently been shown to play a center stage in DED. Th1 cells recognize antigenic peptides in association with MHC class II molecules on the surface of APC, and release pro-inflammatory cytokines that increase vascular permeability and recruit further inflammatory cells to the site of injury. Due to the nonspecific nature of cell recruitment employed by CD4+ Th1 cells, inflammation can be severe with damage to bystander tissue. More recently, Th 17 associated cytokines and IL 17 producing cells have been found in the ocular surface epithelium of dry eye patients and it has been hypothesized that epithelial cells subjected to desiccating conditions promote DC to secrete IL-6, IL-23 and TGF-β, which in turn induce Th17 cells.(Zheng, X. et al.)

3. Leukocyte trafficking

Trafficking signals finely control the movement of distinct subsets of immune cells into and out of specific tissues. Leukocyte extravasation from blood to tissue, including that of APC and T cells, usually occurs through a multistep process, involving adhesion molecules and chemokines. Because the accumulation of leukocytes in tissues contributes to a wide variety of diseases, these 'molecular codes' provide new targets for inhibiting tissue-specific inflammation. However, immune cell migration is also critically important for the delivery of protective immune responses to tissues. Therefore, the challenge lies in identifying trafficking molecules that will specifically inhibit key cell subsets that drive disease processes without affecting the migration of leukocytes required for protective immunity.

Adhesion molecules can be categorized according to their structure or function. Four major families are distinguished structurally: the selectins, the sialomucins, the integrins, and the Ig superfamily. Leukocyte tethering and rolling, mediated typically by three selectins, L-selectin, E-selectin and P-selectin, are the first steps in the process of leukocyte binding to vascular endothelium. Two selectins, P- and E-selectin, are expressed on activated endothelium, whereas L-selectin is found on leukocytes. L-selectin is involved in the homing of T cells to lymphoid tissues but is also expressed on other leukocytes, where it participates in inflammation. E-selectin is expressed on corneal vascular endothelium, whereas P-selectin is expressed on inflamed vascular endothelium and by certain leukocytes. P-selectin glycoprotein ligand-1 (PSGL-1) binds all three selectins and is expressed on peripheral blood DC.

In the cornea, studies in both human and animal models of disease have confirmed that cell adhesion molecules are closely associated with the development of herpetic keratitis, and corneal allograft rejection. P- and E-selectin have been shown to mediate neutrophil recruitment to the cornea in studies using P/E-selectin knockout mice. Integrins are found on most cell types. Two subfamilies are most important for leukocyte migration: the $\alpha 4$ (CD49) and the $\beta 2$ (CD11/CD18) integrins. Four distinct members of $\beta 2$ integrins exist, three of which are expressed by DC. Vascular endothelial ligands for these molecules are members of the immunoglobulin superfamily. Leukocyte arrest in venules requires *in situ* activation of at least one of the four main integrins: VLA-4 (binds to VCAM-1), $\alpha 4\beta 7$ (binds to MadCAM-1), Mac-1(binds to ICAM-1) and LFA-1 (binds to ICAM-1 and 2). VCAM-1 has been shown to be present on monocytes and vascular endothelial cells during corneal inflammation. Arguably the most important ligand for $\beta 2$ integrins is ICAM-1, which is expressed on many cell types and is strongly upregulated upon exposure to inflammatory cytokines in the cornea and on limbal endothelial cells, deletion of which has been shown to suppress corneal graft rejection.

Chemokine receptors regulate leukocyte retention within tissues. The migration of leukocytes to inflammatory sites depends on a cascade of discrete events mediated, in part, by chemokines and their receptors. Numerous chemokines have now been described during inflammation, including CCL3/MIP-1α, CCL4/MIP-1β, and CCL5/RANTES, ligands for CCR1 and CCR5; CCL2/MCP-1, a ligand for CCR2; CCL22/MDC and CCL17/TARC, ligands for CCR4; CCL20/MIP-3α, the ligand for CCR6; CXCL8/IL-8, a ligand for CXCR1 and CXCR2; CXCL1/KC, CXCL2/MIP-2, and CXCL5/ENA-78, ligands for CXCR2; CXCL9 /MIG, CXCL10/IP10 and CXCL11/ITAC, ligands for CXCR3. In addition, constitutively expression of CCLs 2-5,CXCL10, and CCL27/CTACK, a ligand for CCR10 have been described in the normal cornea. Which of these chemokines is relevant in recruitment, retention and egrees of corneal APC, is unclear. Little is known about the constitutive recruitment of DC and macrophage precursors into peripheral tissues in the absence of inflammation. APC function and migratory behavior are related to rapid and coordinated *switching* in chemokine receptor expression by these cells, allowing them to coordinate migratory routes and biological function. During inflammation, CCL2, CCL5, and CXCL8 are produced to attract immature DC that express CXCR4 and CCR4 respectively. In addition, these DC are ideally suited for recruitment to inflammatory sites by their expression of functional receptors for inflammation-induced chemokines, such as CCR1, CCR2, CCR3, CCR5 and CXCR1.

Inflammatory signals induce resident corneal DCs to undergo maturation. Upon maturation, DCs downregulate pattern recognition receptors necessary for surveillance of antigens and upregulate CCR7, a receptor important in the homing of DCs to the lymph nodes. Maturing CCR7+ DCs then enter CCL21-expressing lymphatic vessels and travel to the draining lymph nodes where CCR7 ligands, namely, CCL19/EBI1 ligand chemokine (ELC) and CCL21/secondary lymphoid tissue chemokine (SLC), are produced. In addition, after fluorescein isothiocyanate (FITC) painting (dendritic cell migration assay), CXCR4 inhibition has been shown to impair LC and dermal DC migration to draining LNs, indicating that both CCR7 and CXCR4 make independent contributions to the egress of DCs from resident tissue to the lymph nodes. DC migration into and along afferent lymphatics occurs through a series of steps, including (1) mobilization, (2) detachment, (3) interstitial migration, (4) entry into the afferent lymphatics, and (5) transit via lymph. Recent data have shown that lymphatic endothelial cells upregulate E-selectin, chemokines (CCL5, CCL20, and CXCL5), and adhesion molecules (ICAM-1 and VCAM-1) after cytokine stimulation *in vitro* or *in vivo*. Once in the draining lymph nodes, antigen-loaded mature DCs activate naive T cells, which then proliferate and enter the blood and migrate back to the site of inflammation. In the cornea, CCR5 and CX3CR1, but not CCR1 are partially involved in the recruitment of MHC-II+ LCs. How the central immature LC or stromal APC populations are recruited is not known, although the recently demonstrated constitutive expression of CCR2 on stromal BM-derived cell subsets, implicates a role for this chemokine. Further, both vascular endothelial growth factor (VEGFR)-3 and CCR7 are partially implicated in the egress of stromal DCs. APC recruitment to the cornea is likely complex, highly regulated and dependent on recruitment signals that are either tissue-specific or inflammation-induced, or both.

4. Conclusion

The cornea and ocular surface are constantly exposed to environmental pollutants and irritants, microbes, and other potentially noxious agents. Since from an evolutionary standpoint the scope of the host defense mechanisms against these stimuli should be narrow, that is to say adequately effective to protect the eye against the potential harm from these agents and yet tempered enough not to lead to unwanted damage, the eye has developed many mechanisms to effect and regulate its response to environmental challenges. Identification of the critical pathways of cell migration to and from the cornea will provide new molecular targets for pharmacological intervention in inflammatory, infectious, alloimmune and autoimmune diseases and may lead to novel highly specific strategies for immunotherapy, through modulation of APC and T cell migration and function. Few effective anti-inflammatory drugs have emerged over the last decades in the ophthalmic field and an urgent need for new drugs exists, as many inflammatory diseases are inadequately responsive to current medications.

5. References

Akhtar, J. & Shukla, D. (2009). Viral entry mechanisms: cellular and viral mediators of herpes simplex virus entry. *FEBS J.* 276: 7228-7236.

Alizadeh, H., Niederkorn, J.Y., McCulley, J.P., in: Pepose, J.S., Holland, G.N., Wilhelmus, K.R. (Eds.), Ocular Infection and Immunity, Mosby, St. Louis, 1996, pp. 1062e1071.

Alizadeh H, Apte S, El-Agha MS, Li, L. Hurt, M. Howard, K. Cavanagh, H. D. McCulley, J. P. Niederkorn, J.Y. (2001) Tear IgA and serum IgG antibodies against Acanthamoeba in patients with Acanthamoeba keratitis. *Cornea.* 20:622-627.

Alldredge, O.C. & Krachmer, J.H. (1981). Clinical types of corneal transplant rejection. Their manifestations, frequency, preoperative correlates, and treatment. *Arch Ophthalmol.* 99: 599-604.

Asbell, P.A. & Kamenar, T. (1987). The response of Langerhans cells in the cornea to herpetic keratitis. *Curr Eye Res.* 6: 179-182.

Avery, A.C., Zhao, Z.S., Rodriguez, A., Bikoff, E.K., Soheilian, M., Foster, C.S., & Cantor, H. (1995). Resistance to herpes stromal keratitis conferred by an IgG2a-derived peptide. *Nature.* 376: 431-434.

Babu, J.S., Kanangat, S., & Rouse, B.T. (1995). T cell cytokine mRNA expression during the course of the immunopathologic ocular disease herpetic stromal keratitis. *J Immunol.* 154: 4822-4829.

Babu, J.S., Thomas, J., Kanangat, S., Morrison, L.A., Knipe, D.M., & Rouse, B.T. (1996). Viral replication is required for induction of ocular immunopathology by herpes simplex virus. *J Virol.* 70: 101-107.

Balkwill, F.R. & Burke, F. (1989). The cytokine network. *Immunol Today.* 10: 299-304.

Barabino, S. & Dana, M.R. (2007). Dry eye syndromes. *Chem Immunol Allergy.* 92: 176-184.

Barton, G.M. & Medzhitov, R. (2003). Toll-like receptor signaling pathways. *Science.* 300: 1524-1525.

Bauer, D., Wasmuth, S., Hennig, M., Baehler, H., Steuhl, K.P., & Heiligenhaus, A. (2009). Amniotic membrane transplantation induces apoptosis in T lymphocytes in murine corneas with experimental herpetic stromal keratitis. *Invest Ophthalmol Vis Sci.* 50: 3188-3198.

Bouley, D.M., Kanangat, S., Wire, W., & Rouse, B.T. (1995). Characterization of herpes simplex virus type-1 infection and herpetic stromal keratitis development in IFN-gamma knockout mice. *J Immunol.* 155: 3964-3971.

Brandt, C.R. & Salkowski, C.A. (1992). Activation of NK cells in mice following corneal infection with herpes simplex virus type-1. *Invest Ophthalmol Vis Sci.* 33: 113-120.

Burns, A.R., Li, Z., & Smith, C.W. (2005). Neutrophil migration in the wounded cornea: the role of the keratocyte. *Ocul Surf.* 3: S173-176.

Calonge, M., Enriquez-de-Salamanca, A., Diebold, Y., Gonzalez-Garcia, M.J., Reinoso, R., Herreras, J.M., & Corell, A. (2010). Dry eye disease as an inflammatory disorder. *Ocul Immunol Inflamm.* 18: 244-253.

Campadelli-Fiume, G., Amasio, M., Avitabile, E., Cerretani, A., Forghieri, C., Gianni, T., & Menotti, L. (2007). The multipartite system that mediates entry of herpes simplex virus into the cell. *Rev Med Virol.* 17: 313-326.

Carr, D.J., Harle, P., & Gebhardt, B.M. (2001). The immune response to ocular herpes simplex virus type 1 infection. *Exp Biol Med (Maywood).* 226: 353-366.

Carr, D.J., Wuest, T., & Ash, J. (2008). An increase in herpes simplex virus type 1 in the anterior segment of the eye is linked to a deficiency in NK cell infiltration in mice deficient in CXCR3. *J Interferon Cytokine Res.* 28: 245-251.

Carubelli, R., Nordquist, R.E., & Rowsey, J.J. (1990). Role of active oxygen species in corneal ulceration. Effect of hydrogen peroxide generated in situ. *Cornea.* 9: 161-169.

Chatterjee, S., Lakeman, A.D., Whitley, R.J., & Hunter, E. (1984). Effect of cloned human interferons on the replication of and cell fusion induced by herpes simplex virus. *Virus Res.* 1: 81-87.

Chauhan, S.K., Saban, D.R., Lee, H.K., & Dana, R. (2009). Levels of Foxp3 in regulatory T cells reflect their functional status in transplantation. *J Immunol.* 182: 148-153.

Chen, S.H., Oakes, J.E., & Lausch, R.N. (1994). Synergistic anti-herpes effect of TNF-alpha and IFN-gamma in human corneal epithelial cells compared with that in corneal fibroblasts. *Antiviral Res.* 25: 201-213.

Clarke DW, Alizadeh H, Niederkorn, J.Y. (2005). Failure of Acanthamoeba castellanii to produce intraocular infections. *Invest Ophthalmol Vis Sci.* 46:2472-2478.

Cole, N., Bao, S., Willcox, M., & Husband, A.J. (1999). Expression of interleukin-6 in the cornea in response to infection with different strains of Pseudomonas aeruginosa. *Infect Immun.* 67: 2497-2502.

Cunnusamy, K., Chen, P.W., & Niederkorn, J.Y. (2011). IL-17A-Dependent CD4+CD25+ Regulatory T Cells Promote Immune Privilege of Corneal Allografts. *J Immunol.* 186: 6737-6745.

Daheshia, M., Kanangat, S., & Rouse, B.T. (1998). Production of key molecules by ocular neutrophils early after herpetic infection of the cornea. *Exp Eye Res.* 67: 619-624.

Dana, M.R., Dai, R., Zhu, S., Yamada, J., & Streilein, J.W. (1998). Interleukin-1 receptor antagonist suppresses Langerhans cell activity and promotes ocular immune privilege. *Invest Ophthalmol Vis Sci.* 39: 70-77.

Dana, M.R. & Hamrah, P. (2002). Role of immunity and inflammation in corneal and ocular surface disease associated with dry eye. *Adv Exp Med Biol.* 506: 729-738.

Dana, M.R., Qian, Y., & Hamrah, P. (2000). Twenty-five-year panorama of corneal immunology: emerging concepts in the immunopathogenesis of microbial keratitis, peripheral ulcerative keratitis, and corneal transplant rejection. *Cornea.* 19: 625-643.

Dana, M.R. & Streilein, J.W. (1996). Loss and restoration of immune privilege in eyes with corneal neovascularization. *Invest Ophthalmol Vis Sci.* 37: 2485-2494.

Dana, R. (2007). Comparison of topical interleukin-1 vs tumor necrosis factor-alpha blockade with corticosteroid therapy on murine corneal inflammation, neovascularization, and transplant survival (an American Ophthalmological Society thesis). *Trans Am Ophthalmol Soc.* 105: 330-343.

Dekaris, I., Zhu, S.N., & Dana, M.R. (1999). TNF-alpha regulates corneal Langerhans cell migration. *J Immunol.* 162: 4235-4239.

Dua, H.S. & Azuara-Blanco, A. (1999). Corneal allograft rejection: risk factors, diagnosis, prevention, and treatment. *Indian J Ophthalmol.* 47: 3-9.

Ellison, A.R., Yang, L., Cevallos, A.V., & Margolis, T.P. (2003). Analysis of the herpes simplex virus type 1 UL6 gene in patients with stromal keratitis. *Virology.* 310: 24-28.

Farris, R. (1998). Abnormalities of the tears and treatment of dry eyes. in *The Cornea* (ed. HE Kauffman, B.B., MB McDonald), pp. p109-130. Butterworth-Heinemann, Boston.

Flynn, T.H., Mitchison, N.A., Ono, S.J., & Larkin, D.F. (2008). Aqueous humor alloreactive cell phenotypes, cytokines and chemokines in corneal allograft rejection. *Am J Transplant*. 8: 1537-1543.

Foster, C.S., Rodriguez Garcia, A., Pedroza-Seres, M., Berra, A., Heiligenhaus, A., Soukiasian, S., & Jayaraman, S. (1993). Murine herpes simplex virus keratitis is accentuated by CD4+, V beta 8.2+ Th2 T cells. *Trans Am Ophthalmol Soc*. 91: 325-348; discussion 349-350.

Ghiasi, H., Cai, S., Perng, G.C., Nesburn, A.B., & Wechsler, S.L. (2000). The role of natural killer cells in protection of mice against death and corneal scarring following ocular HSV-1 infection. *Antiviral Res*. 45: 33-45.

Ghiasi, H., Cai, S., Slanina, S.M., Perng, G.C., Nesburn, A.B., & Wechsler, S.L. (1999). The role of interleukin (IL)-2 and IL-4 in herpes simplex virus type 1 ocular replication and eye disease. *J Infect Dis*. 179: 1086-1093.

Griffith, T.S., Brunner, T., Fletcher, S.M., Green, D.R., & Ferguson, T.A. (1995). Fas ligand-induced apoptosis as a mechanism of immune privilege. *Science*. 270: 1189-1192.

Group, T.C.C.T.S.R. (1992). The collaborative corneal transplantation studies (CCTS). Effectiveness of histocompatibility matching in high-risk corneal transplantation. The Collaborative Corneal Transplantation Studies Research Group. *Arch Ophthalmol*. 110: 1392-1403.

Guo, H., Gao, J., & Wu, X. (2011). Toll-like receptor 2 siRNA suppresses corneal inflammation and attenuates Aspergillus fumigatus keratitis in rats. *Immunol Cell Biol*.

Guo, H. & Wu, X. (2009). Innate responses of corneal epithelial cells against Aspergillus fumigatus challenge. *FEMS Immunol Med Microbiol*. 56: 88-93.

Hamrah, P. & Dana, M.R. (2007). Corneal antigen-presenting cells. *Chem Immunol Allergy*. 92: 58-70.

Hamrah, P., Huq, S.O., Liu, Y., Zhang, Q., & Dana, M.R. (2003a). Corneal immunity is mediated by heterogeneous population of antigen-presenting cells. *J Leukoc Biol*. 74: 172-178.

Hamrah, P., Liu, Y., Zhang, Q., & Dana, M.R. (2003b). Alterations in corneal stromal dendritic cell phenotype and distribution in inflammation. *Arch Ophthalmol*. 121: 1132-1140.

Hamrah, P., Liu, Y., Zhang, Q., & Dana, M.R. (2003c). The corneal stroma is endowed with a significant number of resident dendritic cells. *Invest Ophthalmol Vis Sci*. 44: 581-589.

Hamrah, P., Yamagami, S., Liu, Y., Zhang, Q., Vora, S.S., Lu, B., Gerard, C.J., & Dana, M.R. (2007). Deletion of the chemokine receptor CCR1 prolongs corneal allograft survival. *Invest Ophthalmol Vis Sci*. 48: 1228-1236.

Hamrah, P., Zhang, Q., & Dana, M.R. (2002a). Expression of vascular endothelial growth factor receptor-3 (VEGFR-3) in the conjunctiva--a potential link between lymphangiogenesis and leukocyte trafficking on the ocular surface. *Adv Exp Med Biol*. 506: 851-860.

Hamrah, P., Zhang, Q., Liu, Y., & Dana, M.R. (2002b). Novel characterization of MHC class II-negative population of resident corneal Langerhans cell-type dendritic cells. *Invest Ophthalmol Vis Sci*. 43: 639-646.

Hazlett, L.D. (2004). Corneal response to Pseudomonas aeruginosa infection. *Prog Retin Eye Res*. 23: 1-30.

Hazlett, L.D., McClellan, S., Barrett, R., & Rudner, X. (2001). B7/CD28 costimulation is critical in susceptibility to Pseudomonas aeruginosa corneal infection: a comparative study using monoclonal antibody blockade and CD28-deficient mice. *J Immunol.* 166: 1292-1299.

Hazlett, L.D., McClellan, S.A., Rudner, X.L., & Barrett, R.P. (2002). The role of Langerhans cells in Pseudomonas aeruginosa infection. *Invest Ophthalmol Vis Sci.* 43: 189-197.

Hazlett, L.D., Rosen, D.D., & Berk, R.S. (1978). Age-related susceptibility to Pseudomonas aeruginosa ocular infections in mice. *Infect Immun.* 20: 25-29.

Heiligenhaus, A., Bauer, D., Zheng, M., Mrzyk, S., & Steuhl, K.P. (1999). CD4+ T-cell type 1 and type 2 cytokines in the HSV-1 infected cornea. *Graefes Arch Clin Exp Ophthalmol.* 237: 399-406.

Hendricks, R.L. (1997). An immunologist's view of herpes simplex keratitis: Thygeson Lecture 1996, presented at the Ocular Microbiology and Immunology Group meeting, October 26, 1996. *Cornea.* 16: 503-506.

Hendricks, R.L., Janowicz, M., & Tumpey, T.M. (1992a). Critical role of corneal Langerhans cells in the CD4- but not CD8-mediated immunopathology in herpes simplex virus-1-infected mouse corneas. *J Immunol.* 148: 2522-2529.

Hendricks, R.L. & Tumpey, T.M. (1990). Contribution of virus and immune factors to herpes simplex virus type I-induced corneal pathology. *Invest Ophthalmol Vis Sci.* 31: 1929-1939.

Hendricks, R.L., Tumpey, T.M., & Finnegan, A. (1992b). IFN-gamma and IL-2 are protective in the skin but pathologic in the corneas of HSV-1-infected mice. *J Immunol.* 149: 3023-3028.

Hendricks, R.L., Weber, P.C., Taylor, J.L., Koumbis, A., Tumpey, T.M., & Glorioso, J.C. (1991). Endogenously produced interferon alpha protects mice from herpes simplex virus type 1 corneal disease. *J Gen Virol.* 72 (Pt 7): 1601-1610.

Hu, J., Wang, Y., & Xie, L. (2009). Potential role of macrophages in experimental keratomycosis. *Invest Ophthalmol Vis Sci.* 50: 2087-2094.

Huang, X., Barrett, R.P., McClellan, S.A., & Hazlett, L.D. (2005). Silencing Toll-like receptor-9 in Pseudomonas aeruginosa keratitis. *Invest Ophthalmol Vis Sci.* 46: 4209-4216.

Hurt M, Proy V, Niederkorn JY, Alizadeh H. (2003) The interaction of Acanthamoeba castellanii cysts with macrophages and neutrophils. *J Parasitol.* 89:565-572.

Iyer, S.A., Tuli, S.S., & Wagoner, R.C. (2006). Fungal keratitis: emerging trends and treatment outcomes. *Eye Contact Lens.* 32: 267-271.

Jager, M.J., Atherton, S., Bradley, D., & Streilein, J.W. (1991). Herpetic stromal keratitis in mice: less reversibility in the presence of Langerhans cells in the central cornea. *Curr Eye Res.* 10 Suppl: 69-73.

Jager, M.J., Bradley, D., Atherton, S., & Streilein, J.W. (1992). Presence of Langerhans cells in the central cornea linked to the development of ocular herpes in mice. *Exp Eye Res.* 54: 835-841.

Jager, M.J., Bradley, D., & Streilein, J.W. (1995). Immunosuppressive properties of cultured human cornea and ciliary body in normal and pathological conditions. *Transpl Immunol.* 3: 135-142.

Janeway C, T.P., Walport M, Shlomchik M. (2004). *Immunobiology.* Garland Science.

Jayaraman, S., Heiligenhaus, A., Rodriguez, A., Soukiasian, S., Dorf, M.E., & Foster, C.S. (1993). Exacerbation of murine herpes simplex virus-mediated stromal keratitis by Th2 type T cells. *J Immunol.* 151: 5777-5789.

Jin, X., Lin, Z., & Xie, X. (2010). The delayed response of Toll-like receptors may relate to Pseudomonas aeruginosa keratitis exacerbating rapidly at the early stages of infection. *Eur J Clin Microbiol Infect Dis.* 29: 231-238.

Jin, X., Qin, Q., Tu, L., Zhou, X., Lin, Y., & Qu, J. (2007). Toll-like receptors (TLRs) expression and function in response to inactivate hyphae of Fusarium solani in immortalized human corneal epithelial cells. *Mol Vis.* 13: 1953-1961.

Johnson, A.C., Heinzel, F.P., Diaconu, E., Sun, Y., Hise, A.G., Golenbock, D., Lass, J.H., & Pearlman, E. (2005). Activation of toll-like receptor (TLR)2, TLR4, and TLR9 in the mammalian cornea induces MyD88-dependent corneal inflammation. *Invest Ophthalmol Vis Sci.* 46: 589-595.

Jones, D.B. (1973). Early diagnosis and therapy of bacterial corneal ulcers. *Int Ophthalmol Clin.* 13: 1-29.

Jurkunas, U., Behlau, I., & Colby, K. (2009). Fungal keratitis: changing pathogens and risk factors. *Cornea.* 28: 638-643.

Kabashima, K., Banks, T.A., Ansel, K.M., Lu, T.T., Ware, C.F., & Cyster, J.G. (2005). Intrinsic lymphotoxin-beta receptor requirement for homeostasis of lymphoid tissue dendritic cells. *Immunity.* 22: 439-450.

Kennedy, M.C., Rosenbaum, J.T., Brown, J., Planck, S.R., Huang, X., Armstrong, C.A., & Ansel, J.C. (1995). Novel production of interleukin-1 receptor antagonist peptides in normal human cornea. *J Clin Invest.* 95: 82-88.

Kijlstra, A. (1994). The role of cytokines in ocular inflammation. *Br J Ophthalmol.* 78: 885-886.

Kintner, R.L. & Brandt, C.R. (1995). The effect of viral inoculum level and host age on disease incidence, disease severity, and mortality in a murine model of ocular HSV-1 infection. *Curr Eye Res.* 14: 145-152.

Komatsu, K., Miyazaki, D., Morohoshi, K., Kuo, C.H., Kakimaru-Hasegawa, A., Komatsu, N., Namba, S., Haino, M., Matsushima, K., & Inoue, Y. (2008). Pathogenesis of herpetic stromal keratitis in CCR5- and/or CXCR3-deficient mice. *Curr Eye Res.* 33: 736-749.

Kumar RL, Cruzat A, Hamrah P. (2010). Current state of in vivo confocal microscopy in management of microbial keratitis. *Semin Ophthalmol.* 25:166-170.

Kwon, B. & Hazlett, L.D. (1997). Association of CD4+ T cell-dependent keratitis with genetic susceptibility to Pseudomonas aeruginosa ocular infection. *J Immunol.* 159: 6283-6290.

Lee, S., Zheng, M., Kim, B., & Rouse, B.T. (2002). Role of matrix metalloproteinase-9 in angiogenesis caused by ocular infection with herpes simplex virus. *J Clin Invest.* 110: 1105-1111.

Lee, S.K., Choi, B.K., Kang, W.J., Kim, Y.H., Park, H.Y., Kim, K.H., & Kwon, B.S. (2008). MCP-1 derived from stromal keratocyte induces corneal infiltration of CD4+ T cells in herpetic stromal keratitis. *Mol Cells.* 26: 67-73.

Lemp, M.A. (1995). Report of the National Eye Institute/Industry workshop on Clinical Trials in Dry Eyes. *CLAO J.* 21: 221-232.

Li, D.Q., Luo, L., Chen, Z., Kim, H.S., Song, X.J., & Pflugfelder, S.C. (2006). JNK and ERK MAP kinases mediate induction of IL-1beta, TNF-alpha and IL-8 following hyperosmolar stress in human limbal epithelial cells. *Exp Eye Res.* 82: 588-596.

Liu, Y., Hamrah, P., Zhang, Q., Taylor, A.W., & Dana, M.R. (2002). Draining lymph nodes of corneal transplant hosts exhibit evidence for donor major histocompatibility complex (MHC) class II-positive dendritic cells derived from MHC class II-negative grafts. *J Exp Med.* 195: 259-268.

Luo, L., Li, D.Q., Doshi, A., Farley, W., Corrales, R.M., & Pflugfelder, S.C. (2004). Experimental dry eye stimulates production of inflammatory cytokines and MMP-9 and activates MAPK signaling pathways on the ocular surface. *Invest Ophthalmcl Vis Sci.* 45: 4293-4301.

Maguire, M.G., Stark, W.J., Gottsch, J.D., Stulting, R.D., Sugar, A., Fink, N.E., & Schwartz, A. (1994). Risk factors for corneal graft failure and rejection in the collaborative corneal transplantation studies. Collaborative Corneal Transplantation Studies Research Group. *Ophthalmology.* 101: 1536-1547.

Mambula, S.S., Sau, K., Henneke, P., Golenbock, D.T., & Levitz, S.M. (2002). Toll-like receptor (TLR) signaling in response to Aspergillus fumigatus. *J Biol Chem.* 277: 39320-39326.

Merad, M., Manz, M.G., Karsunky, H., Wagers, A., Peters, W., Charo, I., Weissman, I.L., Cyster, J.G., & Engleman, E.G. (2002). Langerhans cells renew in the skin throughout life under steady-state conditions. *Nat Immunol.* 3: 1135-1141.

Meyers-Elliott, R.H. & Chitjian, P.A. (1981). Immunopathogenesis of corneal inflammation in herpes simplex virus stromal keratitis: role of the polymorphonuclear leukocyte. *Invest Ophthalmol Vis Sci.* 20: 784-798.

Miller, J.K., Laycock, K.A., Nash, M.M., & Pepose, J.S. (1993). Corneal Langerhans cell dynamics after herpes simplex virus reactivation. *Invest Ophthalmol Vis Sci.* 34: 2282-2290.

Miller, R.L., Meng, T.C., & Tomai, M.A. (2008). The antiviral activity of Toll-like receptor 7 and 7/8 agonists. *Drug News Perspect.* 21: 69-87.

Naik, S.H., Metcalf, D., van Nieuwenhuijze, A., Wicks, I., Wu, L., O'Keeffe, M., & Shortman, K. (2006). Intrasplenic steady-state dendritic cell precursors that are distinct from monocytes. *Nat Immunol.* 7: 663-671.

Netea, M.G., Van Der Graaf, C.A., Vonk, A.G., Verschueren, I., Van Der Meer, J.W., & Kullberg, B.J. (2002). The role of toll-like receptor (TLR) 2 and TLR4 in the host defense against disseminated candidiasis. *J Infect Dis.* 185: 1483-1489.

Netea, M.G., Warris, A., Van der Meer, J.W., Fenton, M.J., Verver-Janssen, T.J., Jacobs, L.E., Andresen, T., Verweij, P.E., & Kullberg, B.J. (2003). Aspergillus fumigatus evades immune recognition during germination through loss of toll-like receptor-4-mediated signal transduction. *J Infect Dis.* 188: 320-326.

Newell, C.K., Martin, S., Sendele, D., Mercadal, C.M., & Rouse, B.T. (1989a). Herpes simplex virus-induced stromal keratitis: role of T-lymphocyte subsets in immunopathology. *J Virol.* 63: 769-775.

Newell, C.K., Sendele, D., & Rouse, B.T. (1989b). Effects of CD4+ and CD8+ T-lymphocyte depletion on the induction and expression of herpes simplex stromal keratitis. *Reg Immunol.* 2: 366-369.

Nicas, T.I. & Iglewski, B.H. (1985). The contribution of exoproducts to virulence of Pseudomonas aeruginosa. *Can J Microbiol.* 31: 387-392.

Niederkorn, J.Y. (1990). Immune privilege and immune regulation in the eye. *Adv Immunol.* 48: 191-226.

Niederkorn, J.Y. (1999). The immunology of corneal transplantation. *Dev Ophthalmol.* 30: 129-140.

Niederkorn JY, Alizadeh H, Leher H, McCulley JP. (1999) The pathogenesis of Acanthamoeba keratitis.*Microbes Infect.* 1:437-443.

Niederkorn, J.Y. (2002). Immunology and immunomodulation of corneal transplantation. *Int Rev Immunol.* 21: 173-196.

Niederkorn, J.Y., Peeler, J.S., Ross, J., & Callanan, D. (1989). The immunogenic privilege of corneal allografts. *Reg Immunol.* 2: 117-124.

Niemialtowski, M.G. & Rouse, B.T. (1992a). Phenotypic and functional studies on ocular T cells during herpetic infections of the eye. *J Immunol.* 148: 1864-1870.

Niemialtowski, M.G. & Rouse, B.T. (1992b). Predominance of Th1 cells in ocular tissues during herpetic stromal keratitis. *J Immunol.* 149: 3035-3039.

O'Callaghan, R.J., Engel, L.S., Hobden, J.A., Callegan, M.C., Green, L.C., & Hill, J.M. (1996). Pseudomonas keratitis. The role of an uncharacterized exoprotein, protease IV, in corneal virulence. *Invest Ophthalmol Vis Sci.* 37: 534-543.

O'Keeffe, M., Hochrein, H., Vremec, D., Scott, B., Hertzog, P., Tatarczuch, L., & Shortman, K. (2003). Dendritic cell precursor populations of mouse blood: identification of the murine homologues of human blood plasmacytoid pre-DC2 and CD11c+ DC1 precursors. *Blood.* 101: 1453-1459.

Pepose, J.S. (1991). Herpes simplex keratitis: role of viral infection versus immune response. *Surv Ophthalmol.* 35: 345-352.

Pepose, J.S., Gardner, K.M., Nestor, M.S., Foos, R.Y., & Pettit, T.H. (1985). Detection of HLA class I and II antigens in rejected human corneal allografts. *Ophthalmology.* 92: 1480-1484.

Pflugfelder, S.C. (1998). Advances in the diagnosis and management of keratoconjunctivitis sicca. *Curr Opin Ophthalmol.* 9: 50-53.

Redfern, R.L. & McDermott, A.M. (2010). Toll-like receptors in ocular surface disease. *Exp Eye Res.* 90: 679-687.

Russell, R.G., Nasisse, M.P., Larsen, H.S., & Rouse, B.T. (1984). Role of T-lymphocytes in the pathogenesis of herpetic stromal keratitis. *Invest Ophthalmol Vis Sci.* 25: 938-944.

Sankaridurg, P.R., Rao, G.N., Rao, H.N., Sweeney, D.F., & Holden, B.A. (2000). ATPase-positive dendritic cells in the limbal and corneal epithelium of guinea pigs after extended wear of hydrogel lenses. *Cornea.* 19: 374-377.

Schang, L.M., Phillips, J., & Schaffer, P.A. (1998). Requirement for cellular cyclin-dependent kinases in herpes simplex virus replication and transcription. *J Virol.* 72: 5626-5637.

Schang, L.M., Rosenberg, A., & Schaffer, P.A. (2000). Roscovitine, a specific inhibitor of cellular cyclin-dependent kinases, inhibits herpes simplex virus DNA synthesis in the presence of viral early proteins. *J Virol.* 74: 2107-2120.

Schaumberg, D.A., Sullivan, D.A., Buring, J.E., & Dana, M.R. (2003). Prevalence of dry eye syndrome among US women. *Am J Ophthalmol.* 136: 318-326.

Shukla, D., Liu, J., Blaiklock, P., Shworak, N.W., Bai, X., Esko, J.D., Cohen, G.H., Eisenberg, R.J., Rosenberg, R.D., & Spear, P.G. (1999). A novel role for 3-O-sulfated heparan sulfate in herpes simplex virus 1 entry. *Cell.* 99: 13-22.

Shukla, D. & Spear, P.G. (2001). Herpesviruses and heparan sulfate: an intimate relationship in aid of viral entry. *J Clin Invest.* 108: 503-510.

Smith, P.M., Wolcott, R.M., Chervenak, R., & Jennings, S.R. (1994). Control of acute cutaneous herpes simplex virus infection: T cell-mediated viral clearance is dependent upon interferon-gamma (IFN-gamma). *Virology.* 202: 76-88.

Spear, P.G. (2004). Herpes simplex virus: receptors and ligands for cell entry. *Cell Microbiol.* 6: 401-410.

Stern, M.E., Beuerman, R.W., Fox, R.I., Gao, J., Mircheff, A.K., & Pflugfelder, S.C. (1998). The pathology of dry eye: the interaction between the ocular surface and lacrimal glands. *Cornea.* 17: 584-589.

Stern, M.E., Gao, J., Siemasko, K.F., Beuerman, R.W., & Pflugfelder, S.C. (2004). The role of the lacrimal functional unit in the pathophysiology of dry eye. *Exp Eye Res.* 78: 409-416.

Stewart GL, Kim I, Shupe K, Alizadeh, H. Silvany, R. McCulley, J. P. Niederkorn, J. Y. (1992) Chemotactic response of macrophages to Acanthamoeba castellanii antigen and antibody-dependent macrophage-mediated killing of the parasite. *J Parasito..* ;78:849-855.

Streilein, J.W. (1993). Tissue barriers, immunosuppressive microenvironments, and privileged sites: the eye's point of view. *Reg Immunol.* 5: 253-268.

Streilein, J.W. (1995). Immunological non-responsiveness and acquisition of tolerance in relation to immune privilege in the eye. *Eye (Lond).* 9 (Pt 2): 236-240.

Streilein, J.W. (1999). Immunobiology and immunopathology of corneal transplantation. *Chem Immunol.* 73: 186-206.

Streilein, J.W., Bradley, D., Sano, Y., & Sonoda, Y. (1996). Immunosuppressive properties of tissues obtained from eyes with experimentally manipulated corneas. *Invest Ophthalmol Vis Sci.* 37: 413-424.

Streilein, J.W., Dana, M.R., & Ksander, B.R. (1997). Immunity causing blindness: five different paths to herpes stromal keratitis. *Immunol Today.* 18: 443-449.

Streilein, J.W., Toews, G.B., & Bergstresser, P.R. (1979). Corneal allografts fail to express Ia antigens. *Nature.* 282: 326-327.

Stuart, P.M., Griffith, T.S., Usui, N., Pepose, J., Yu, X., & Ferguson, T.A. (1997). CD95 ligard (FasL)-induced apoptosis is necessary for corneal allograft survival. *J Clin Invest.* 99: 396-402.

Sun, Y., Chandra, J., Mukherjee, P., Szczotka-Flynn, L., Ghannoum, M.A., & Pearlman, E. (2010). A murine model of contact lens-associated fusarium keratitis. *Invest Ophthalmol Vis Sci.* 51: 1511-1516.

Sun, Y., Karmakar, M., Roy, S., Ramadan, R.T., Williams, S.R., Howell, S., Shive, C.L., Han, Y., Stopford, C.M., Rietsch, A., & Pearlman, E. TLR4 and TLR5 on corneal macrophages regulate Pseudomonas aeruginosa keratitis by signaling through MyD88-dependent and -independent pathways. *J Immunol.* 185: 4272-4283.

Tang, Q. & Bluestone, J.A. (2008). The Foxp3+ regulatory T cell: a jack of all trades, master of regulation. *Nat Immunol.* 9: 239-244.

Tarabishy, A.B., Aldabagh, B., Sun, Y., Imamura, Y., Mukherjee, P.K., Lass, J.H., Ghannoum, M.A., & Pearlman, E. (2008). MyD88 regulation of Fusarium keratitis is dependent on TLR4 and IL-1R1 but not TLR2. *J Immunol.* 181: 593-600.

Thiel, M.A., Kaufmann, C., Coster, D.J., & Williams, K.A. (2009). Antibody-based immunosuppressive agents for corneal transplantation. *Eye (Lond).* 23: 1962-1965.

Thomas, J., Gangappa, S., Kanangat, S., & Rouse, B.T. (1997). On the essential involvement of neutrophils in the immunopathologic disease: herpetic stromal keratitis. *J Immunol.* 158: 1383-1391.

Thomas, J., Kanangat, S., & Rouse, B.T. (1998). Herpes simplex virus replication-induced expression of chemokines and proinflammatory cytokines in the eye: implications in herpetic stromal keratitis. *J Interferon Cytokine Res.* 18: 681-690.

Thomas, J. & Rouse, B.T. (1997). Immunopathogenesis of herpetic ocular disease. *Immunol Res.* 16: 375-386.

Thomas, P.A. & Geraldine, P. (2007). Infectious keratitis. *Curr Opin Infect Dis.* 20: 129-141.

Torres, P.F. & Kijlstra, A. (2001). The role of cytokines in corneal immunopathology. *Ocul Immunol Inflamm.* 9: 9-24.

Traver, D., Akashi, K., Manz, M., Merad, M., Miyamoto, T., Engleman, E.G., & Weissman, I.L. (2000). Development of CD8alpha-positive dendritic cells from a common myeloid progenitor. *Science.* 290: 2152-2154.

Trinkaus-Randall, V., Leibowitz, H.M., Ryan, W.J., & Kupferman, A. (1991). Quantification of stromal destruction in the inflamed cornea. *Invest Ophthalmol Vis Sci.* 32: 603-609.

Tullo, A.B., Shimeld, C., Blyth, W.A., Hill, T.J., & Easty, D.L. (1983). Ocular infection with herpes simplex virus in nonimmune and immune mice. *Arch Ophthalmol.* 101: 961-964.

Tumpey, T.M., Chen, S.H., Oakes, J.E., & Lausch, R.N. (1996). Neutrophil-mediated suppression of virus replication after herpes simplex virus type 1 infection of the murine cornea. *J Virol.* 70: 898-904.

Tumpey, T.M., Cheng, H., Cook, D.N., Smithies, O., Oakes, J.E., & Lausch, R.N. (1998). Absence of macrophage inflammatory protein-1alpha prevents the development of blinding herpes stromal keratitis. *J Virol.* 72: 3705-3710.

Van Horn, D.L., Davis, S.D., Hyndiuk, R.A., & Alpren, T.V. (1978). Pathogenesis of experimental Pseudomonas keratitis in the guinea pig: bacteriologic, clinical, and microscopic observations. *Invest Ophthalmol Vis Sci.* 17: 1076-1086.

Van Klink F, Taylor WM, Alizadeh H, Jager MJ, van Rooijen N, Niederkorn JY. (1996) The role of macrophages in Acanthamoeba keratitis. *Invest Ophthalmol Vis Sci.* 37:1271-1281.

Verjans, G.M., Remeijer, L., Mooy, C.M., & Osterhaus, A.D. (2000). Herpes simplex virus-specific T cells infiltrate the cornea of patients with herpetic stromal keratitis: no evidence for autoreactive T cells. *Invest Ophthalmol Vis Sci.* 41: 2607-2612.

Weiss, S.J. (1989). Tissue destruction by neutrophils. *N Engl J Med.* 320: 365-376.

Whitley, R.J. & Roizman, B. (2001). Herpes simplex virus infections. *Lancet.* 357: 1513-1518.

Wolpe, S.D., Davatelis, G., Sherry, B., Beutler, B., Hesse, D.G., Nguyen, H.T., Moldawer, L.L., Nathan, C.F., Lowry, S.F., & Cerami, A. (1988). Macrophages secrete a novel heparin-binding protein with inflammatory and neutrophil chemokinetic properties. *J Exp Med.* 167: 570-581.

Wolpe, S.D., Sherry, B., Juers, D., Davatelis, G., Yurt, R.W., & Cerami, A. (1989). Identification and characterization of macrophage inflammatory protein 2. *Proc Natl Acad Sci U S A.* 86: 612-616.

WorkShop, I.D.E. (2007a). The definition and classification of dry eye disease: report of the Definition and Classification Subcommittee of the International Dry Eye WorkShop (2007). *Ocul Surf.* 5: 75-92.

WorkShop, I.D.E. (2007b). The epidemiology of dry eye disease: report of the Epidemiology Subcommittee of the International Dry Eye WorkShop (2007). *Ocul Surf.* 5: 93-107.

Wu, L., D'Amico, A., Hochrein, H., O'Keeffe, M., Shortman, K., & Lucas, K. (2001). Development of thymic and splenic dendritic cell populations from different hemopoietic precursors. *Blood*. 98: 3376-3382.

Wuest, T.R. & Carr, D.J. (2008). Dysregulation of CXCR3 signaling due to CXCL10 deficiency impairs the antiviral response to herpes simplex virus 1 infection. *J Immunol*. 181: 7985-7993.

Yamagami, S., Hamrah, P., Zhang, Q., Liu, Y., Huq, S., & Dana, M.R. (2005). Early ocular chemokine gene expression and leukocyte infiltration after high-risk corneal transplantation. *Mol Vis*. 11: 632-640.

Yamagami, S., Isobe, M., & Tsuru, T. (2000). Characterization of cytokine profiles in corneal allograft with anti-adhesion therapy. *Transplantation*. 69: 1655-1659.

Yamagami, S., Miyazaki, D., Ono, S.J., & Dana, M.R. (1999). Differential chemokine gene expression in corneal transplant rejection. *Invest Ophthalmol Vis Sci*. 40: 2892-2897.

Yildiz, E.H., Abdalla, Y.F., Elsahn, A.F., Rapuano, C.J., Hammersmith, K.M., Laibson, P.R., & Cohen, E.J. (2010). Update on fungal keratitis from 1999 to 2008. *Cornea*. 29: 1406-1411.

Youker, K., Smith, C.W., Anderson, D.C., Miller, D., Michael, L.H., Rossen, R.D., & Entman, M.L. (1992). Neutrophil adherence to isolated adult cardiac myocytes. Induction by cardiac lymph collected during ischemia and reperfusion. *J Clin Invest*. 89: 602-609.

Yuan, X. & Wilhelmus, K.R. (2009). Corneal neovascularization during experimental fungal keratitis. *Mol Vis*. 15: 1988-1996.

Zhao, Z.S., Granucci, F., Yeh, L., Schaffer, P.A., & Cantor, H. (1998). Molecular mimicry by herpes simplex virus-type 1: autoimmune disease after viral infection. *Science*. 279: 1344-1347.

Zheng, M., Deshpande, S., Lee, S., Ferrara, N., & Rouse, B.T. (2001). Contribution of vascular endothelial growth factor in the neovascularization process during the pathogenesis of herpetic stromal keratitis. *J Virol*. 75: 9828-9835.

Zheng, X., de Paiva, C.S., Li, D.Q., Farley, W.J., & Pflugfelder, S.C. Desiccating stress promotion of Th17 differentiation by ocular surface tissues through a dendritic cell-mediated pathway. *Invest Ophthalmol Vis Sci*. 51: 3083-3091.

Zhou, Z., Wu, M., Barrett, R.P., McClellan, S.A., Zhang, Y., & Hazlett, L.D. (2010). Role of the Fas pathway in Pseudomonas aeruginosa keratitis. *Invest Ophthalmol Vis Sci*. 51: 2537-2547.

Zhu, S., Dekaris, I., Duncker, G., & Dana, M.R. (1999). Early expression of proinflammatory cytokines interleukin-1 and tumor necrosis factor-alpha after corneal transplantation. *J Interferon Cytokine Res*. 19: 661-669.

Zhu, S.N. & Dana, M.R. (1999). Expression of cell adhesion molecules on limbal and neovascular endothelium in corneal inflammatory neovascularization. *Invest Ophthalmol Vis Sci*. 40: 1427-1434.

5

Corneal Surgical Techniques

Miroslav Vukosavljević, Milorad Milivojević and Mirko Resan
Eye Clinic, Military Medical Academy, Belgrade,
Serbia

1. Introduction

1.1 History of corneal refractive surgery

There is a long history of corneal refractive surgery. Leonardo Da Vinci in 1508 said the theory of refractive errors. The first systematic analysis of the nature and results of refractive errors came from Francis Cornelius Donders. His classic treatise, "On the anomalies of accommodation and refraction of the eye", outlined the fundamental principles of physiological optics. Ironically, in this treatise, Donders railed against surgical attempts to correct refractive errors by altering the corneal shape. In 1885 Hjalmar Schiotz performed corneal incision to correct astigmatism. Modern refractive surgery extended corneal reshaping to treat myopia and astigmatism. Throughout the 1930s and 1940s, Sato published several reports, describing his attempts to refine incisional refractive surgery with anterior and posterior corneal incisions. The Russian ophthalmologist, Fyodorov later developed a systematic process of anterior radial keratotomy and treated thousands of myopic patients with greater predictability. Lamellar surgery was first introduced by Jose Barraquer. He invented keratoplasty procedures that involved the transplantation of corneal tissue of a size different from the host size to alter the curvature of cornea. He also invented a series of lamellar procedures and developed a formula that represented the relationship between the added corneal thickness and the change in refractive power, later called Barraquer's law of thickness. The transition from incisional to ablative laser refractive surgery arose with the development of Excimer laser technology. Excimer lasers use argon fluoride gases to emit ultraviolet laser pulses. Taboda and Archibald reported the use of the Excimer laser to reshape the corneal epithelium in 1981. In 1983, Trokel and colleagues showed how the Excimer laser could be used to ablate bovine corneal stroma. In 1985, Seiler did the first Excimer laser treatment in a blind eye. He later did the first Excimer laser astigmatic keratotomy. In 1989, McDonald and colleagues did the first photorefractive keratectomy on a seeing eye with myopia. Jose Barraquer's pioneering work, including the use of lamellar procedures to subtract corneal stromal tissue and the development of the first microkerotomes, set the stage for laser in situ keratomileusis (LASIK) surgery. Ruiz and Rowsey modified Barraquer's technique to perform keratomileusis in situ with a geared automated microkeratome. In the early 1990s, Pallikaris and colleagues and Buratto and colleagues independently described a technique that combined two existing technologies: the microkeratome and the Excimer laser. Pallikaris coined the term LASIK for this new technique, which has become a widely used refractive technique worldwide (1).

1.2 Introduction

Astigmatism is a unique refractive error that causes reduced visual acuity and produces symptoms of glare, monocular diplopia, asthenopia, and distortion. The control and correction of astigmatism has been a topic of great interest to cataract, refractive and corneal surgeons.

Corneal refractive surgical techniques that can correct astigmatism are: incisional surgical techniques, such as arcuate keratotomy and limbal relaxing incisions; laser-assisted *in situ* keratomileusis (LASIK); and surface ablation techniques, such as photorefractive keratectomy (PRK), *trans*-epithelial PRK (tPRK), laser-assisted subepithelial keratomileusis (LASEK), epi-LASIK and Intralase.

Arcuate keratotomy is an incisional surgical technique in which arcuate incisions of approximately 95% depth are made in the corneal midperipheral 7,0 mm zone placed in the steep meridian(s). Arcuate keratotomy was used to correct naturally occuring astigmatism, but it is now used primarily to correct postkeratoplasty astigmatism. Limbal relaxing incisions are incisions set at approximately 600 μm depth, or 50 μm less than the thinnest pachymetry at the limbus, and placed just anterior to the limbus. Limbal relaxing incisions are used to manage astigmatism during or after phacoemulsification and intraocular lens (IOL) implantation (2).

LASIK is a lamellar laser refractive surgical technique in which the Excimer laser ablation is done under a partial-thickness lamellar corneal flap. The lamellar flap could be made with a microkeratome or with a femtosecond laser. The microkeratome uses an oscillating blade to cut the flap after immobilization of the cornea with a suction ring. Microkeratomes from several companies cut the lamellar flaps with either superior or nasal hinges, and can cut to depths of 100–200 μm. A femtosecond laser has been developed that can etch lamellar flaps within the cornea stroma at a desired corneal depth. The femtosecond laser provides more accuracy in flap thickness than previous methods; the microkeratome cuts can vary widely in depth. The ablation might either correct sphere and cylinder error, or is wavefront-guided. After the ablation has been completed, the stromal bed is irrigated and the corneal flap is repositioned (3).

Surface ablation is a generic term referring to the application of Excimer laser directly on the anterior stromal surface. The epithelium is removed in order for the Excimer laser to be applied to the stroma. There are several ways in which the epithelium can be separated from Bowmans layer. The epithelium can be fashioned as a flap and replaced (as in LASEK and epi-LASIK) or removed (as in PRK). Surface ablation techniques are continuously evolving in order to achieve better results with faster visual recovery and less pain (4).

LASIK and PRK are the most commonly used refractive surgical methods worldwide.

2. Laser in situ keratomileusis (LASIK)

Laser in situ keratomileusis (LASIK) is the most commonly used refractive surgical method worldwide. This method employs two technologies: Excimer laser and microkeratome. Excimer (acronym for excited dimer) laser is an ultraviolet gas laser (argon-fluoride, ArF) with wavelength of 193 nm, which achieves photoablative effect on tissue of corneal stroma.

First, microkeratome cuts through the cornea and make intrastromal flap on hinge. Flap has a diameter from 8 to 10 mm and its thickness can be 100-180 µm, but usually 100-130 µm (about 15-35% of total corneal thickness). Then the flap is lifted and the corneal stroma exposed to the Excimer laser, and stroma is remodeled according to the type of ametropia and its values. On the end of Excimer laser the flap is repositioned and for a short time have stable position without of need for sutures (5). Postoperative visual rehabilitation is rapid. Sixteen hours after LASIK the majority of patients are reaching 97% of the preoperative best corrected visual acuity (6).

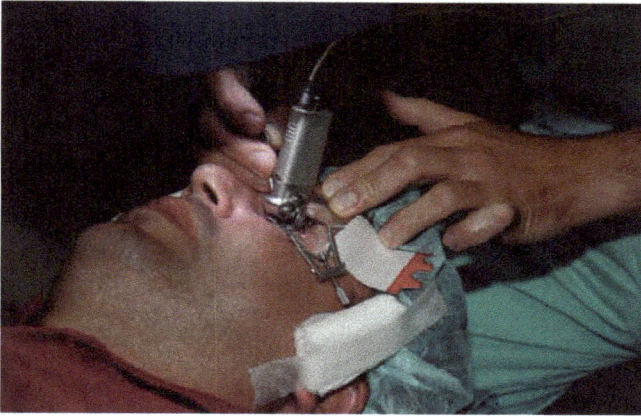

Fig. 1. Placing of suction ring and microkeratome on the eye (5).

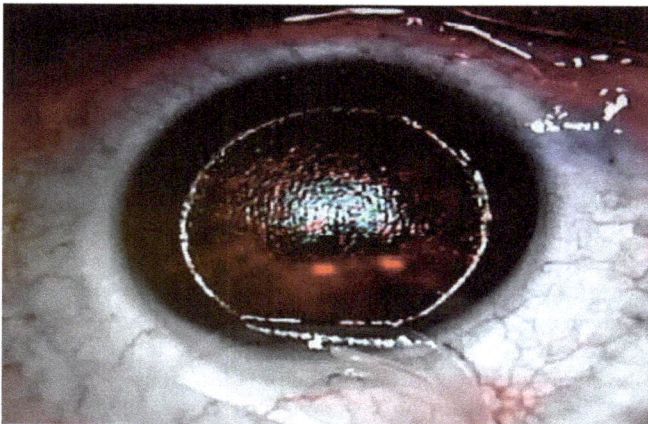

Fig. 2. Flap is created and corneal stroma prepared for Excimer laser ablation (5).

The American Academy of Ophthalmology (AAO) recommended the indications for LASIK: myopia up to - 10 Dsph, hyperopia up to + 4 Dsph, and astigmatism up to 4 Dcyl (7).

The contraindications for Excimer laser refractive surgery including LASIK and PRK are general and ophthalmic. General are: immunological diseases (autoimmune, collagen vascular, immune deficiency); pregnancy or breast feeding; the tendency to form keloids; diabetes; and systemic administration of isotretionin or amiodarone. Ophthalmic are: dry eye; neurotrophic keratitis; herpes zoster ophthalmicus / keratitis herpetica; glaucoma; ectatic corneal dystrophy (keratoconus, keratoglobus); highly irregular astigmatism; uveitis, diabetic retinopathy; progressive retinal disease and previously performed radial keratotomy (8).

The complications of LASIK include: intraoperative and postoperative complications. The intraoperative complications or flap related complications (9) are: wrong ablation, flap loss, buttonhole flap (hole in the flap), thin flap, brief flap, free cap (flap amputation), corneal bleeding, epithelial defects and corneal perforation (very rare). The postoperative complications (10) are: infections, dislocation of the flap, flap folding (striae), diffuse lamellar keratitis (sands of the Sahara), epithelial ingrowth, corneal ectasia, regression, intraflap fluid accumulation and paradoxical hypotony.

Each candidate for LASIK should be at least 21 years of age and must have a stable refractive error in the period of two years. Preoperative evaluation of each candidate includes: general and ophthalmic history; autorefractokeratometry; uncorrected visual acuity (UCVA) and best corrected visual acuity (BCVA); Schirmer test; review of the eye anterior segment on slit-lamp; applanation tonometry; review of the eye fundus in a wide pupil; imaging of corneal topography and aberrometry. The following formula to evaluate whether a candidate can safely perform LASIK is:

Central pachymetry – flap thickness - ablation depth = residual stromal thickness of the cornea

As a limit value for residual stromal thickness of the cornea (residual stromal bed) after cutting and effects of Excimer laser 300 μm are taken; as a critical value for steep corneal meridian (steep K) <39 or > 47 D are taken; as a limit value for elevation of the posterior corneal surface 50 μm are taken (5).

Numerous studies confirm the effectiveness of LASIK for the correction of astigmatism. Stojanovic and Nitter evaluated safety, efficacy, predictability, and stability in the treatment of myopic astigmatism with LASIK and PRK using the 200 Hz flying-spot technology of the Excimer laser. This retrospective study included 110 eyes treated with LASIK and 87 eyes treated with PRK that were available for evaluation at 6 and 12 months. The mean preoperative spherical equivalent (SE) was −5.35 diopters (D) ± 2.50 (SD) (range −1.13 to −11.88 D) in the LASIK eyes and −4.72 ± 2.82 D (range −1.00 to −15.50 D) in the PRK eyes. The treated astigmatism was 4.00 D in both groups. None of the eyes lost 2 or more lines of best spectacle-corrected visual acuity. Seventy-seven percent of the LASIK eyes and 78% of the PRK eyes achieved an uncorrected visual acuity of 20/20 or better; 98% in both groups achieved 20/40 or better. In conclusion, Excimer laser was safe, effective, and predictable and with LASIK and PRK the results are stable when treating low to moderate myopia and astigmatism up to 4.0 D (11). Ditzen et al evaluated safety, predictability, efficacy, and stability of LASIK for spherical hyperopia and hyperopia with astigmatism. This retrospective study analyzed the results of 23 eyes of 23 patients who had LASIK for spherical hyperopia (preoperative astigmatism ≤0.75 D) and 44 eyes of 44 patients who had LASIK for hyperopia with astigmatism. In group 1 (spherical hyperopia), mean preoperative spherical equivalent refraction was +4.88 ± 2.13 D (range +2.13 to +9.63 D); in group 2 (hyperopic astigmatism), +4.33 ± 2.15 D (range +0.50 to +9.50 D). One year after LASIK, mean spherical equivalent refraction was +0.30 ± 0.90 D (range -0.75 to +2.50 D) in group 1 and +0.29 ± 1.27 D (range -3.25 to +3.25 D) in group 2. In group 1, no eyes lost two or more lines, and one eye (6%) lost one line of best spectacle-corrected visual acuity at 1 year. In group 2, one eye (4%) lost one line and one eye (4%) lost more than two lines at 1 year. Uncorrected visual acuity of 20/40 or better was achieved in 83% (group 1) vs. 62% (group 2) at 1 year. In conclusion, LASIK seemed to be safe and effective for hyperopia and hyperopia with astigmatism for corrections up to +6.00 D (12). Albarran-Diego et al evaluated bitoric LASIK for the correction of mixed astigmatism. This prospective study included 28 eyes of 21 patients with mixed astigmatism who had bitoric LASIK. Six months after bitoric LASIK, the mean UCVA was 0.70 ± 0.23 (SD). The percentage of eyes with a UCVA of 20/40 or better was 78.6% and of 20/20, 21.4%. There was a statistically significant increase in the mean BCVA from 0.71 ± 0.19 before surgery to 0.83 ± 0.15 at 6 months. Three eyes (10.7%) lost 1 line of BCVA. The mean preoperative astigmatism of −4.04 ± 1.13 diopters (D) was reduced to −0.67 ± 0.79 D after surgery (13).

3. Photorefractive keratectomy (PRK)

Photorefractive keratectomy (PRK) is still a successful method in certain indications and now is used worldwide as PRK or as its modification - LASEK and EpiLASIK. All methods for its performance require use of Excimer laser (14).

PRK is superficial ablative method because the Excimer laser thinner and reshapes the anterior part of the corneal stroma just below Bowman's membrane. This provides greater residual stromal thickness, and thus strengthens the biomechanical strength of the cornea. But, ablation of front stroma, especially through a layer of Bowman's membrane, causing aggressive response in wound healing, which may result in frequent appearance of subepithelial clouding (haze) and scarring compared with LASIK. Recovery after PRK is slower and more painful compared with LASIK. One to four days after the intervention most of the patients have a transient low-intensity pain. Postoperative visual rehabilitation is a little longer and lasts several weeks (1,15).

Certain situations may favor PRK over LASIK in particular safety issues due to the absence of flap related complications in PRK. These situations include: predisposition for contact injury (e.g. those involved in martial arts or boxing); anterior basement membrane (BM) dystrophy; epithelial sloughing during LASIK in the fellow eye; thin corneas in which the residual stromal bed would be less than 250–300 mm; deep set eyes or a small palpebral aperture (poor exposure for the microkeratome); previous surgery involving the conjunctiva (e.g. glaucoma drainage bleb, scleral buckle); and moderate dry eye before surgery. In addition, flat (< 41 D) or steep corneas (> 48 D), with the risk of free, thin, incomplete or buttonholed flaps, may be better suited to PRK. It is desirable to avoid suction and iatrogenically raising the IOP during LASIK, as in patients with glaucoma or a risk of poor optic nerve perfusion, PRK procedure would be preferred (15).

In PRK the first step is corneal epithelium removing (mechanically with knife-hockey or rotating brush; or by chemical abrasion with 20% ethanol), then the corneal stroma is exposed to the effects of Excimer laser which thins and reshapes it according to the type of ametropia and its values and after that therapeutic soft contact lens is applied for 5 days.

The American Academy of Ophthalmology (AAO) recommended the next indications for PRK: myopia up to – 8 Dsph, hyperopia up to + 4 Dsph, and astigmatism up to 4 Dcyl (7). Large corrections (ablation depth greater than 100 µm) are considered for adjunctive 0,02% mitomycin C (MMC) because of the increased risk of postoperative haze and regression (16).

Complications of PRK include: subepithelial haze, corneal scarring, ectasia and regression.

Each candidate for PRK should be at least 21 years of age and must have a stable refractive error in the period of two years. Preoperative evaluation of each candidate includes: general and ophthalmic history; autorefractokeratometry; uncorrected visual acuity (UCVA) and best corrected visual acuity (BCVA) in each eye; Schirmer test; examination of the eye anterior segment on slit-lamp; applanation tonometry; examination of the eye fundus in a wide pupil; imaging of corneal topography and aberrometry. As a limit value for residual stromal thickness of the cornea (residual stromal bed) is 300 µm. The critical value for steep corneal meridian (steep K) is <39 or > 47 D and the limit value for elevation of the posterior corneal surface is 50 µm (5).

Numerous studies have investigated the effectiveness of PRK in the correction of astigmatism. Haw and Manche evaluated the safety and efficacy of PRK for the treatment of primary compound myopic astigmatism. Ninety three eyes from 56 patients with a mean spherical equivalent of −4.98 ± 1.80 diopters (range, −1.75 to −8.5) underwent photoastigmatic refractive keratectomy and were followed for 2 years. Fifty-six eyes (94.9%) had an uncorrected visual acuity of 20/40 or greater, whereas 34 eyes (57.6 %) demonstrated an uncorrected visual acuity of 20/20 or greater. One eye (1.7%) lost 2 or more lines of best spectacle-corrected visual acuity (17). Nagy et al evaluated the results of PRK using Gaussian flying spot technology in the treatment of hyperopia and hyperopic astigmatism. Two hundred eyes were evaluated with 12-month follow-up. Eyes were divided into four groups: group 1 (spherical hyperopia up to +3.50 D and astigmatism less than 1.00 D, n=62); group 2 (hyperopia up to +3.50 D and astigmatism of 1.00 D or more, n=44); group 3 (hyperopia greater than +3.50 D and astigmatism less than 1.00 D, n=56); and group 4 (hyperopia greater than +3.50 D and astigmatism of 1.00 D or more, n=38). In group 1, 82.2% (51/62 eyes) were within ±0.50 D of target refraction; 88.7% (55/62 eyes) had 20/20 or better uncorrected visual acuity; 1.6% (1/62 eye) lost two or more lines. In group 2, 68.1% (30/44 eyes) were within ±0.50 D; 77.2% (34/44 eyes) had 20/20 or better uncorrected visual acuity; 9.1% (4/44 eyes) lost two or more lines of spectacle-corrected visual acuity. In group 3, 76.8% (43/56 eyes) were within ±0.50 D; 78.6% (44/56 eyes) had 20/20 or better uncorrected visual acuity; 5.4% (3/56 eyes) lost two or more lines of spectacle-corrected visual acuity. In group 4, 42% (16/38 eyes) were within ±0.50 D; 60.5% (23/38 eyes) had 20/20 or better uncorrected visual acuity; 15.8% (6/38 eyes) lost two or more Snellen lines. In conclusion PRK was most safe and effective for low hyperopia (18).

4. Trans-epithelial photorefractive keratectomy (tPRK)

In this method, the Excimer laser is used to ablate the epithelium in addition to then ablating the underlying stroma. The cornea undergoes an epithelial ablation within a fixed diameter. The operating room lights are turned off as blue fluorescent light is emitted whereas epithelium is ablated. Once the blue fluorescence disappears, this indicates that the epithelium has been removed. Accuracy with this method is dependent upon regular epithelial thickness across the diameter treatment zone and also similar epithelial thicknesses between different eyes. This technique can produce variable results when laser surface enhancement is proposed after previous refractive surgery due to areas of epithelial hyperplasia causing variable epithelial thickness (15).

5. Laser-assisted subepithelial keratomileusis (LASEK)

LASEK is a surgical procedure that combines certain elements of both LASIK and PRK to improve the risk/benefit ratio. Diluted alcohol is used to loosen the epithelial adhesion to the corneal stroma. The loosened epithelium is moved aside from the treatment zone as a hinged sheet. Laser ablation of the subepithelial stroma is performed before the epithelial sheet is returned to its original position. The main rationale for combining elements of LASIK and PRK to LASEK is to avoid the flap-related LASIK complications and the slow visual recovery and haze risk of PRK. LASEK may avoid several of the inherent complications, including free caps, incomplete pass of the microkeratome, flap wrinkles, epithelial ingrowth, flap melt, interface debris, corneal ectasia, and diffuse lamellar keratitis, after LASIK and postoperative pain, subepithelial haze, and slow visual rehabilitation after PRK. Current ophthalmic literature does not provide the specific indications, visual outcomes, complications, and limitations of LASEK (19). Bilgihan et al. evaluated the efficacy, predictability, and safety of LASEK for treatment of high myopia with astigmatism. LASEK was performed in 61 eyes of 36 consecutive patients with myopic spherical equivalent refraction of -6.00 to -10.00 D using the Aesculap-Meditec MEL60 Excimer laser. Ninety-six percent of eyes achieved 20/40 or better uncorrected visual acuity (UCVA) at 1 month. At 12 months, 64% of eyes achieved 20/20 and 92% achieved 20/40 or better UCVA. Two eyes lost 2 lines of best spectacle-corrected visual acuity (BSCVA) at 6 or 12 months. Accuracy of correction was ±0.50 D from emmetropia in 82% of eyes, and ±1.00 D in 90% at 12 months (20). Taneri et al evaluated the visual outcomes and complications in low to moderate levels of myopia and astigmatism treated with LASEK. One hundred seventy-one eyes of 105 patients were studied. Preoperatively, the mean spherical equivalent was -2.99 diopters (D) ± 1.43 (SD) and the mean cylinder -0.78 ± 0.73 D. One week postoperatively, 96% of eyes had a UCVA of 20/40 or better but definitive visual recovery took more than 4 weeks in some eyes. Approximately 95% of eyes were within ±1.0 D of emmetropia after 4 to 52 weeks; the remaining 5% did not show major deviations. At 4 to 52 weeks, only 1 eye was overcorrected by more than 1.0 D of manifest refraction (21).

6. Epithelial laser in situ keratomileusis (Epi-LASIK)

Epi-LASIK has proved to be a suitable procedure, especially in patients with active lifestyles or occupations, eyes with thin corneas without ectatic disorders, and patients with moderate dry-eye syndrome. In epi-LASIK, an epithelial flap is created with the help of a special microkeratome. The epithelial flap is repositioned on the cornea after photoablation. It has been postulated that compared with conventional laser-assisted subepithelial keratectomy (LASEK), in which an epithelial flap is created after the epithelium is exposed to an alcohol solution, cell viability of the epithelial sheet is better in epi-LASIK surgery, in which mechanical separation is performed with a microkeratome. The quality of the epithelial separation is crucial for the success of the procedure because stromal lacerations or remaining islands of basal epithelial cells would reduce the optical quality of the cornea after photoablation (22).

Factor	PRK	LASEK	EPI-LASIK	LASIK
Range of correction	Low to moderately high			Low to moderately high
Postoperative pain	Mild to moderate 24–72 hours			Minimum 12 hours
Postoperative medications	1–3 months			1 week
Functional vision recovery	3 to 7 days			<24 hours
Refractive stability achieved	3 weeks to 3 months			1 week to 3 months
Specific complications	Haze formation, scarring	Haze formation, scarring	Haze formation, scarring, incomplete epithelial flap, stromal incursions	Free caps, incomplete pass of microkeratome, flap wrinkles, epithelial ingrowth, flap melt, interface debris, corneal ectasia, diffuse lamellar keratitis
Dry-eye sensitive	1 to 6 months			1 to 12 months
Thin corneas or wide pupils	Often not contraindicated			May be contraindicated depending on amount of intended correction
Special (relative) indications	Thin corneal pachymetry, wide scotopic pupil, LASIK complications in fellow eye, predisposition to trauma, keratoconus suspect (irregular astigmatism), glaucoma suspect, recurrent erosion syndrome, dry-eye syndrome, basement membrane disease			Concern about postoperative pain, requirement of rapid visual recovery
Special (relative) contraindications	Concern about postoperative pain, requirement of rapid visual recovery	Concern about postoperative pain, requirement of rapid visual recovery	Concern about postoperative pain, requirement of rapid visual recovery, glaucoma, scleral buckle, deep-set eyes, small palpebral fissure	Thin corneas, wide pupils, recurrent erosion syndrome, glaucoma, scleral buckle, deep-set eyes, small palpebral fissure

Fig. 3. Widely accepted relative differences between PRK, LASEK, epi-LASIK, and LASIK (23).

7. Femtosecond laser in laser in situ keratomileusis

In the early 1960s, Barraquer introduced the concept of lamellar refractive procedures. In the 1990s, Pallikaris et al. and Buratto et al. conceived of techniques combining lamellar procedures with Excimer laser ablation. These advances led to the development of modern laser in situ keratomileusis (LASIK) procedures. LASIK has several advantages over PRK when performed properly in appropriate eyes. These include faster visual recovery, less discomfort after surgery, and milder and more predictable wound healing with less risk for corneal stromal opacity (haze). Lamellar corneal flap formation is the critical step in successful LASIK surgery. Improper flap formation, including improper flap geometry, decentration, irregularity of the cut, and epithelial damage, can lead to myriad LASIK complications. Considerable progress has been made over the years in producing safer instruments for LASIK flap formation since the Automated Corneal Shaper was adapted to LASIK. Thus, more reliable and safer mechanical microkeratomes contributed to the explosive growth of refractive surgery over the past 15 years. Despite these advances, complications such as incomplete or partial flaps, free flaps, buttonholes, and small irregular flaps continue to plague refractive surgeons who perform LASIK with a microkeratome. There are also significant limitations to the eyes that can safely have lamellar flap formation performed with a mechanical microkeratome, including corneas that are too steep (likely to have buttonhole flaps), too flat (likely to have small diameter flaps), or relatively thin (more likely to have low residual stromal bed) (Fig. 4).

Decentered flaps
Irregular-shaped flaps
Incomplete flaps
Button-hole flaps
Flap laceration
Epithelial defects
Limited hinge location, 1 or 2 sites per head (nasal or superior)
Poor flap thickness predictability, SD of flap thickness ± 20 to
    40 μm
Wide range of flap thickness for a given attempted thickness
    (up to 200 μm range)
Achieved mean thickness less than the labeled head
Sensitive to preoperative corneal curvature: steeper corneas
    create thinner flaps
Sensitive to preoperative corneal thickness: thicker corneas
    create thicker flaps[20,21]
Meniscus-shaped flaps: thinner centrally than peripherally
Highly variable hinge length
Flap thickness dependent on translation speed: faster
    translation creates thinner flaps
Blade quality affects results: second eye use of same blade
    associated with thinner flaps
Gap width of microkeratome head variable affecting flap
    thickness predictability
Anterior chamber perforation (older models)

Fig. 4. Corneal complications reported with conventional microkeratomes (24).

The femtosecond laser became available for LASIK flap formation approximately 10 years ago. Since the early femtosecond laser models were introduced, considerable progress has been made in improving flap geometry and limiting complications of LASIK performed with the laser. This has led to increasing popularity of LASIK performed with the femtosecond laser, to the point that different sources estimate that 30% to 50% of LASIK procedures in the United States in 2008 were performed using a femtosecond laser. Recently, new femtosecond laser models were introduced. These include the Femtec (20/10 Perfect Vision AG), the Femto LDV (Zeimer Group), the Visu-Max (Carl Zeiss Meditec) and commonly used IntraLase 60 kHz femtosecond laser (Abbott Medical Optics, Inc.). All 4 commercially available femtosecond laser systems use ultrashort pulses of laser and produce corneal tissue cutting using a photodisruption process. To create the lamellar flap, the IntraLase laser generates pulses of femtosecond laser at a near-infrared (1053 nm) wavelength and delivers closely spaced 3 mm spots, which are focused at variable depths to photodisrupt stromal tissue. When a high peak power is reached, hot plasma is generated, initiating a process of tissue ionization that is commonly called laser-induced optical breakdown. The hot plasma expands in shock waves and creates an intrastromal cavitation bubble composed primarily of water and carbon dioxide. Multiple cavitation bubbles coalesce, and an intrastromal cleavage plane is created. The laser delivers a series of pulses in a specified pattern to create the lamellar intrastromal cut and then extends the cleavage to the surface with a side cut to complete the flap (25). Stonecipher et al. reported the refractive results after LASIK for high myopia and cylinder at one center with one surgeon comparing two laser platforms. A total of 206 eyes of 121 patients were treated for –6.00 to –12.00 diopters (D) of spherical equivalent refractive error with up to 3.00 D of cylinder. All eyes underwent LASIK with the ALLEGRETTO WAVE 200-Hz (n=141) or 400-Hz (n=65) laser (Alcon Laboratories Inc). Corneal flaps were created with the IntraLase femtosecond laser (Abbott Medical Optics) at an intended thickness of 100 or 110 μm in all cases. At 3- and 6-month follow-up in the 200-Hz group, 77% (109/141) and 86% (121/141) of eyes, respectively, were within ±0.50 D of intended correction. In the 400-Hz group, 98.5% (64/65) and 100% (65/65) of eyes were within ±50 D of intended correction at 3 and 6 months postoperatively. At 3- and 6-month follow-up, 84% (119/141) and 77% (109/141) of eyes, respectively, in the 200-Hz group and 80% (52/65) and 92% (60/65) of eyes, respectively, in the 400-Hz group had 20/20 or better uncorrected distance visual acuity. At 6-month follow-up, refractive predictability and visual acuity were statistically superior in eyes in the 400-Hz group (chi square, P<.01). No eyes underwent retreatment as a secondary procedure during the time of analysis (26).

8. Refractive laser surgery in children

The use of Excimer laser vision correction in children is controversial because their eyes and refractive state continue to change. More studies on the growing eye and the effect of Excimer laser on the pediatric corneal endothelium are needed before the effect of refractive surgery in the pediatric age group can be fully understood (27).

Traditional methods of correcting and rehabilitating the refractive status of children with high myopia, myopic anisometropic amblyopia, hyperopia, hyperopic anisometropic amblyopia or significant astigmatism include glasses and contact lenses combined with some form of occlusion or optical penalization therapy. However, some children may not improve with these traditional forms of treatment because of aniseikonia, compliance issues, or both. This is especially true when children have concurrent medical diagnoses such as autism, cerebral palsy, developmental delay, Down syndrome, or other associated ocular disorders (eg, corneal, retinal, and optic nerve problems). So, in such children traditional optical refractive correction is often not successful (28, 29).

In the past ten years, refractive laser surgery techniques have been shown to be a good last-resort treatment in children who have failed with traditional treatment approaches. There are numerous reports of the successful performance of PRK, LASIK and LASEK in children when conventional therapy failed.

Autrata and Rehurek evaluated the visual and refractive results of multizonal PRK for high myopic anisometropia and contact-lens intolerance in children. Twenty-one patients aged 7 to 15 years with high myopic anisometropia had multizonal PRK in the more myopic eye and were retrospectively analyzed. The scanning-slit Nidek EC-5000 Excimer laser was used. The safety, efficacy, predictability, and stability of the procedure were evaluated. Long-term binocular vision outcome was analyzed. All patients completed a 4-year follow-up. The mean preoperative spherical equivalent (SE) refraction was - 8.93 diopters (D) ± 1.39 (SD) (range - 6.75 to - 11.75 D) and the mean postoperative SE was – 1.66 ± 0.68 D (range -

0.50 to - 2.75 D). The mean preoperative uncorrected visual acuity (UCVA) of 0.034 ± 0.016 increased to 0.35 ± 0.15 postoperatively. The mean preoperative best spectacle-corrected visual acuity (BSCVA) was 0.53 ± 0.19 and changed to 0.64 ± 0.16 postoperatively. No eye lost a line of BSCVA; 9 eyes gained 1 line, and 5 eyes gained 2 lines. No eye had + 3 haze. There were no significant complications. In conclusion, PRK was safe and effective in correcting high myopic anisometropia in children who were contact-lens intolerant (30).

Yin et al. assessed the efficacy of LASIK in facilitating amblyopia management of children from 6 to 14 years old, with high hyperopic and myopic anisometropia. Between 2000 and 2005, 42 children with high hyperopic anisometropic amblyopia and 32 children with high myopic anisometropic amblyopia underwent LASIK to reduce their anisometropia. LASIK was performed under topical or general anesthesia. Follow-up ranged from 6 months to 3 years, the averages of which were 17,45 months in the hyperopic group and 18,31 months in myopic group. Hyperopic anisometropia correction ranged from + 3.50 D to + 7.75 D, and the mean postoperative anisometropia was +0.56 ± 0.75 D at 3 years. Myopic anisometropia correction ranged from -15.75 to - 5.00 D and the mean postoperative anisometropia at 3 years was - 2.20 ± 1.05 D. The best-corrected visual acuity for distance and reading in the myopic group improved from 0.4 ± 0.25 and 0.58 ± 0.27, respectively, before surgery to 0.59 ± 0.28 and 0.96 ± 0.35, respectively, 3 years after surgery. In the hyperopic group, best-corrected visual acuity for distance and reading improved from 0.23 ± 0.21 and 0.34 ± 0.32, respectively, before surgery to 0.53 ± 0.31 and 0.80 ± 0.33, respectively, 3 years after surgery. Study shows that LASIK is an alternative method for correcting high hyperopic and myopic anisometropia. The proportion of patients who had stereopsis increased from 19.1% preoperatively to 46.7% postoperatively in the hyperopic group and from 19% to 89% in the myopic group. In conclusion, LASIK reduced high hyperopic and myopic anisometropia in children, thus facilitating amblyopia management and improving their visual acuity and stereopsis (31).

Astle et al. assessed the refractive, visual acuity, and binocular results of LASEK for anisomyopia, anisohyperopia, and anisoastigmatia in children with various levels of amblyopia secondary to the anisometropic causes. Retrospective review was of 53 children with anisometropia who had LASEK to correct the refractive difference between eyes. All LASEK procedures were performed using general anesthesia. Patients were divided into 3 groups according to their anisometropia as follows: myopic difference greater than 3.00 diopters (D), astigmatic difference greater than 1.50 D, and hyperopic difference greater than 3.50 D. The children were followed for at least 1 year. The mean age at treatment was 8.4 years (range 10 months to 16 years). The mean preoperative anisometropic difference was 6.98 D in the entire group, 9.48 D in the anisomyopic group, 3.13 D in the anisoastigmatic group, and 5.50 D in the anisohyperopic group. One year after LASEK, the mean anisometropic difference decreased to 1.81 D, 2.43 D, 0.74 D, and 2.33 D, respectively, and 54% of all eyes were within ± 1.00 D of the fellow eye, 68% were within ± 2.00 D, and 80% were within ± 3.00 D. Preoperative visual acuity and binocular vision could be measured in 33 children. Postoperatively, 63.6% of children had an improvement in best corrected visual acuity (BCVA) and the remainder had no noted change. No patient had a reduction in BCVA or a loss in fusional ability after LASEK. Of the 33 children, 39.4% had positive stereopsis preoperatively and 87.9% had positive stereopsis 1 year after LASEK. In conclusion, LASEK is an effective surgical alternative to improve visual acuity in anisometropic children unable to tolerate conventional methods of treatment or in whom these methods fail (32).

9. References

[1] Sakimoto T, Rosenblatt MI, Azar DT. Laser eye surgery for refractive errors. The Lancet 2006; 367 (9520): 1432-1447.

[2] American Academy of Ophthalmology. Incisional Corneal Surgery. In: American Academy of Ophthalmology. Refractive surgery, Section 13, 2010-2011. Singapore: American Academy of Ophthalmology; 2010. p. 67-71.

[3] American Academy of Ophthalmology. Photoablation. In: American Academy of Ophthalmology. Refractive surgery, Section 13, 2010-2011. Singapore: American Academy of Ophthalmology; 2010. p. 109-146.

[4] American Academy of Ophthalmology. Photoablation. In: American Academy of Ophthalmology. Refractive surgery, Section 13, 2010-2011. Singapore: American Academy of Ophthalmology; 2010. p. 92-109.

[5] Vukosavljević M, Milivojević M, Resan M, Cerović V. Laser in situ keratomyleusis (LASIK) for correction of myopia and hypermetropia – our one year experience Vojnosanitet Pregl 2009; 66 (12): 979–984.

[6] Giessler S, Duncker GIW. Short-term visual rehabilitation after LASIK. Graefes Arch Clin Exp Ophthalmol 2001; 239 (8): 603-608.

[7] American Academy of Ophthalmology. Patient Evaluation. In: American Academy of Ophthalmology. Refractive surgery, Section 13, 2010-2011. Singapore: American Academy of Ophthalmology; 2010. p. 41-58.

[8] Young JA, Kornmehl EW. Preoperative evaluation for refractive surgery. In: Yanoff M, Duker JS. Ophthalmology. St. Louis: Mosby; 2004. p. 133-136.

[9] Probst LE. Intraoperative complications. In: Probst LE. Lasik: a color atlas and surgical synopsis. Thorofare, NJ: Slack Incorporated; 2001. p. 211-232.

[10] Probst LE. Early and late postoperative complications. In: Probst LE. Lasik: a color atlas and surgical synopsis. Thorofare, NJ: Slack Incorporated; 2001. p. 257-297.

[11] Stojanovic A, Nitter TA. 200 Hz flying-spot technology of the LaserSight LSX excimer laser in the treatment of myopic astigmatism: six and 12 month outcomes of laser in situ keratomileusis and photorefractive keratectomy. J Cataract Refract Surg 2001; 27 (8): 1263- 1277.

[12] Ditzen K, Fiedler J, Pieger S. Laser in situ Keratomileusis for Hyperopia and Hyperopic Astigmatism Using the Meditec MEL 70 Spot Scanner. J Refract Surg 2002; 18: 430-434.

[13] Albarran-Diego C, Munoz G, Montes-Mico R, Alio JL. Bitoric laser in situ keratomileusis for astigmatism. J Cataract Refract Surg 2004; 30 (7): 1471-1478.

[14] Grabner G. Die entwicklung der refraktiven chirurgie. Spektrum Augenheilkd 2009; 23 (3): 187–192.

[15] Reynolds A, Moore JE, Naroo SA, Moore CBT, Shah S. Excimer laser surface ablation – a review. Clin Experiment Ophthalmol 2010; 38 (2): 168-182.

[16] Hashemi H, Taheri SM, Fotouhi A, Kheiltash A. Evaluation of the prophylactic use of mitomycin C to inhibit haze formation after photorefractive keratectomy in high myopia: a prospective clinical study. BMC Ophthalmol 2004; 4: 12.

[17] Haw WW, Manche EE. Photorefractive keratectomy for compound myopic astigmatism. Am J Ophthalmol 2000; 130 (1): 12-19.

[18] Nagy ZZ, Munkacsy G, Popper M. Photorefractive Keratectomy Using the Meditec MEL 70 G-scan Laser for Hyperopia and Hyperopic Astigmatism. J Refract Surg 2002; 18: 542-550.

[19] Taneri S, Zieske JD, Azar DT. Evolution, techniques, clinical outcomes and pathophysiology of LASEK : review of the literature. Surv Ophthalmol 2004; 49: 576–602.

[20] Bilgihan K, Hondur A, Hasanreisoglu B. Laser subepithelial keratomileusis for myopia of -6 to -10 diopters with astigmatism with the MEL60 laser. J Refract Surg 2004; 20: 121-126.

[21] Taneri S, Feit R, Azar DT. Safety, efficacy, and stability indices of LASEK correction in moderate myopia and astigmatism. J Cataract Refract Surg 2004; 30: 2130-2137.

[22] Herrmann WA, Hillenkamp J, Hufendiek K et al. Epilaser in situ keratomileusis: comparative evaluation of epithelial separation with 3 microkeratomes. J Cataract Refract Surg 2008; 34: 1761–1766.

[23] Taneri S, Weisberg M, Azar DT. Surface ablation techniques. J Cataract Refract Surg 2011; 37: 392–408.

[24] Binder PS. One thousand consecutive IntraLase laser in situ keratomileusis flaps. J Cataract Refract Surg 2006; 32: 962–969.

[25] Saloma MQ, Wilson SE. Femtosecond laser in laser in situ keratomileusis. J Cataract Refract Surg 2010; 36: 1024–1032.

[26] Stonecipher KG, Kezirian GM, Stonecipher M. LASIK for -6.00 to -12.00 D of myopia with up to 3.00 D of cylinder using the ALLEGRETTO WAVE: 3- and 6-month results with the 200- and 400-Hz platforms. J Refract Surg 2010; 26: 814-818.

[27] American Academy of Ophthalmology. Refractive Surgery in Ocular and Systemic Disease. In: American Academy of Ophthalmology. Refractive surgery, Section 13, 2010-2011. Singapore: American Academy of Ophthalmology; 2010. p. 203-222.

[28] Astle WF, Huang PT, Ereifej I, Paszuk A. Laser-assisted subepithelial keratectomy for bilateral hyperopia and hyperopic anisometropic amblyopia in children. J Cataract Refract Surg 2010; 36:260–267.

[29] Astle WF, Fawcett SL, Huang PT, Alewenah O, Ingram A. Long-term outcomes of photorefractive keratectomy and laser-assisted subepithelial keratectomy in children J Cataract Refract Surg 2008; 34: 411–416.

[30] Autrata R, Rehurek J. Clinical results of excimer laser photorefractive keratectomy for high myopic anisometropia in children: Four-year follow-up. J Cataract Refract Surg 2003; 29: 694–702.

[31] Yin ZQ, Wang H, Yu T, Ren Q, Chen Li. Facilitation of amblyopia management by laser in situ keratomileusis in high anisometropic hyperopic and myopic children. J AAPOS 2007; 11: 571–576.

[32] Astle WF, Rahmat J, Ingram AD, Huang PT. Laser-assisted subepithelial keratectomy for anisometropic amblyopia in children: Outcomes at 1 year. J Cataract Refract Surg 2007; 33: 2028–2034.

6

Recent Advances in Mucosal Immunology and Ocular Surface Diseases

De-Quan Li[1,*], Zuguo Liu[2], Zhijie Li[1,3], Zhichong Wang[4] and Hong Qi[5]
[1]Ocular Surface Center, Cullen Eye Institute, Department of Ophthalmology,
Baylor College of Medicine, Houston, TX,
[2]Xiamen Eye Institute, Xiamen University, Xiamen,
[3]Key Laboratory for Regenerative Medicine of Ministry of Education and
Department of Ophthalmology, Jinan University, Guangzhou,
[4]State Key Laboratory of Ophthalmology, Zhongshan Ophthalmic Center,
Sun Yat-sen University, Guangzhou,
[5]Department of Ophthalmology, Peking University Third Hospital, Beijing,
[1]USA
[2,3,4,5]China

1. Introduction

The mucosa, a mucus-secreting membrane, is linings of surface and cavities that are exposed to the external environment and internal organs. The mucosal immune system has a unique anatomy and physiology, which provides protection to an organism's various mucous membranes from invasion by potentially pathogenic microbes. It provides three main functions: protecting the mucus membrane against infection, preventing the uptake of antigens, microorganisms, and other foreign materials, and moderating the organism's immune response to that material. The mucosal epithelium forms the initial interface between the environment and host, and functions not only as a barrier but also as a sensor providing bidirectional communication with other resident mucosal lymphoid cells with the capacity to respond to pathogenic microbes and other injurious agents.

It has become increasingly clear that epithelial cells play important roles not only in host defense and inflammation, but also in regulation of immune responses. The mammalian immune system is comprised of two branches, the innate immune system and the adaptive immune system, that work in tandem to provide resistance to infection. The innate immune cells, represented primarily by monocytes, macrophages, dendritic cells and granulocytes, are the first line of host defense and are responsible for immediate recognition and control of microbial invasion. In contrast, the adaptive immune system, represented by B and T lymphocytes, has a delayed response, which is characterized by clonal expansion of cells that bind to a highly specific antigen and have immunological memory [1]. Substantial new evidence now indicates that epithelial cells are central participants, as initiators, mediators and regulators, in the innate and adaptive immune responses, as well as in the transition from innate immunity to adaptive immunity.

---

* Corresponding Author

This new concept has been recently generated from studies mainly in skin and airway epithelial cells. In addition to its function as a physical barrier, human skin has been shown to be an important immune organ displaying various defense mechanisms, which can be divided into three major functional compartments: natural epithelial defense, innate immunity and antigen-elicited adaptive immunity [2-4]. Airway epithelial cells have been recognized to be at the interface of innate and adaptive immunity [5-7]. Airway epithelial cells produce antimicrobial host defense molecules and proinflammatory cytokines and chemokines in response to microbial pathogens. Recruitment of immune cells, including dendritic cells, T cells and B cells into the proximity of epithelium results in the enhancement of adaptive immunity through interactions with epithelial cells. Epithelial cells are also responsible for mucus production in both protective immune responses and allergic airway inflammatory diseases. The crucial roles of epithelial cells in the innate and adaptive immune responses for host defense have also been recognized in other epithelia, including gastrointestinal mucosa [8-10] and ocular surface [11-13]. This chapter is focused on recent advances of this new concept that mucosal epithelium plays a central role in initiating and regulating innate and adaptive immune responses in ocular inflammatory diseases, based on literature review and our new findings. These novel breakthroughs in mucosal immunology would facilitate new therapeutic strategies for treating ocular inflammatory diseases.

2. Toll-like receptors and ocular mucosal innate immunity

The innate immune response relies on evolutionarily ancient germline-encoded receptors, the pattern recognition receptors (PRRs) [14], which recognize highly conserved microbial structures (Table 1). PRRs recognize microbial components, known as pathogen-associated molecular patterns. A breakthrough in the understanding of the ability of innate immune system to rapidly recognize pathogens occurred with the discovery of the Toll-like receptors (TLRs), which is the most important family among the PRRs. At least 10 human TLRs have been identified to date. Each TLR has unique ligand specificity. In general, TLRs 1, 2, 4, 5 and 6 present on the cell plasma membrane and respond to a variety of components of bacteria and fungi (Table 1); and TLRs 3, 7, 8 and 9 mainly present on endosomal membranes inside cells and recognize viral nucleic acids [12]. Among 4 types of transmembrane proteins structurally, TLRs are single-pass type I transmembrane proteins with leucine rich repeats in the extracellular domain for ligand recognition, and a Toll/IL-1 receptor (TIR) domain in the cytoplasmic portion for intracellular signaling [12, 15-17]. TLRs are expressed on immune cells that are most likely to first encounter microbes, such as neutrophils, monocytes, macrophages, and dendritic cells [15]. Ligand recognition by TLRs facilitates the dimerisation of TLRs that triggers the activation of signaling pathways, which originates from the cytoplasmic TIR domain, and culminates in the activation of the nuclear transcription factor NF-κB (nuclear factor kappa-light-chain-enhancer of activated B cells), which leads to the expression of pro-inflammatory molecules, such as TNF-α, IL-1β, IL-6 [16, 18-20]. In addition to innate immune cells, an array of TLRs is expressed by epithelial cells at interfaces between host and environment including that of the skin [2, 21], respiratory tract [5, 6], gastrointestinal tract [9], and ocular surface [12, 13]. Strategic expression of TLRs at such host/environment interfaces appears to play an important role in the first line of defense against microbial invasion at these sites.

TLR	Microbial components	Ligands used for study
TLR1/TLR2	Triacylated lipopeptide (LP)	Pam3CSK4 (1-100 µg/ml)
TLR2*	Bacterial lipoprotein	
	Peptidoglycan	peptidoglycan-BS (1-50 µg/ml)
	lipoteichoic acid	LTA-SA (0.1-10 µg/ml)
	Zymosan (fungi)	Zymosan (1-100 µg/ml)
TLR3	Double stranded RNA (viruses dsRNA)	Poly I:C (5-50 µg/ml)
TLR4	LPS (Gram negative bacteria)	LPS (1-50 µg/ml)
	Bacterial HSP60	
	Respiratory syncytial virus coat protein	
TLR5	Flagellin (flagellated bacteria)	Flagellin-ST (1-25 µg/ml)
TLR6/TLR2	Diacylated lipopeptides	FSL-1 (0.1-10 µg/ml)
TLR7	Imidazoquinolone antiviral drug	Imiquimod (R837, 1-50 µg/ml)
TLR8	Single stranded RNA (viruses ssRNA)	ssRNA40 (0.1-10 µg/ml)
	Imidazoquinolone antiviral drug	
TLR9	Unmethylated CpG motifs of bacterial DNA	C-CpG-ODN (1-50 µg/ml)
TLR10	Unknown	

* TLR2 forms heterodimers with TLR1 and TLR6: TLR1 associates with TLR2 to recognize tri-acyl lipopeptides; TLR6/TLR2 heterodimer recognizes diacyl lipopeptides.

Table 1. Human Toll-like receptors (TLRs) and their microbial ligands

Ocular mucosal epithelial cells have been identified to express an array of functional TLRs [12, 13]. The production of pro-inflammatory cytokines, chemokines and antimicrobial peptides is stimulated via TLR2 by corneal epithelial cells exposed to yeast zymosan [22] and peptidoglycan of Staphylococcus aureus [23]. This pathway may have a role in the pathogenesis of Gram positive bacterial keratitis. Signaling through TLR9 appears important in P. aeruginosa keratitis, and silencing TLR9 signaling reduces inflammation, but likely contributes to decreased bacterial killing in the cornea [24]. Stimulation of TLR3 can induce the expression of proinflammatory cytokines, chemokines and antiviral genes that help to defend the cornea against viral infection [25, 26]. However, the distinctive role of ligand-stimulated TLR signaling in epithelium on regulation of innate and adaptive immunity remains to be elucidated.

3. Ocular epithelial cytokine TSLP links innate and adaptive immunity via Th2 inflammatory responses

Compelling evidence has been recently provided that thymic stromal lymphopoietin (TSLP) represents a key initiator of allergic inflammation at the interface of epithelial and dendritic cells, and TSLP may have a determinant role in the initiation and maintenance of the allergic immune response in atopic dermatitis and asthma [27-31]. Skin-derived TSLP was found to trigger progression from epidermal-barrier defects to asthma, the atopic march, in mice [31, 32].

TSLP is a 140-amino acid IL-7-like 4-helix bundle cytokine that was first isolated from a murine thymic stromal cell line and shown to support B-cell development in the absence of IL-7 [33]. Mouse and human TSLP share a poor homology of 43% amino acid identity. The human TSLP gene is localized in chromosome 5q22, not far from the gene cluster encoding for all the Th2 cytokines, IL-4, IL-5 and IL-13 [34]. The TSLP receptor (TSLPR) complex consists of a TSLP binding chain and the IL-7 receptor α chain (IL-7Rα). Like TSLP, human and mouse TSLPR share approximately 40% amino acid identity. By interacting with the heterodimeric receptor TSLPR/IL-7Rα, TSLP appears to initiate phosphorylation of signal transducer and activator of transcription (STAT) 3 and STAT-5 [27, 35].

It was demonstrated that epithelial cell-derived TSLP could strongly activate human myeloid dendritic cells to mature dendritic cells that produce OX40 ligand (OX40L) in the absence of IL-12 to induce an inflammatory Th2 response characterized by high level of pro-inflammatory cytokine TNF-α with low level of anti-inflammatory cytokine IL-10, distinct from the regulatory Th2 responses characterized by low TNF-α and high IL-10 production [27, 28]. This suggests that TSLP represents a key initiator of allergic inflammation at the interface of epithelial cells and dendritic cells. TSLP was also demonstrated to direct the innate phase of allergic immune responses through activating mast cells. Therefore, TSLP and OX40L may represent important targets for intervention in the initiation of allergic inflammatory responses.

Epithelial cells appear to be the major potential producer of TSLP in both mice and humans, although fibroblasts, smooth muscle cells, and mast cells all have the potential to produce TSLP [35, 36]. The expression of TSLP by epithelial cells has been recently shown to be stimulated by microbial ligands, inflammatory and Th2 cytokines [37-39]. Using ocular mucosal epithelium as a model, Li and associates [40] have evaluated the expression and production of TSLP by primary human corneal epithelial cells in response to 11 extracted or synthetic microbial components that are ligands of TLRs 1-9 (Table 1). As shown in Figure 1A, TSLP expression and production were found to be largely induced by the ligands to TLRs 3, 5 and 6, which were polyinosinic-polycytidylic acid (polyI:C), flagellin and FSL-1, respectively, representing viral dsRNA and the bacterial components flagellin and lipopeptides. PolyI:C and flagellin, the major TSLP inducers, stimulated TSLP production to 67- and 19-fold, respectively. The TSLP mRNA reached the peak levels rapidly in 4 hours in response to these ligands. The specificity of this response was confirmed when respective antibody against TLR3 or TLR5 significantly blocked TSLP expression induced by polyI:C and flagellin, respectively. The pattern of TLR-dependant TSLP induction indicates that human corneal epithelial cells are able to rapidly initiate an innate immune response to virus or bacteria through TLR-mediated pathways. TSLP was also moderately induced by pro-inflammatory cytokines at both mRNA and protein levels. TNF-α or IL-1β induced a concentration dependent increase in the TSLP mRNA and protein, but their stimulatory effects were much weaker than that of polyI:C and flagellin, which stimulated TSLP protein production over 15- and 4-fold higher, respectively, than TNF-α. These data suggest that TSLP induction is mainly through a TLR-dependant innate immune response to microbes in human ocular epithelium.

IL-4 and IL-13, the major cytokines secreted by Th2 cells, not only moderately induced TSLP mRNA and protein, but also strongly synergized with microbial ligands, such as polyI:C, or pro-inflammatory cytokine TNF-α to promote TSLP expression and production (Figure 1B). This synergized induction of TSLP was further confirmed in an ex vivo experiment model using fresh human corneal epithelial tissues (Figure 1C). These findings demonstrate that adaptive immunity-derived Th2 cytokines are capable of amplifying the TSLP expression and production by the corneal epithelium, which in turn has the capability of priming Th2 cell differentiation through dendritic cell activation [27, 28]. These findings suggest that blocking TSLP could be a novel strategy for treatment of allergic diseases or other TSLP-driven conditions.

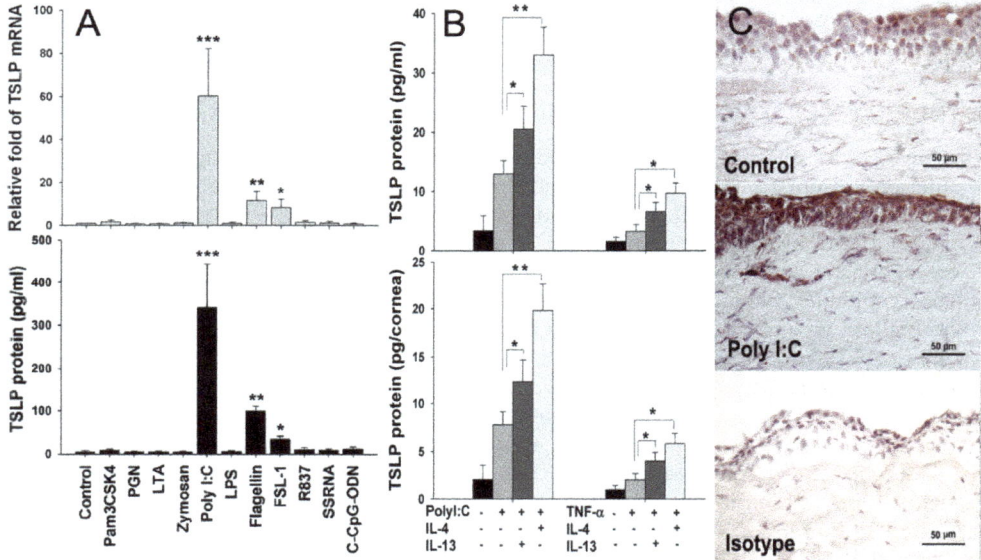

Fig. 1. TLR-mediated induction of TSLP by microbial ligands, TNF-α and Th2 cytokines. **A**. TSLP induction in HCECs. The confluent primary HCECs were incubated with 50μg/ml polyI:C or 10μg/ml of Pam_3CSK_4, peptidoglycan (PGN), LTA, Zymosan, LPS, flagellin, FSL-1, R837, single stranded RNA (ssRNA40) or C-CpG-ODN for 4 hours for TSLP mRNA expression by RT-qPCR, or for 48 hours for TSLP protein in the culture supernatants by ELISA; **B**. TSLP induction in an ex vivo model of human corneal tissues. A fresh corneoscleral tissue was cut into 4 equal size pieces. Each quarter of corneal tissue was placed into a well of 8-chamber slides in 150 μl of serum-free SHEM medium without or with polyI:C (50 μg/ml) or TNF-α (20 ng/ml) in the presence of IL-4 or IL-13 (100 ng/ml) for 24 hours. The culture supernatants were used for TSLP ELISA. Results shown are mean ± SD of 3 independent experiments. * $p < 0.05$; ** $p < 0.01$; *** $P < 0.001$. **C**. The corneal tissues were prepared for cryosections for TSLP immunohistochemical staining with isotype IgG as negative control.

Although the recognition of different ligands by specific TLRs leads to activation of an intracellular signaling cascade in a myeloid differentiation primary response gene 88 (MyD88)-dependent or independent fashion, all TLRs share NF-κB signal transduction pathways for activation of the transcription factors [20]. TNF-α is also well known to promote activation of the NF-κB signaling pathway [41]. TSLP induction has been observed through NF-κB activation in airway epithelial cells [30] and synovial fibroblasts [42]. As evaluated by Western blot analysis and immunofluorescent staining, NF-κB was found to be dramatically activated in corneal epithelial cells exposed to polyI:C, flagellin or TNF-α for 4 hours. This activation was evidenced by nuclear translocation of p65 protein, one of the two proteins in NF-κB heterodimer. This p65 nuclear translocation and TSLP induction, stimulated by polyI:C, flagellin or TNF-α were markedly blocked by TLR3, TLR5 or TNF-α specific antibody, respectively, and also by quinazoline, a NF-κB activation inhibitor [40]. These findings confirm that TSLP is mainly induced by microbial components, proinflammatory cytokines and Th2 cytokines in human corneal epithelial cells via TLR and NF-κB signaling pathways, suggesting that epithelium-derived TSLP links the innate and adaptive immune responses,

4. TSLP/OX40L/OX40 signaling initiates Th2-dominant allergic conjunctivitis

Allergic diseases like seasonal allergy, asthma, atopic dermatitis, affect up to 20-30% of the population in industrialized countries, and up to 50% of these individuals reporting ocular allergic manifestations [43-45]. The incidence of allergies has increased steadily over the past 30 years. Th2-dominant hypersensitivity is a major contributor to allergic inflammatory diseases, but the underlining mechanism for initiation of this adaptive immune disorder by mucosal epithelia remains a relative mystery. The molecular triggers for Th2 allergic inflammation were not clear until studies identified a novel epithelium-derived pro-allergic cytokine TSLP, which activates myeloid dendritic cells (DCs) to produce OX40 ligand (OX40L) that triggers a Th2 inflammatory response. TSLP has been identified as a key initiator in the development of human allergic disease [31, 46, 47], including asthma, atopic dermatitis and allergic conjunctivitis, a triad of common atopic IgE-dependent allergic diseases [48]. The direct link between TSLP expression and the pathogenesis of atopic dermatitis and asthma in vivo has been demonstrated [29]. TSLP was found to be highly expressed by keratinocytes in skin lesions of atopic dermatitis and was associated with dendritic cell activation in situ [49]. Evidence associating TSLP with human asthma has also been reported [29, 32]. Patients suffering from one member of the triad often show symptoms of one or both of the other members, suggesting a common genetic or initiating element in these diseases [31].

Using a well characterized murine model of experimental allergic conjunctivitis (EAC) induced by short ragweed (SRW) pollen [50, 51], Li and colleagues observed that the repeated topical challenges with ragweed pollen allergen generated typical signs of allergic conjunctivitis in the pollen-sensitized BALB/c mice, which developed lid edema, conjunctival redness, chemosis, and tearing, as well as frequent scratching of the eye lids [52]. They found that TSLP mRNA expression was significantly upregulated in the corneal and conjunctival epithelia from mice sensitized and challenged with pollen when compared with phosphate buffered saline (PBS) alone and untreated normal controls. Immunohistochemical staining confirmed an increase in TSLP production in the eyes challenged with SRW pollen. As shown in Figure 2A, the corneal and conjunctival epithelia in EAC BALB/c mice displayed much stronger TSLP staining throughout the entire epithelium, especially the superficial epithelial layers of the conjunctiva, than the PBS-treated control. These data indicate the stimulated TSLP mRNA expression and protein production by ocular surface epithelia in the SRW-induced EAC murine model.

The accumulation of CD11c positive (CD11c+) dendritic cells on the ocular surface was detected in this EAC model by reverse transcription and quantitative real-time polymerase

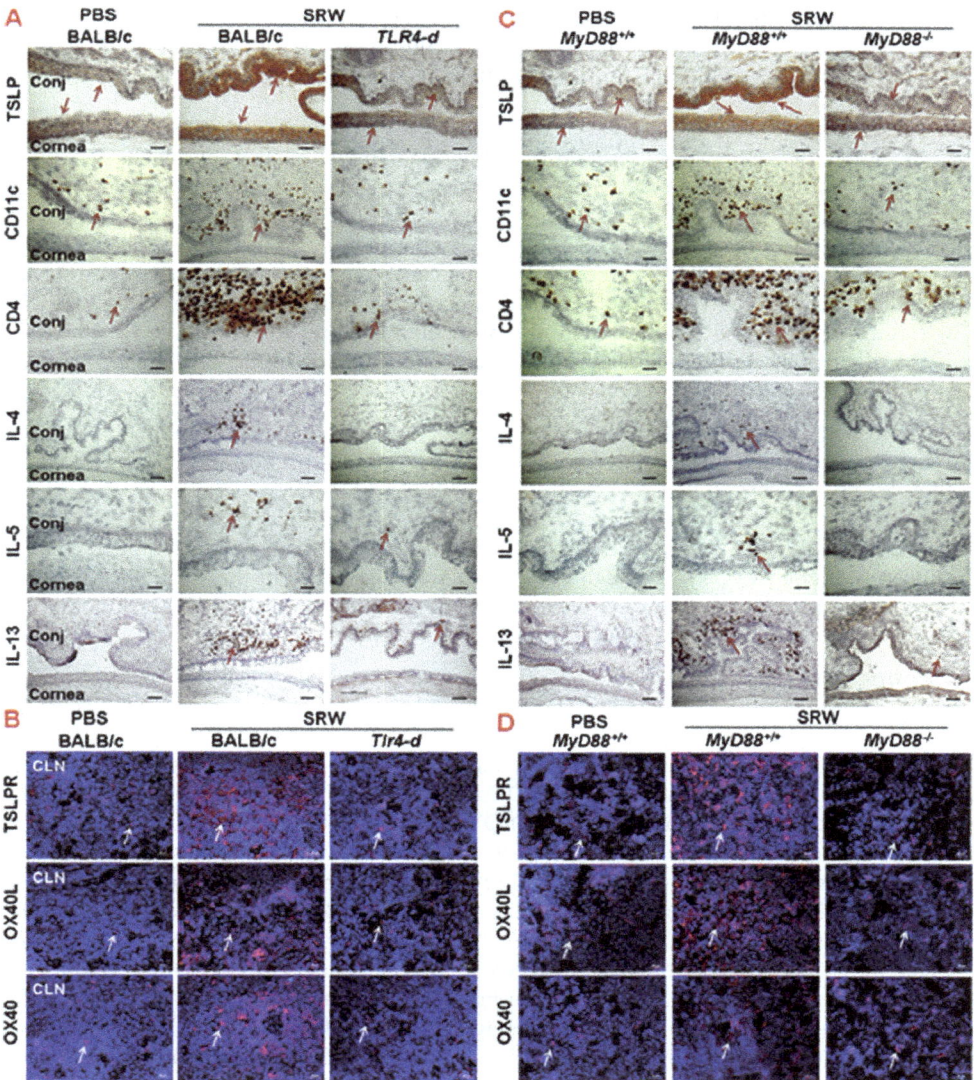

Fig. 2. The stimulated production of TSLP signaling proteins and Th2-dominant inflammation in SRW-induced EAC model requires TLR4 and MyD88. **Top panel**: The representative images showing immunohistochemical staining of epithelial TSLP, markers for dendritic (CD11c) and T cells (CD4), and Th2 cytokines (IL-4, IL-5 and IL-13) on cornea and conjunctiva (Conj) of wild type and *Tlr4* deficient BALB/c mice challenged by SRW pollen, with PBS-treated mice as controls (**A**), and of C57BL/6 based wild type *MyD88+/+* and knockout *MyD88-/-* mice challenged by SRW pollen, with PBS-treated mice as controls (**C**). **Bottom panel**: The representative images showing immunofluorescent staining of TSLP activated signals, TSLPR, OX40L and OX40 on cervical lymph nodes (CLN) of wild type and

Tlr4 deficient BALB/c mice challenged by SRW pollen with PBS-treated mice as controls (**B**), and of C57BL/6 based wild type *MyD88*$^{+/+}$ and knockout *MyD88*$^{-/-}$ mice challenged by SRW pollen, with PBS-treated mice as controls (**D**). Bar: 20μm; Arrows: red or red brown positive staining signals.

chain reaction (RT-qPCR) and immunostaining. The increased mRNA levels of CD11c, TSLPR and OX40L were observed in ocular surface, especially in conjunctival tissues, where their transcripts increased to 4-10 fold, respectively (P< 0.05 or <0.01), from SRW pollen-challenged mice, compared with PBS controls. The large amount of CD11c$^+$ dendritic cells was accumulated in the ocular surface of the pollen challenged eyes, primarily in the stroma subjacent to the conjunctival epithelia, in EAC mice, but not in the control mice treated with PBS (Figure 2A). These results suggest that ocular surface was infiltrated with TSLP activated dendritic cells that express TSLPR and produce OX40L in the EAC mice.

Th2-dominant inflammatory response was clearly observed on ocular surface in the mice challenged by pollen. The infiltration of T lymphocytes was evidenced by the increased CD4 mRNA expression and a markedly increased number of CD4 immunopositive (CD4$^+$) cells in the ocular surface, especially in the conjunctiva, of EAC mice (Figure 2A), when compared with PBS control mice. These CD4$^+$ T cells appear to be Th2 lineage because the transcripts of three key Th2 cytokines, IL-4, IL-5 and IL-13, were all found to be expressed at significantly higher levels in corneal and conjunctival tissues from the EAC mice than the PBS controls. Immunostaining data confirmed that the IL-4, IL-5 and IL-13-producing Th2 cells were largely infiltrated in conjunctival stroma (Figure 2A).

To confirm the TSLP signaling in SRW pollen-induced EAC mice, the ocular surface draining cervical lymph nodes (CLN) were collected for evaluation (Figure 3A). Compared with PBS controls, the mRNA levels of TSLPR and OX40L were significantly stimulated to 7.5 and 4.1 fold respectively (both P<0.01) while CD11c expression only slightly increased in CLN from EAC mice, indicating CD11c$^+$ DCs were markedly activated by ocular surface epithelia-derived TSLP. The mRNA levels of OX40 (3.4 fold, P<0.05) and Th2 cytokines, IL-4, IL-5 and IL-13 (13.2, 12.8 and 5.5 fold, respectively, all P<0.01), significantly increased while CD4 expression was not changed in the CLN from EAC mice, indicating naive CD4$^+$ T cells were largely differentiated to Th2 cells that might be primed by OX40L produced by TSLP activated dendritic cells [28]. The increased TSLPR$^+$, OX40L$^+$ and OX40$^+$ cells in the draining CLN of the pollen challenged EAC mice were further confirmed by immunofluorescent staining that showed dramatically increased immunoreactivity of these 3 signaling proteins at cell membrane and cytoplasm in CLN (Figure 2B). All these results demonstrate that TSLP/OX40L/OX40 signaling plays a critical role in the development of Th2-dominant allergic inflammation in pollen induced EAC model in BALB/c mice, suggesting that TSLP signaling molecules could be novel therapeutic targets to treat allergic inflammatory disease.

5. Cutting edge breakthrough: Short ragweed pollen triggers ocular allergic inflammation through TLR4-dependent innate immune response

Although there have been numerous studies on the development of allergen-induced inflammation, the mechanisms leading to resolution of allergic inflammation remain poorly understood. This represents an important knowledge gap and potential challenge because failure to resolve allergen driven inflammation potentially leads to recurrent or chronic allergic diseases. Pollen, a ubiquitous allergen, affects a large population of allergic patients. Pollen is the trigger of seasonal rhinitis, conjunctivitis and asthma, as well as an exacerbating factor of atopic dermatitis. However, the underlying molecular mechanism by which pollen induces Th2-dominant allergic inflammation via epithelial innate immunity pathways is largely unknown. Substantial evidence now indicates that epithelial cells are central participants in innate and adaptive immune responses [4, 5, 7]. Based on the observation that we and other groups have made [40, 53, 54] that TSLP is mainly induced via TLR mediated innate response in epithelia exposed to microbial products, we hypothesized that pollen, such as Ambrosia artemisiifolia short ragweed (SRW), the most widespread plant in North America, may serve as a functional TLR4 agonist that induces production of a proallergic cytokine TSLP via innate immune response to trigger Th2-dominant allergic inflammation. To uncover the novel phenomenon and molecular signaling pathways involved in pollen induced allergic inflammation, a comprehensive set of experiments has been conducted using a well-characterized murine model of allergic conjunctivitis induced by SRW pollen in BALB/c, TLR4 deficient and MyD88 knockout mice, as well as a murine topical ocular surface challenge model and a culture model of primary human corneal epithelial cells exposed to an aqueous extract of defatted SRW pollen.

TLR-mediated TSLP induction has been recognized [39, 53, 54]. We have demonstrated that TSLP was largely induced by specific TLR ligands in human corneal epithelial cells [40]. MyD88 is a universal adapter protein necessary for response to all TLRs except TLR3 [55, 56]. *Tlr4*-deficient (*Tlr4*-d, C.C3-Tlr4Lps-d/J) and MyD88 knockout (*MyD88*-/-) mice have been used to identify TLR4 mediated signaling [57, 58]. To explore whether SRW pollen stimulates TSLP through TLR4-dependent innate response, we sensitized and topically challenged the wild-type BALB/c, *Tlr4*-d (Jackson Laboratory, Bar Harbor, ME) and *MyD88*-/- mice (gifts from Dr. Shizuo Akira, Research Institute for Microbial Disease, Osaka University, Japan) with SRW pollen.

Compared with wild-type BALB/c mice, the ocular allergic signs, stimulated TSLP/OX40L/OX40 signaling and Th2-dominant inflammatory response by ocular mucosa, especially conjunctival tissues, were dramatically reduced or eliminated in BALB/c based *Tlr4*-d mice. As shown in Figure 3A, the mRNA levels of TSLP, OX40L, OX40 and Th2 cytokines (IL-4, IL-5 and IL-13) were significantly stimulated in cornea, conjunctiva and draining CLN from wild-type BALB/c, but not in those from *Tlr4*-d mice. The immunostaining results confirmed that SRW pollen did not stimulate TSLP and its downstream molecules or a Th2 response in ocular mucosal tissues (Figure. 2A) and draining CLN (Figure. 2B) of *Tlr4*-d mice. These findings suggest that TLR4-dependent TSLP signaling was involved in the SRW pollen induced allergic inflammation.

The SRW topical challenges triggered the typical allergic signs and scratching behavior in wild type *MyD88*+/+ mice, although less severe than BALB/c mice. The expression of TSLP and its signaling molecules, TSLPR, OX40L and OX40, as well as Th2 cytokines IL-4, IL-5 and IL-13 was significantly stimulated in the cornea, conjunctiva and CLN from SRW challenged wild type *MyD88*+/+ mice at both mRNA (Figure. 3B) and protein levels (Figure 2C, 2D). Clinical allergic signs and stimulated production of TSLP signaling molecules (TSLPR, OX40L and OX40) and Th2 cytokines (IL-4, IL-5 and IL-13) were dramatically reduced or eliminated in SRW challenged *MyD88*-/- mice as evaluated by RT-qPCR (Figure

3B) and immunostaining (Figure 2C, 2D). These findings suggest that MyD88 pathway is involved in the TLR4-dependent TSLP signaling induced by SRW pollen.

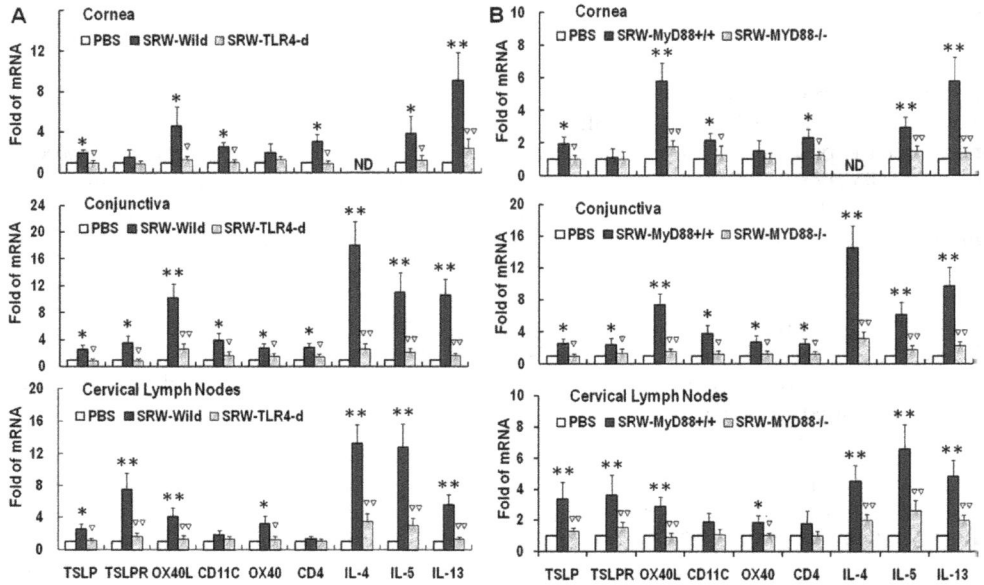

Fig. 3. The stimulated expression of TSLP signaling molecules and Th2 cytokines in SRW-induced EAC model requires TLR4 and MyD88. The mRNA expression of proallergic cytokine TSLP, its downstream signals in dendritic (TSLPR, OX40L, & CD11c) and T cells (OX40 & CD4), as well as Th2 cytokines (IL-4, IL-5 and IL-13) by corneal epithelium, conjunctiva and cervical lymph nodes in wild type and *Tlr4* deficient BALB/c mice sensitized and topically challenged by SRW with PBS-treated mice as controls (**A**), and in C57BL/6 based wild type *MyD88+/+* and knockout *MyD88-/-* mice, sensitized and topically challenged by SRW pollen, with PBS-treated mice as controls (**B**). The mRNA levels are presented as relative fold in EAC mice over the controls, which were evaluated by RT and real-time qPCR using TaqMan gene expression assay system with GAPDH as an internal control. Results shown are the Mean ± SD of four independent experiments. *P<0.05, **P<0.01; n=4, compared with PBS controls; ▽P<0.05, ▽▽P<0.01, n=4, compared with wild type mice.

To confirm that SRW pollen directly stimulates TSLP production by ocular mucosal epithelia through TLR4-dependent innate immunity pathway, we created a topical challenge murine model using an aqueous extract of defatted SRW pollen (SRWe) at 150μg/5μl/eye for 4-24 hours. TSLP mRNA was induced as early as 4 hours and reached peak levels at 8 hours, and TSLP protein levels increased in 24 hours in ocular epithelia exposed to SRWe. As shown in Figure 4 A & B, SRWe significantly stimulated TSLP mRNA by 2 fold in corneal and conjunctival epithelia (Both P<0.05), and its protein levels by 3.2 fold (from 150.2±37.6 pg/mg cellular protein to 480.00±89.6 pg/mg) in cornea epithelia and 2.2 fold (from 128.6±29.8 pg/mg to 281.6±19.3 pg/mg) in conjunctiva in BALB/c mice when compared with untreated or PBS-treated controls. The SRWe-stimulated TSLP were significantly decreased at both mRNA and protein levels by TLR4 blocker, a rat anti-mouse TLR4 antibody, but not by its isotype rat IgG2a.

The SRWe topical challenge did not increase TSLP mRNA (Figure 4C) and protein levels (Figure 4D) in corneal and conjunctival epithelia of $Tlr4$-d mice. Similarly, a TLR4 agonist lipopolysaccharides (LPS, $5\mu g/5\mu l$/eye) stimulated TSLP production by corneal and conjunctival epithelia in BALB/c mice, but not in $Tlr4$-d mice. Furthermore, we applied this topical challenge model to MyD88 knockout mice and their wild type controls. SRWe

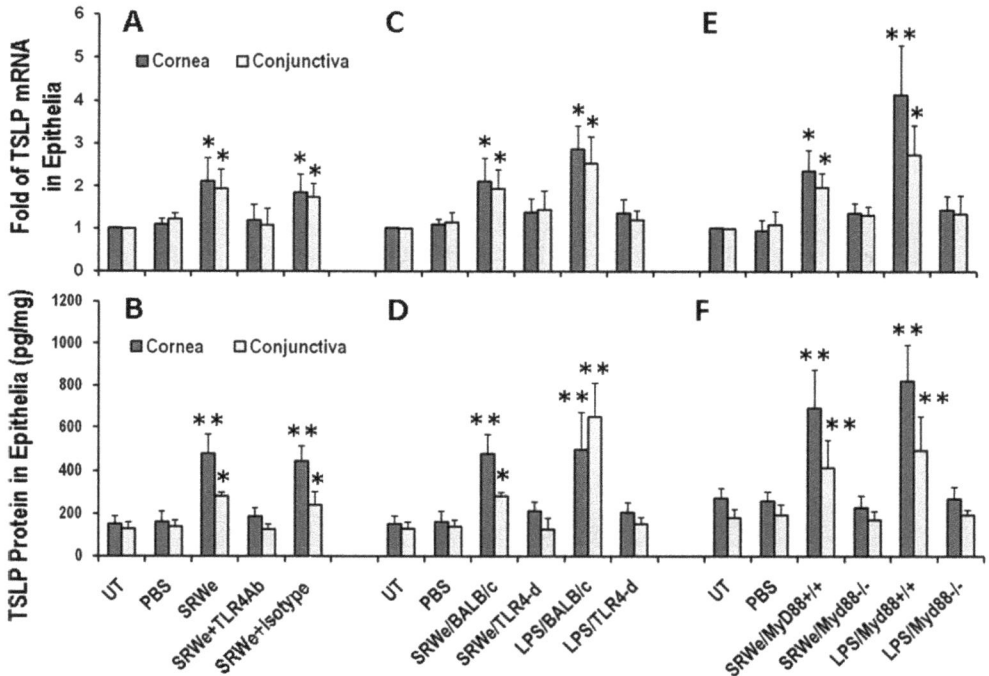

Fig. 4. Aqueous extract of defatted SRW pollen (SRWe) induces TSLP expression and production by murine ocular surface epithelia through TLR4- and MyD88-dependent innate immunity pathway. A, B. BALB/c mice were topically instilled with SRWe at $150\mu g/5\mu l$/eye for 6 or 24 hours for TSLP mRNA (A) or protein (B) respectively, without or with pre-instilled rat anti-mouse TLR4 antibody ($1\mu g/5\mu l$/eye) or its isotype rat IgG2a. Untreated (UT) and PBS-treated mice were used as controls. Corneal epithelium and conjunctiva were harvested for TSLP mRNA and protein by RT-qPCR and ELISA respectively. C, D. TSLP mRNA (C) and protein (D) induction by topically challenged SRWe or LPS ($5\mu g/5\mu l$/eye) in wild type and $Tlr4$-d BALB/C mice, with untreated or PBS-treated mice as controls. E, F. TSLP mRNA (E) and protein (F) induction by topically challenged SRWe or LPS in wild type $MyD88^{+/+}$ and knockout $MyD88^{-/-}$ mice, with untreated or PBS-treated mice as controls. Results shown are the Mean ± SD of four independent experiments. *$P<0.05$, **$P<0.01$; n=4, compared with PBS controls.

promoted TSLP production by ocular epithelia at both mRNA (Figure 4E) and protein levels (Figure 4F) only in $MyD88^{+/+}$ mice, but not in $MyD88^{-/-}$ mice, a similar pattern to that observed following LPS topical challenge. Taken together, these data demonstrated that SRWe directly stimulates TSLP production by ocular mucosal epithelia via a TLR4-dependent innate pathway.

To explore whether this phenomenon occurs in humans, we investigated TSLP expression in human corneal epithelium. TSLP mRNA was upregulated at 4 hours and its protein was detected at 24 hours in human corneal epithelial cells (HCECs) exposed to SRWe, which is consistent with our previous report [40]. TSLP induction at mRNA (Figure 5A) and protein levels (Figure 5B) was concentration-dependently stimulated by SRWe in primary HCECs. TSLP protein was barely detectable (4.83±1.60 pg/ml) in the supernatant of normal HCEC cultures. SRWe at 10µg/ml increased the TSLP protein to 48.92±4.23 pg/ml ($P<0.01$), the levels comparable to that stimulated by 10ng/ml of TNF-α in HCECs [40]. The SRWe (10µg/ml)-stimulated TSLP mRNA was significantly blocked by pre-incubation of cells with 10µg/ml of neutralizing monoclonal antibody against human TLR4, but not by its isotype mouse IgG2a k (Figure 5C). Furthermore, SRWe stimulated TSLP expression was also significantly inhibited by quinazoline, a NF-κB Activation Inhibitor (Figure 5C). These findings were confirmed by detection of increased TSLP protein levels as shown in Figure 5D. These data demonstrate that SRW induces TSLP production in human corneal epithelial cells through TLR4 and NF-κB innate signaling pathways.

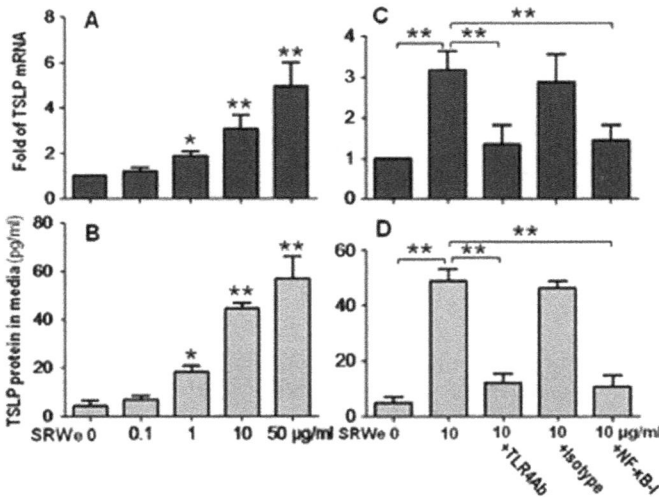

Fig. 5. SRWe induces TSLP expression and production by human corneal epithelial cells (HCECs) through TLR4 and NF-κB signaling pathways. **A, B**. Confluent cultures of primary HCECs were treated with 0.1 to 50 µg/ml of SRWe for 4 hours for TSLP mRNA or 48 hours for TSLP protein in the supernatants. **C, D**. HCECs were pre-incubated with mouse TLR4 antibody (10µg/ml), isotype mouse IgG2a k, or NF-κB activation inhibitor quinazoline (NFkB-I, 10µM) for 1 hour before adding 10µg/ml SRWe for 4 hours for TSLP mRNA or 48 hours for TSLP protein in the supernatants. Results shown are the Mean ± SD of four independent experiments. *$P<0.05$, **$P<0.01$; n=4.

Traditionally, TLRs recognize conserved microbial components as ligands or agonists. Recent studies have revealed that TLR4 recognizes a wider variety of ligands than previous thought. In addition to its first identified ligand, bacterial LPS, TLR4 was found to recognize certain viral proteins such as the F protein from respiratory syncytial virus and mouse mammary tumor virus. Not limited to pathogen-associated molecular patterns (PAMP), TLR4 responds to human endogenous structural proteins derived from tissue injury or during inflammation, the damage-associated molecular patterns (DAMP), such as type III repeat extra domain A of fibronectin, oligosaccharides of hyaluronic acid, human heat-shock protein Hsp60 and Hsp70 (see review [59]). A few reports have revealed the potential for protein extracts from plants and herbs to activate TLR4, such as taxol, an antitumor agent derived from the Yew plant [60], and aqueous extract of Rhodiola imbricata rhizome, a medicinal plant [61].

In conclusion, we have for the first time uncovered a novel phenomenon and a unknown mechanism that short ragweed pollen, serving as a functional TLR4 agonist, induces TSLP/OX40L/OX40 signaling to trigger Th2-dominant allergic inflammation via TLR4-dependent innate immunity pathways [62]. These novel findings shed light on the understanding of innate mucosal epithelial immunity involved in allergic inflammation, and may create new therapeutic targets to cure allergic disease.

6. Epithelium-derived interleukin 33 initiates allergic inflammation

The IL-1 receptor family has several members, including the classical IL-1 receptor (IL-1R) and the IL-18 receptor (IL-18R). In 1989, one member of the family, ST2, a protein encoded by IL-1 receptor-like 1 (IL-1RL1) gene, was identified as an orphan receptor [63]. Investigation into the function of ST2 revealed its participation in inflammatory processes, particularly regarding mast cells, type 2 CD4+ T helper cells and the production of Th2-associated cytokines. In fact, ST2 was characterized as a specific cellular marker that differentiated Th2 from Th1 T cells. Clinical and experimental observations led to the association of ST2 with disease entities such as asthma, pulmonary fibrosis, rheumatoid arthritis, collagen vascular diseases and septic shock [64]. In 2005, the discovery of IL-33 as a ST2 ligand provided new insights into ST2 signaling [65]. By binding to ST2 receptor, IL-33 can activate Th2 cells and mast cells to secrete the proinflammatory and Th2 cytokines and chemokines that lead to severe pathological changes in mucosal organs [66].

IL-33 is produced mainly by epithelial and endothelial cells, fibroblast, and others [66-68]. IL-33 expression has been found to be up-regulated by stimulation with inflammatory cytokines, TNF-α and IL-1β [69]. However, the expression and regulation of IL-33 by mucosal surface epithelia has not been well elucidated. Using fresh donor corneal tissues and primary HCECs, we recently observed that IL-33 is mainly expressed by epithelium and largely induced by microbial products through TLR and NF-κB signaling pathways [70]. The findings suggest that the mucosal epithelial cell-derived cytokine IL-33 may play an important role in allergic inflammatory diseases through innate immune responses.

As shown in Figure 6A, IL-33 expression and production were largely induced by polyI:C, lipopolysaccharides (LPS), flagellin, FSL-1 and R837, the ligands for TLR3, -4, -5, -6 and -7, representing viral dsRNA and the bacterial components flagellin and lipopeptides, respectively. PolyI:C and flagellin were major IL-33 inducers, stimulating IL-33 production by 7- and 4-fold, respectively, with the peak mRNA levels at 8 hours by HCECs. The IL-33 induction by these 2 ligands was further confirmed using an ex vivo donor corneal tissue model (Figure 6B). The specificity of TLR-dependent response by HCECs was also confirmed when an antibody against TLR3 or TLR5 significantly inhibited IL-33 expression by polyI:C or flagellin respectively (Figure 6C). The pattern of TLR-dependent IL-33 induction indicates that HCECs are able to rapidly initiate an innate immune response to virus or bacteria, and play an important role in allergic inflammatory disease.

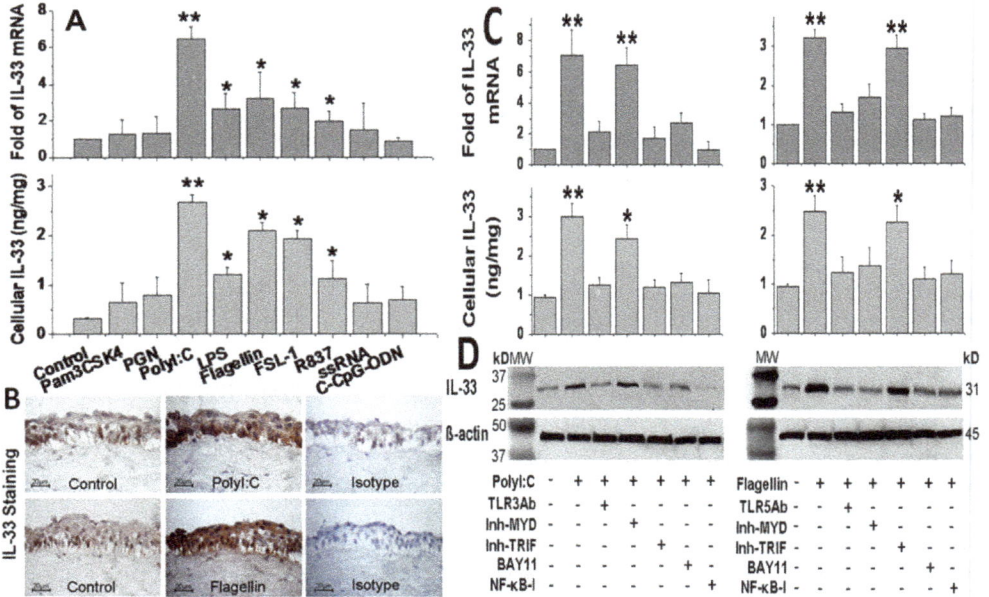

Fig. 6. TLR-dependent induction of IL-33 by microbial ligands in human corneal epithelium. **A.** IL-33 mRNA and protein levels induced by primary human corneal epithelial cells (HCECs) exposed to 50μg/ml polyI:C or 10μg/ml of Pam3CSK4, peptidoglycan (PGN), polyI:C, LPS, flagellin, FSL-1, R-837, ssRNA40 or C-CpG-ODN for 8 or 48 hours, evaluated by quantitative real-time PCR or ELISA, respectively. Results shown are the mean ± SD of four independent experiments. *P< 0.05; **P < 0.01. **B.** The immunohistochemical staining showing IL-33 induction in an ex vivo human corneal tissues by polyI:C (50μg/ml) or flagellin (10μg/ml) for 24 hours with isotype IgG as a negative control. **C.** TLR and NF-κB signaling pathways involved in IL-33 induction by polyI:C or flagellin in HCECs exposed to polyI:C (50μg/mL) or flagellin (10μg/mL) in the absence or presence of preincubated rabbit TLR3Ab (10μg/mL), TLR5Ab (10μg/mL), BAY11-7082 (10μM) or quinazoline (10μM) for 1 hour, and Pepinh-MYD (40μM) or Pepinh-TRIF (40μM) for 6 hours. The cultures treated by ligands for 8 hours for IL-33 mRNA, or for 48 hours for IL-33 protein by ELISA and by Western blot with β-actin as control (**D**). Results shown are the mean ± SD of four independent experiments. *P< 0.05; **P < 0.01.

IL-33 is an extracellular inflammatory cytokine while it also acts as a nuclear transcription factor [71]. It has been shown that IL-33 is mainly localized to the nucleus of endothelial cells and bound to chromatin. IL-33 mRNA is primarily translated and synthesized in vivo as a 30-kDa precursor, a pro-IL-33 protein. As a member of IL-1 super family and like IL-1 and

IL-18, pro-IL-33 protein sequence does not have a signal peptide that directs it for secretion via the ER–Golgi pathway [66, 72]. Like pro-IL-1β, human pro-IL-33 was reported to be cleaved by caspase-1 to generate active form, an 18-kDa fragment (mature IL-33), which is sufficient to activate signaling via the IL-33 receptor ST2. Recombinant mature IL-33 has been known to induce Th2-associated cytokines and inflammatory cytokines via its receptor, ST2 [72, 73]. However, processing of pro-IL-33 in vivo has not been clarified yet. It is not clear whether caspase-1 cleavage of pro-IL-33 occurs in vivo and whether, as for IL-1β, this cleavage is a prerequisite for IL-33 secretion and bioactivity.

Our data have showed that no significantly changes of IL-33 protein levels can be detected by ELISA in the culture supernatants, other than in cell lysate, of the HCECs. IL-33 protein levels significantly increased in the cell lysate, but not in the culture supernatants, of HCECs exposed to polyI:C or flagellin for 24-48 hours, when compared with the untreated control. However, the stimulated cellular IL-33 protein was released outside the cells into culture supernatant after co-incubation with ATP for additional 30 minutes, as evaluated by ELISA and Western blot analysis [70]. The finding supports a notion that caspase 1-dependant activation may involved in the release and secretion of IL-33 protein since ATP has been known to activate caspase-1 through triggering the P2X7 receptor [74]. Further studies are necessary to clarify the underlining mechanism.

As shown in Figure 6C evaluated by RT-qPCR and ELISA, as well as in Figure 6D by Western blotting, synthetic dsRNA polyI:C-induced IL-33 mRNA expression and protein production were markedly blocked by TLR3 antibody and TIR-domain-containing adaptor inducing interferon (TRIF) inhibitory peptide (Pepinh-TRIF), but not by TLR5 antibody or MyD88 inhibitory peptide (Pepinh-MYD), while extracted bacterial component flagellin-induced IL-33 production was dramatically suppressed by TLR5 antibody and Pepinh-MYD, but not by TLR3 antibody or Pepinh-TRIF, in corneal epithelial cells. The stimulated IL-33 induction by polyI:C or flagellin were also significantly blocked by IκB-α inhibitor BAY11-7082 or NF-κB activation inhibitor quinazoline. Further study has shown that NF-κB was dramatically activated with p65 protein nuclear translocation in corneal epithelial cells exposed to polyI:C or flagellin for 4 hours, as evaluated by Western blot analysis and immunofluorescent staining. BAY 11 selectively inhibits the phosphorylation and degradation of IκB-α, blocked the nuclear translocation of NF-κB p65 protein. NF-κB activation inhibitor quinazoline also blocked the p65 nuclear translocation. These findings demonstrate a novel phenomenon that a newly defined pro-allergic cytokine IL-33 is largely induced by microbial components through TLR and NF-κB signaling pathways in human corneal epithelium. This suggests that human ocular mucosal epithelium plays an important role in initiating Th2-dominant allergic inflammation via innate immune responses.

In a clinical study, we have tested conjunctival impression cytology specimens obtained from 8 patients with active atopic conjunctivitis and 8 normal subjects by RT-qPCR (Figure 7). The mRNA levels of TSLP, TSLPR, OX40L, OX40, IL-33 and ST2 were found to be significantly elevated in the atopic group compared with the normal control subjects, suggesting a potential role of TSLP/TSLPR/OX40L/OX40 and IL-33/ST2 signaling pathways in allergic conjunctivitis (Figure 7A). In SRW pollen induced EAC mice, the transcripts and proteins of IL-33, ST2, and IL-1 receptor accessory protein (IL1RAP) were also found to be significantly increased in the corneal epithelium, conjunctiva and CLN, as evaluated by RT-qPCR (Figure 7B) and immunostaining (Figure 7C). IL-33, ST2 and TLRs could become novel biomarkers and molecular targets for the intervention to treat allergic inflammatory diseases.

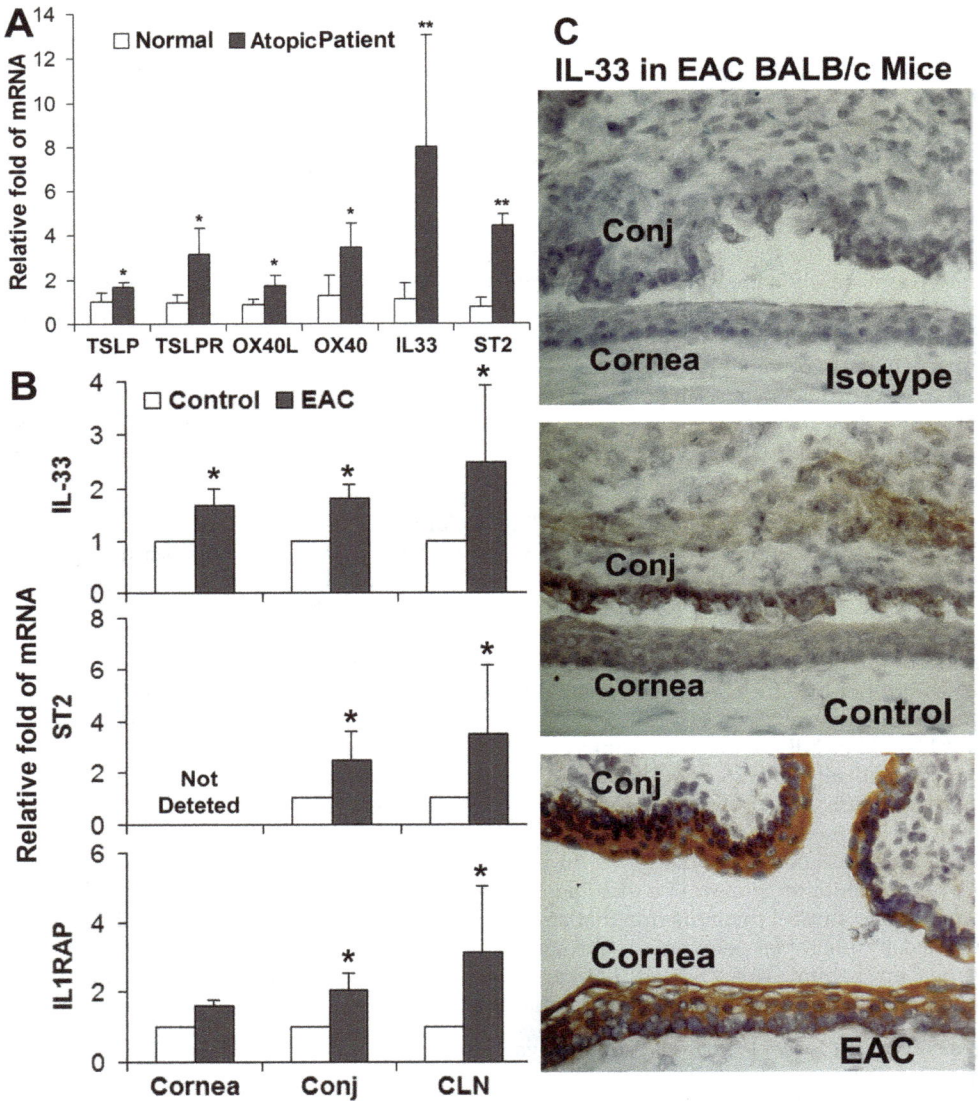

Fig. 7. The role of IL-33 in allergic disease. **A.** Elevated mRNA levels of TSLP and IL-33 signaling molecules in conjunctiva of atopic patients compared with normal subjects by RT-qPCR. * $P<0.05$, **$P<0.01$, n=8. **B.** The mRNA levels of IL-33, ST2 and IL1RAP in corneal epithelium (Cornea), conjunctiva (Conj) and cervical lymph nodes (CLN) of in BALB/c mice with PBS-treated mice as controls. * $P<0.05$, n=3. **C.** Immunostaining images showing the stimulated IL-33 in ocular surface of EAC BALB/c mice with untreated mouse control and isotype IgG negative control.

7. Th17 pathway links innate and adaptive immunity

Th17 has been recently identified as a new T helper cell subset. CD4+ T helper (Th) cells now include three different types based on their cytokine signatures: interferon-γ (IFN-γ)-secreting Th1, IL-4, -5, and -13-secreting Th2 [75], and IL-17-producing Th17 cells [76]. Th17 cells have been recognized to be key effector T cells in a variety of human inflammatory and autoimmune diseases as well as experimental animal models [77, 78]. The IL-17 family includes 6 members (IL17A-F). IL-17A (also known as IL-17) and IL-17F are the founding members of the IL-17 cytokine family. The genes encoding IL-17A and IL-17F are localized in the same chromosomal region in mice and in humans. But IL-17F has significantly weaker biological activity than IL-17A [79, 80]. IL-17E, also known as IL-25, is produced by Th2 cells and mast cells. In contrast, IL-17B, IL-17C and IL-17D have not been well investigated [81, 82]. The receptor for IL-17A (IL-17R or IL-17RA) is a single-pass transmembrane protein of approximately 130 kDa. Four additional receptors (IL-17RB-RE) have been identified, but are not well characterized. IL-17RC was recently identified to be a receptor for IL-17F [83]. It has been reported that Th17 cells also produce IL-22 [84, 85] and CC-chemokine attractant ligand 20 (CCL20) [86] in mice and humans. Therefore, distinct from Th1 and Th2 cells, Th17 cells produce a unique and expanding array of pro-inflammatory cytokines.

Compelling evidence has demonstrated that the differentiation of Th17 cells from naïve CD4+ T cells is initiated by cytokines IL-6 or TGF-β, and expanded by cytokines IL-23, IL-1β and IL-21. IL-6 or TGF-β was proposed as a major initiator necessary for Th17 differentiation [87-89]. IL-23 was the first cytokine shown to selectively regulate IL-17 expression [90, 91], but it might not be required for the initial differentiation of Th17 cells in vivo [92]. Recently, IL-1β was found to promote Th17 cell development and proliferation in the presence of TGF-β and IL-6 [88]. IL-21, produced by activated T cells and natural killer (NK) cells [93], may be required for full commitment of Th17 cells [94, 95]. Hence IL-23, IL-1β and IL-21 may possibly maintain and expand the differentiated Th17 cells in the presence of IL-6 and TGF-β [88]. Furthermore, STAT3 has been found to mediate the initiation of Th17 cell differentiation by these inducing cytokines [87]. Activation of STAT3 induces the expression of retinoic-acid-receptor-related orphan receptor-α (RORα) and RORγt [96], two transcription factors that promote the Th17-cell-associated gene-expression program, leading to the production of IL-17, IL-17F, IL-22 and CCL20.

Using peripheral CD4+ T cell isolated from mouse spleen and cervical lymph nodes, our team evaluated the differential effects of these inducing cytokines in promoting Th17 differentiation [97]. The results showed that IL-6 and TGF-β1, only minimally induced IL-17 production at both mRNA and protein levels. In the presence of IL-6 and TGF-β1, IL-23 was the strongest stimulator of the Th17 signature cytokines IL-17A and IL-17F, IL-22, and chemokine CCL20, as well as STAT3 among the 3 expanding cytokines IL-23, IL-1β and IL-21. In the 4 cytokine system, IL-1β stimulated much higher levels of IL-17 family cytokines, 1.5-2 fold greater than IL-21 in the presence of TGF-β1, IL-6 and IL-23. These findings suggest that TGF-β1 and IL-6 initiate low level differentiation of Th17 cells; and their maintenance and development need other expanding factors, among which IL-23 plays a potent role and IL-1β amplifies this expansion further in Th17 differentiation [97].

A variety of mucosal epithelia have been found to produce Th17 inducing cytokines, including TGF-β1, IL-6, IL-23, and IL-1β [98, 99]. IL-1β is a well recognized proinflammatory cytokine produced by mucosal epithelia in response to stress, infection or wounding. In an attempt to mimic known stressors of the ocular surface, we measured production of Th17 inducing cytokines in cultured HCECs in response to hyperosmotic stress, microbial components and inflammatory cytokines.

The ocular surface epithelium is subjected to hyperosmotic stress in dry eye conditions. Exposure of human epithelial cells to hyperosmotic stress has been noted to activate mitogen-activated protein kinase pathways and stimulate production of pro-inflammatory cytokines, such as IL-1β, TNF-α, and IL-8 [100]. We have also observed that TGF-β1, IL-6 and IL-23 were highly induced in the corneal epithelium in response to hyperosmotic stress.

We evaluated the expression and production of Th17-inducing cytokines by HCECs in response to 9 extracted or synthetic microbial components that are ligands of TLRs 1-9, respectively. TGF-β1, IL-6, IL-23, and IL-1β expression and production were found to be largely induced by polyI: C, flagellin, and R837, the respective ligands for TLRs3, 5 and 7, representing viral or bacterial infections. Among these TLR agonists, polyI:C was the strongest stimulator of Th17 inducing cytokines by HCECs.

Hyperosmotic stress and microbial components also promoted production of pro-inflammatory cytokines including TNF-α, which plays an important role in ocular surface disease [100, 101]. Consequently, TNF-α stimulus was found to markedly induce TGF-β1, IL-6, IL-23, and IL-1β.

Based on our findings that among TLR ligands, polyI:C is the potent stimulator of Th17 inducing cytokines, and that TNF-α is a representative pro-inflammatory factor, we evaluated the Th17 inducing capacity of conditioned media (CM) of HCECs treated with polyI:C and TNF-α [97]. It has been observed that Th17 cell differentiation was significantly stimulated in CD4+ T cells exposed to the 50% conditioned media of HCECs challenged by polyI:C (CM-polyI:C) or TNF-α (CM-TNF-α) when compared with media from untreated cultures.

As shown in Figure 8A-E, the mRNA levels of IL-17A, IL-17F, IL-22, CCL-20 and STAT3 were significantly higher in CD4+ T cells treated with CM-polyI:C or CM-TNF-α for 4 days compared with the control medium or conditioned media of HCEC culture without any stressors (CM-Control, all $P<0.05$, n=3). IL-17 protein levels in the supernatants of CD4+ T cells exposed to CM-polyI:C or CM-TNF-α for 4 days (Figure 8F) were also significantly higher than the media (both $P<0.01$, n=3) and CM ($P<0.05$, n=3) controls. Furthermore, the number of IL-17-producing cells differentiated from CD4+ T cells, determined by ELISPOT bioassay (Figure 8G, 8H), displayed the same pattern to the induction of IL-17 mRNA and protein. The numbers of IL-17-producing cells were stimulated by CM-polyI:C or CM-TNF-α, to the levels similar to that seen in the 3-cytokine system (TGF-β1+IL-6+IL-23), suggesting that cytokines in the conditioned media of HCECs exposed to polyI:C or TNF-α were capable to promote Th17 cell expansion to levels induced by IL-6+TGF-β1+IL-23. It suggests that the Th17 cells can be indeed promoted by factors produced by corneal epithelium in response to a variety of inflammatory stimuli [97].

8. Th17-mediated inflammation in dry eye

Dry eye is the second most common problem of patients seeking eye care, and is characterized by eye irritation symptoms and blurred vision. The prevalence of dry eye

G. The number of IL-17-producing cells

Control   3 Cytokines   CM-Control   CM-PolyI:C   CM-TNF-α

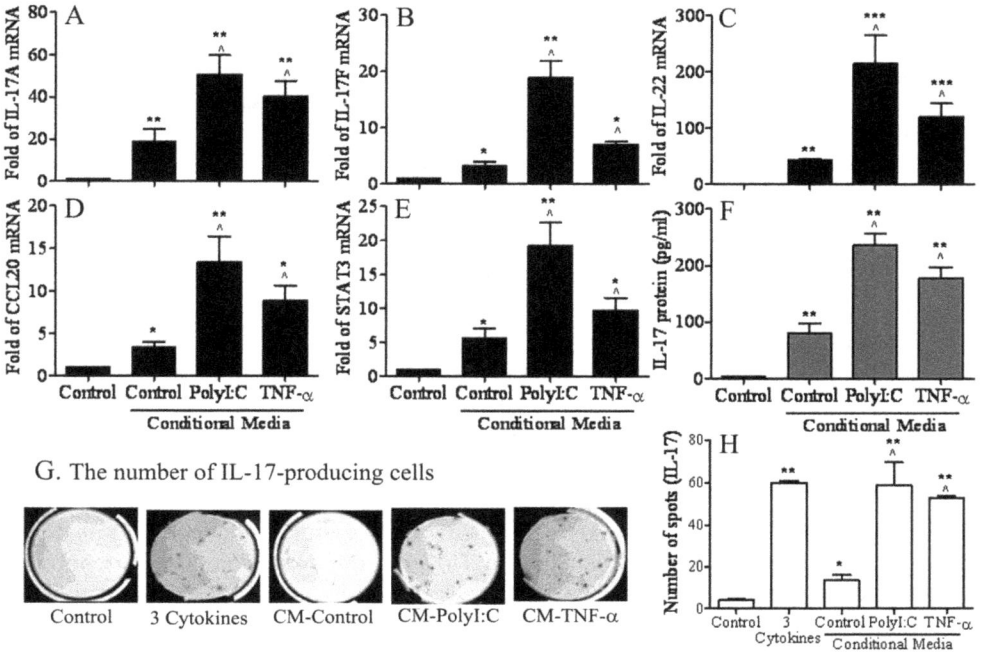

Fig. 8. Induction of Th17 differentiation of murine CD4+ T cells cultured in RPMI media containing 50% conditioned media (CM) of HCECs. **A-E.** Real-time PCR data showing the relative fold of mRNA of Th17 associated cytokines (IL-17A, IL-17F, IL-22, CCL-20) and regulator STAT3 in CD4+ T cells incubated for 4 days with 50% of conditioned media of HCECs irritated by polyI:C (CM-PolyI:C) or TNF-α (CM-TNF-α) for 48 hrs. **F.** Luminex immunobead assay showing IL-17 concentration in the supernatant of CD4+ T cells receiving the same treatment for 4 days. **G & H.** ELISPOT bioassay showing the spots/3x10^5 cells/well, representing the numbers of IL-17-producing T cells, in CD4+ T cells treated with CM-PolyI:C, CM-TNF-α, or 3 cytokines (TGF-β1+IL-6+IL-23) for 7 days. Results shown are mean ± SD of 3-5 independent experiments. *, $P < 0.05$; **, $P < 0.01$; ***, $P < 0.001$ each treated groups vs. media control. ^, $P < 0.05$; ^^, $P < 0.01$; ^^^, $P < 0.001$ CM-PolyI:C or CM-TNF-α groups vs. CM-control group.

increases with age, 6% at the age of 40, and 15-25% in the population over the age of 65. Among dry eye patients, 11% have been estimated to have the systemic autoimmune condition Sjögren's syndrome, a severe and potentially blinding condition. Dry eye is a potent stimulus of both innate and adaptive immune systems. At the nexus of the dry eye inflammatory/immune response is the dynamic interplay between the ocular surface epithelia and bone marrow derived immune cells. On the one hand, the ocular surface epithelial cells play a key initiating role in this inflammatory reaction, while on the other hand they are targets of cytokines that are produced by activated T cells that are recruited to the ocular surface in response to dry eye.

Dry eye has been demonstrated to cause inflammation of the ocular surface, evidenced by increased levels of inflammatory cytokines (IL-1, IL-6, and TNF-α) in the tear fluid, corneal and conjunctival epithelium, and an increased infiltration of dendritic cells and T lymphocytes in the conjunctiva [102-105]. Recently, increased levels of IL-17, IL-23 and IL-6 were found in saliva and salivary glands biopsies obtained from patients with the severe autoimmune dry eye condition, Sjögren's syndrome [106]. The increased matrix metalloproteinase (MMP) 9 and disrupted barrier function were observed in human [107] and murine dry eye [108]. Recently, our group has found increased expression of Th17 associated cytokines and IL-17-producing cells in human and experimental murine dry eye [108, 109]. Increased expression of Th17 cytokine IL-17A was observed in corneal and conjunctival epithelia of the dry eye mice. Since IL-17A is produced by T cells, not by epithelial cells, the Th17 reaction of the ocular surface is likely due to CD4+ T cells, which have previously been found to infiltrate ocular surface tissues following experimental desiccating stress [110, 111]. Antibody neutralization of IL-17 ameliorated experimental dry eye-induced corneal epithelial barrier dysfunction and decreased the expression of MMP-3 and -9 [108]. These findings provide clear evidence that changes in the ocular surface environment, such as Th17-inducing cytokines, following desiccating stress are capable of inducing Th17 differentiation [112], which plays an important role in dry eye disease.

Th17 differentiation was also found to be mediated through a dendritic cell-mediated pathway. DCs have an important function in Th17 cell differentiation. They are antigen-presenting cells specialized to activate CD4+ T cells and through their interaction with CD4+ T cells to initiate primary immune responses. Furthermore, when primed, certain DCs express a high-level of Th17 inducing cytokines, including IL-6, TGF-β, IL-23 and IL-1 [113].

We found that efficient differentiation of CD4+ T cells to IL-17 producers required the combination of ocular surface epithelium from dry eye mice and dendritic cells. CD4+ T cells that were co-cultured with ocular epithelial explants from desiccating stress-induced dry eye mice and dendritic cells were found to express increased mRNA levels of Th17 cytokines (IL-17A, IL-17F, IL-22) and chemokine (C-C motif) ligand 20 (CCL20) (Figure 9A), as well as to produce and release IL-17A (Figure 9B & 9D), but not Th1 cytokine IFN-γ (Figure 9C). Exposure of dendritic cells to conditioned media from ocular surface explants of dry eye mice did not sufficiently activate these cells to promote T cell differentiation. The possible explanations for these findings include the need for direct contact between these cells, more efficient activation of cytokines such as TGF-β1 produced by the ocular surface epithelial cells or insufficient concentrations of Th17 inducing factors in the explants conditioned media.

The transcription factor RORγt was identified as a candidate master regulator that drives Th17 cell lineage differentiation [96]. Expression of RORγt is induced by TGF-β or IL-6, and overexpression of γt was found to promote Th17-cell differentiation when both Th1- and Th2-cell differentiations were blocked. In a model of experimental autoimmune encephalomyelitis, mice with RORγt-deficient T cells were found to have attenuated autoimmune disease and lacked tissue-infiltrating Th17 cells [96]. We found robust up-regulation (up to 100 fold) of the level of Th17 cell transcription factor-RORγt in T cells co-cultured with desiccated ocular surface tissues and dendritic cells (Figure 9E). This provides further evidence of the potent Th17 prone environment induced by desiccation.

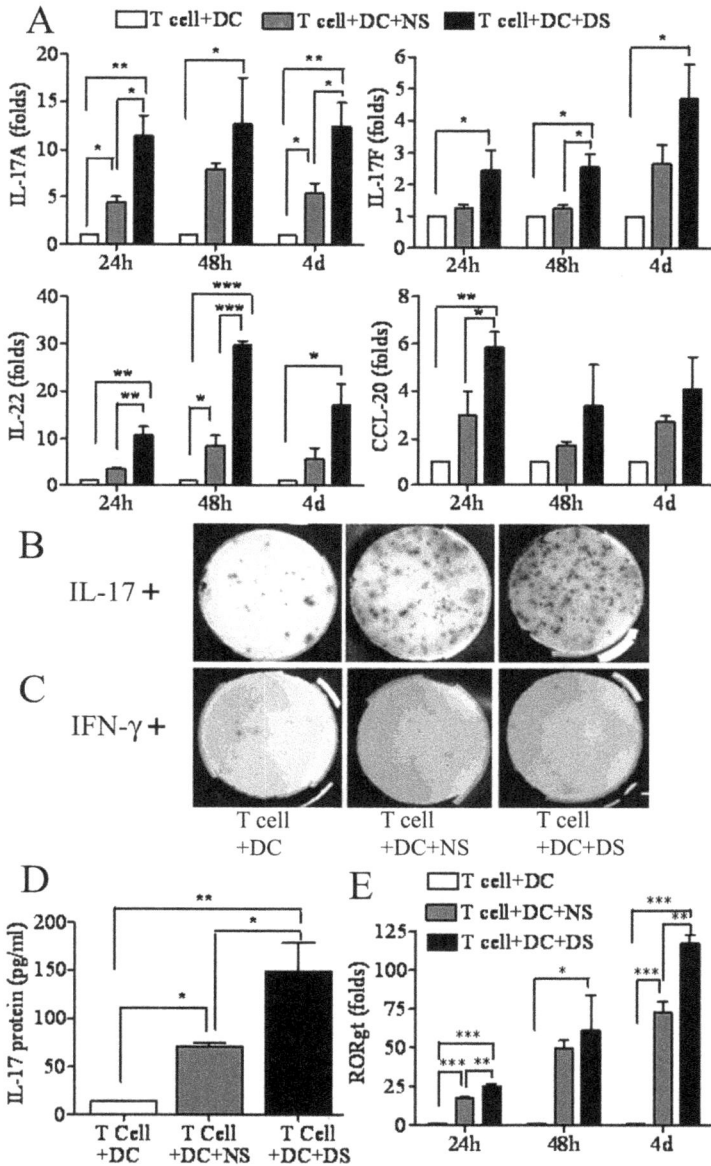

Fig. 9. Th17 differentiation of CD4+ T cells induced by the co-culture with dendritic cells (DCs) in the presence of cornea and conjunctival tissues of C57BL/6 mice subjected to desiccating stress. A. Real-time PCR data showing the relative mRNA expression (x-fold) of Th17 cytokines (IL-17A, IL-17F, IL-22, CCL-20) in CD4+ T cells (3×10^5 cells/ well) co-cultured for 1, 2, 4 days with DCs (T cell+DC), or with DCs and cornea and conjunctival explants from non-stressed control mice (T cell+DC+NS) or from mice desiccating stressed for 10-day (T

cell+DC+DS), (n=4). B & C. ELISPOT bioassay showing the numbers of IL-17 or IFN-γ-
producing cells in these 3 groups. D. IL-17 concentration in the supernatant of CD4+ T cells co-
cultured with DCs for 4 days in absence or presence of corneal and conjunctival explants from
non-stressed and 10 day desiccating stressed mice. E. Real-time PCR showing the relative
mRNA expression of RORγt in CD4+ T cells co-cultured for 1, 2, 4 days in 3 conditions. Data
are presented as mean ± SD of 3 or 4 independent experiments. *P<0.05, **P<0.01, ***P<0.001.

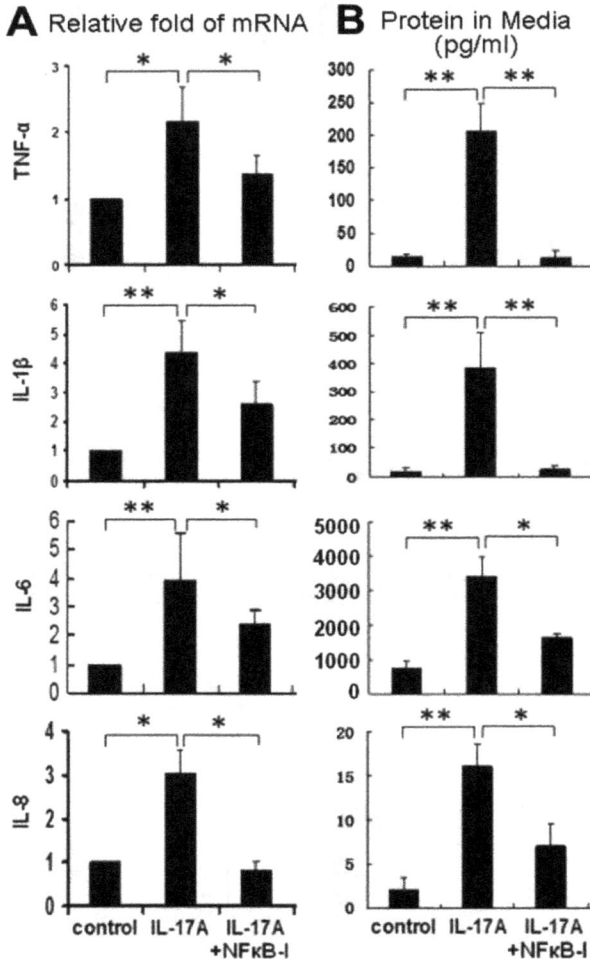

Fig. 10. The inflammatory effects of IL-17 on HCECs. Primary HCECs ($5×10^5$ cells/well)
were treated with recombinant human IL-17A at 10 ng/ml for 4-48 hours with or without
NF-κB activation inhibitor quinazoline (NFκB-I, 5μM). The pro-inflammatory cytokines
(TNF-α, IL-1β and IL-6) and chemokine IL-8 were measured by RT-qPCR for mRNA (**A**) and
by ELISA or Luminex immunobead assays in culture supernatants (**B**). Results shown are
mean ± SD of 4 independent experiments. * $P < 0.05$, ** $P< 0.01$.

IL-17 producing T cells are distinct from Th1 cells. Analysis of the expression of transcription factors showed clearly that IL-17-producing T cells expressed neither GATA-3 nor T-bet and its target Hlx, which were typically expressed by IFN-γ-producing Th1 cells [88]. In the T cells co-cultured with desiccated ocular surface tissues and dendritic cells, we observed the lower expression of Th1 associated factors (IL-2, T-bet) and Th2 associated factors (IL-4, IL-13, GATA-3). There was no change in production of IFN-γ and IL-12 transcripts as well as in the number of IFN-γ-producing $CD4^+T$ cells in this co-culture system. Taken together, these findings indicate that desiccating stress may selectively promote the Th17 pathway, a finding that is consistent with the increased level of IL-17 in dry eye disease [108].

IL-17 initiates pro-inflammatory effects by binding to the IL-17 receptor (IL-17R), which is expressed by a variety of cell types including epithelial, endothelial, and fibroblastic stromal cells [81, 114]. As shown in Figure 10, recombinant human IL-17A (10 ng/ml) significantly increased mRNA levels (2-4 fold) of proinflammatory cytokines (TNF-α, IL-1β and IL-6) and chemokine IL-8 expressed by HCECs. These stimulatory responses to IL-17A were confirmed by 4-7 fold increases at protein levels. The stimulated production of these inflammatory cytokines and chemokine was significantly suppressed at both mRNA (all $P<0.05$, n=4) and protein levels ($P<0.05$ or 0.01) by NF-κB activation inhibitor quinazoline [115], indicating NF-κB pathway is involved in the inflammatory effect of IL-17 on mucosal epithelium.

These findings demonstrate that desiccating stress stimulates the expression and production of Th17 inducing cytokines by corneal and conjunctival epithelia, and that desiccation creates an environment promoting Th17 differentiation through a dendritic cell-mediated pathway. We hypothesize that Th17 inducing cytokines produced by the ocular epithelium may participate in Th17 differentiation in three ways: (1) activation of immature dendritic cells on the ocular surface; (2) direct transfer to the lymph node in lymphatic liquid; or (3) direct promotion of differentiated Th17 cells that infiltrate the ocular surface.

9. Conclusion

This chapter focused on recent breakthroughs in ocular mucosal immunology, including the discoveries of TLR signaling in innate immunity, novel epithelium-derived pro-allergic cytokines TSLP and IL-33, and a new Th17 cell population in adaptive immunity. One of important breakthroughs is a discovery of a novel mechanism by which short ragweed pollen, serving as a functional TLR4 agonist, induces TSLP/OX40L/OX40 signaling to trigger Th2-dominant allergic inflammation via TLR4-dependent innate immunity pathways. All these advances provide compelling evidence that mucosal epithelium actively participate, as initiators, mediators and regulators, in innate and adaptive immune responses for host defense, in addition to physical barrier function. These novel signaling molecules may be critical for allergic, inflammatory and autoimmune diseases on mucosal ocular surface, and may become potential molecular targets for new therapies to treat these ocular diseases.

10. Abbreviations used in this chapter

CLN: cervical lymph nodes; **DAMP**: damage-associated molecular patterns; **DC**: dendritic cell; **dsRNA**: double stranded RNA; **EAC**: experimental allergic conjunctivitis; **HCECs**:

human corneal epithelial cells; **IL**: interleukin; **MyD88**: myeloid differentiation primary response gene 88; *MyD88-/-*: *MyD88* knockout mice; **LPS**: lipopolysaccharide; **NF-κB**: nuclear factor kappa B; **PBS**: phosphate buffered saline; **PGN**: peptidoglycan; **PAMP**: pathogen-associated molecular patterns; **PCR**: polymerase chain reaction; **polyI:C**: polyinosinic-polycytidylic acid; **PRR**: pattern recognition receptor; **R837**: imiquimod; **RT-qPCR**: reverse transcription and quantitative real-time PCR; **ROR**: retinoic-acid-receptor-related orphan receptor; **SRW**: short ragweed; **SRWe**: aqueous extract of defatted short ragweed pollen; **ssRNA**: single stranded RNA; **TGF-β**: transforming growth factor; **Th1**: T helper cell type 1; **Th17**: T helper cell producing IL-17 family; **Th2**: T helper cell type 2; **TLR**: Toll-like receptor; *Tlr4-d*: *Tlr4* gene deficient; **TRIF**: TIR-domain-containing adaptor inducing interferon; **TSLP**: thymic stromal lymphopoietin; **TSLPR**: TSLP receptor.

11. References

[1] Hoebe K, Janssen E, Beutler B. The interface between innate and adaptive immunity. *Nat Immunol*. 2004;5:971-974.

[2] Meyer T, Stockfleth E, Christophers E. Immune response profiles in human skin. *Br J Dermatol*. 2007;157 Suppl 2:1-7.

[3] Buchau AS, Gallo RL. Innate immunity and antimicrobial defense systems in psoriasis. *Clin Dermatol*. 2007;25:616-624.

[4] Wollenberg A, Klein E. Current aspects of innate and adaptive immunity in atopic dermatitis. *Clin Rev Allergy Immunol*. 2007;33:35-44.

[5] Kato A, Schleimer RP. Beyond inflammation: airway epithelial cells are at the interface of innate and adaptive immunity. *Curr Opin Immunol*. 2007;19:711-720.

[6] Mayer AK, Dalpke AH. Regulation of local immunity by airway epithelial cells. *Arch Immunol Ther Exp (Warsz)*. 2007;55:353-362.

[7] Schleimer RP, Kato A, Kern R, Kuperman D, Avila PC. Epithelium: at the interface of innate and adaptive immune responses. *J Allergy Clin Immunol*. 2007;120:1279-1284.

[8] Muller CA, Autenrieth IB, Peschel A. Innate defenses of the intestinal epithelial barrier. *Cell Mol Life Sci*. 2005;62:1297-1307.

[9] Ishihara S, Rumi MA, Ortega-Cava CF, Kazumori H, Kadowaki Y, Ishimura N, Kinoshita Y. Therapeutic targeting of toll-like receptors in gastrointestinal inflammation. *Curr Pharm Des*. 2006;12:4215-4228.

[10] Sharma R, Young C, Neu J. Molecular modulation of intestinal epithelial barrier: contribution of microbiota. *J Biomed Biotechnol*. 2010;2010:305879.

[11] Hazlett LD. Role of innate and adaptive immunity in the pathogenesis of keratitis. *Ocul Immunol Inflamm*. 2005;13:133-138.

[12] Kumar A, Yu FS. Toll-like receptors and corneal innate immunity. *Curr Mol Med*. 2006;6:327-337.

[13] Chang JH, McCluskey PJ, Wakefield D. Toll-like receptors in ocular immunity and the immunopathogenesis of inflammatory eye disease. *Br J Ophthalmol*. 2006;90:103-108.

[14] Akira S, Uematsu S, Takeuchi O. Pathogen recognition and innate immunity. *Cell*. 2006;124:783-801.

[15] Takeda K, Kaisho T, Akira S. Toll-like receptors. *Annu Rev Immunol*. 2003;21:335-376.

[16] Trinchieri G, Sher A. Cooperation of Toll-like receptor signals in innate immune defence. *Nat Rev Immunol*. 2007;7:179-190.

[17] Gay NJ, Gangloff M. Structure and function of Toll receptors and their ligands. *Annu Rev Biochem*. 2007;76:141-165.

[18] Vercammen E, Staal J, Beyaert R. Sensing of viral infection and activation of innate immunity by toll-like receptor 3. *Clin Microbiol Rev.* 2008;21:13-25.

[19] Liu J, Buckley JM, Redmond HP, Wang JH. ST2 negatively regulates TLR2 signaling, but is not required for bacterial lipoprotein-induced tolerance. *J Immunol.* 2010;184:5802-5808.

[20] Kawai T, Akira S. Signaling to NF-kappaB by Toll-like receptors. *Trends Mol Med.* 2007;13:460-469.

[21] Miller LS, Modlin RL. Toll-like receptors in the skin. *Semin Immunopathol.* 2007;29:15-26.

[22] Li DQ, Zhou N, Zhang L, Ma P, Pflugfelder SC. Suppressive effects of azithromycin on zymosan-induced production of proinflammatory mediators by human corneal epithelial cells. *Invest Ophthalmol Vis Sci.* 2010;51:5623-5629.

[23] Kumar A, Zhang J, Yu FS. Innate immune response of corneal epithelial cells to Staphylococcus aureus infection: role of peptidoglycan in stimulating proinflammatory cytokine secretion. *Invest Ophthalmol Vis Sci.* 2004;45:3513-3522.

[24] Huang X, Barrett RP, McClellan SA, Hazlett LD. Silencing Toll-like receptor-9 in Pseudomonas aeruginosa keratitis. *Invest Ophthalmol Vis Sci.* 2005;46:4209-4216.

[25] Kumar A, Zhang J, Yu FS. Toll-like receptor 3 agonist poly(I:C)-induced antiviral response in human corneal epithelial cells. *Immunology.* 2006;117:11-21.

[26] Ueta M, Hamuro J, Kiyono H, Kinoshita S. Triggering of TLR3 by polyI:C in human corneal epithelial cells to induce inflammatory cytokines. *Biochem Biophys Res Commun.* 2005;331:285-294.

[27] Liu YJ. Thymic stromal lymphopoietin and OX40 ligand pathway in the initiation of dendritic cell-mediated allergic inflammation. *J Allergy Clin Immunol.* 2007;120:238-244.

[28] Liu YJ, Soumelis V, Watanabe N, Ito T, Wang YH, Malefyt RW, Omori M, Zhou B, Ziegler SF. TSLP: an epithelial cell cytokine that regulates T cell differentiation by conditioning dendritic cell maturation. *Annu Rev Immunol.* 2007;25:193-219.

[29] Holgate ST. The epithelium takes centre stage in asthma and atopic dermatitis. *Trends Immunol.* 2007;28:248-251.

[30] Lee HC, Ziegler SF. Inducible expression of the proallergic cytokine thymic stromal lymphopoietin in airway epithelial cells is controlled by NFkappaB. *Proc Natl Acad Sci USA.* 2007;104:914-919.

[31] Demehri S, Morimoto M, Holtzman MJ, Kopan R. Skin-derived TSLP triggers progression from epidermal-barrier defects to asthma. *PLoS Biol.* 2009;7:e1000067.

[32] Zhang Z, Hener P, Frossard N, Kato S, Metzger D, Li M, Chambon P. Thymic stromal lymphopoietin overproduced by keratinocytes in mouse skin aggravates experimental asthma. *Proc Natl Acad Sci U S A.* 2009;106:1536-1541.

[33] Sims JE, Williams DE, Morrissey PJ, Garka K, Foxworthe D, Price V, Friend SL, Farr A, Bedell MA, Jenkins NA, Copeland NG, Grabstein K, Paxton RJ. Molecular cloning and biological characterization of a novel murine lymphoid growth factor. *J Exp Med.* 2000;192:671-680.

[34] Quentmeier H, Drexler HG, Fleckenstein D, Zaborski M, Armstrong A, Sims JE, Lyman SD. Cloning of human thymic stromal lymphopoietin (TSLP) and signaling mechanisms leading to proliferation. *Leukemia.* 2001;15:1286-1292.

[35] Reche PA, Soumelis V, Gorman DM, Clifford T, Liu M, Travis M, Zurawski SM, Johnston J, Liu YJ, Spits H, de Waal MR, Kastelein RA, Bazan JF. Human thymic stromal lymphopoietin preferentially stimulates myeloid cells. *J Immunol.* 2001;167:336-343.

[36] Soumelis V, Reche PA, Kanzler H, Yuan W, Edward G, Homey B, Gilliet M, Ho S, Antonenko S, Lauerma A, Smith K, Gorman D, Zurawski S, Abrams J, Menon S, McClanahan T, de Waal-Malefyt RR, Bazan F, Kastelein RA, Liu YJ. Human epithelial cells trigger dendritic cell mediated allergic inflammation by producing TSLP. *Nat Immunol.* 2002;3:673-680.

[37] Allakhverdi Z, Comeau MR, Jessup HK, Yoon BR, Brewer A, Chartier S, Paquette N, Ziegler SF, Sarfati M, Delespesse G. Thymic stromal lymphopoietin is released by human epithelial cells in response to microbes, trauma, or inflammation and potently activates mast cells. *J Exp Med.* 2007;204:253-258.

[38] Bogiatzi SI, Fernandez I, Bichet JC, Marloie-Provost MA, Volpe E, Sastre X, Soumelis V. Cutting Edge: Proinflammatory and Th2 cytokines synergize to induce thymic stromal lymphopoietin production by human skin keratinocytes. *J Immunol.* 2007;178:3373-3377.

[39] Kato A, Favoreto S Jr, Avila PC, Schleimer RP. TLR3- and Th2 cytokine-dependent production of thymic stromal lymphopoietin in human airway epithelial cells. *J Immunol.* 2007;179:1080-1087.

[40] Ma P, Bian F, Wang Z, Zheng X, Chotikavanich S, Pflugfelder SC, Li DQ. Human corneal epithelium-derived thymic stromal lymphopoietin links the innate and adaptive immune responses via TLRs and Th2 cytokines. *Invest Ophthalmol Vis Sci.* 2009;50:2702-2709.

[41] Mohan RR, Mohan RR, Kim WJ, Wilson SE. Modulation of TNF-alpha-induced apoptosis in corneal fibroblasts by transcription factor NF-kappaB. *Invest Ophthalmol Vis Sci.* 2000;41:1327-1336.

[42] Ozawa T, Koyama K, Ando T, Ohnuma Y, Hatsushika K, Ohba T, Sugiyama H, Hamada Y, Ogawa H, Okumura K, Nakao A. Thymic stromal lymphopoietin secretion of synovial fibroblasts is positively and negatively regulated by Toll-like receptors/nuclear factor-kappaB pathway and interferon-gamma/dexamethasone. *Mod Rheumatol.* 2007;17:459-463.

[43] Stern ME, Siemasko KF, Niederkorn JY. The Th1/Th2 paradigm in ocular allergy. *Curr Opin Allergy Clin Immunol.* 2005;5:446-450.

[44] Niederkorn JY. Immune regulatory mechanisms in allergic conjunctivitis: insights from mouse models. *Curr Opin Allergy Clin Immunol.* 2008;8:472-476.

[45] Buc M, Dzurilla M, Vrlik M, Bucova M. Immunopathogenesis of bronchial asthma. *Arch Immunol Ther Exp (Warsz).* 2009;57:331-344.

[46] Ying S, O'Connor B, Ratoff J, Meng Q, Fang C, Cousins D, Zhang G, Gu S, Gao Z, Shamji B, Edwards MJ, Lee TH, Corrigan CJ. Expression and cellular provenance of thymic stromal lymphopoietin and chemokines in patients with severe asthma and chronic obstructive pulmonary disease. *J Immunol.* 2008;181:2790-2798.

[47] Matsuda A, Ebihara N, Yokoi N, Kawasaki S, Tanioka H, Inatomi T, de Waal MR, Hamuro J, Kinoshita S, Murakami A. Functional role of thymic stromal lymphopoietin in chronic allergic keratoconjunctivitis. *Invest Ophthalmol Vis Sci.* 2010;51:151-155.

[48] Kay AB. Allergy and allergic diseases. First of two parts. *N Engl J Med.* 2001;344:30-37.

[49] Komine M. Analysis of the mechanism for the development of allergic skin inflammation and the application for its treatment:keratinocytes in atopic dermatitis - their pathogenic involvement. *J Pharmacol Sci.* 2009;110:260-264.

[50] Magone MT, Chan CC, Rizzo LV, Kozhich AT, Whitcup SM. A novel murine model of allergic conjunctivitis. *Clin Immunol Immunopathol.* 1998;87:75-84.

[51] Stern ME, Siemasko K, Gao J, Duong A, Beauregard C, Calder V, Niederkorn JY. Role of interferon-gamma in a mouse model of allergic conjunctivitis. *Invest Ophthalmol Vis Sci.* 2005;46:3239-3246.

[52] Zheng X, Ma P, de Paiva CS, Cunningham MA, Hwang CS, Pflugfelder SC, Li DQ. TSLP and downstream molecules in experimental mouse allergic conjunctivitis. *Invest Ophthalmol Vis Sci.* 2010;51:3076-3082.

[53] Le TA, Takai T, Vu AT, Kinoshita H, Chen X, Ikeda S, Ogawa H, Okumura K. Flagellin Induces the Expression of Thymic Stromal Lymphopoietin in Human Keratinocytes via Toll-Like Receptor 5. *Int Arch Allergy Immunol.* 2010;155:31-37.

[54] Kinoshita H, Takai T, Le TA, Kamijo S, Wang XL, Ushio H, Hara M, Kawasaki J, Vu AT, Ogawa T, Gunawan H, Ikeda S, Okumura K, Ogawa H. Cytokine milieu modulates release of thymic stromal lymphopoietin from human keratinocytes stimulated with double-stranded RNA. *J Allergy Clin Immunol.* 2009;123:179-186.

[55] Johnson AC, Heinzel FP, Diaconu E, Sun Y, Hise AG, Golenbock D, Lass JH, Pearlman E. Activation of toll-like receptor (TLR)2, TLR4, and TLR9 in the mammalian cornea induces MyD88-dependent corneal inflammation. *Invest Ophthalmol Vis Sci.* 2005;46:589-595.

[56] Piggott DA, Eisenbarth SC, Xu L, Constant SL, Huleatt JW, Herrick CA, Bottomly K. MyD88-dependent induction of allergic Th2 responses to intranasal antigen. *J Clin Invest.* 2005;115:459-467.

[57] Akira S, Hoshino K, Kaisho T. The role of Toll-like receptors and MyD88 in innate immune responses. *J Endotoxin Res.* 2000;6:383-387.

[58] Tsuji RF, Hoshino K, Noro Y, Tsuji NM, Kurokawa T, Masuda T, Akira S, Nowak B. Suppression of allergic reaction by lambda-carrageenan: toll-like receptor 4/MyD88-dependent and -independent modulation of immunity. *Clin Exp Allergy.* 2003;33:249-258.

[59] Fasciano S, Li L. Intervention of Toll-like receptor-mediated human innate immunity and inflammation by synthetic compounds and naturally occurring products. *Curr Med Chem.* 2006;13:1389-1395.

[60] Kawasaki K, Akashi S, Shimazu R, Yoshida T, Miyake K, Nishijima M. Mouse toll-like receptor 4.MD-2 complex mediates lipopolysaccharide-mimetic signal transduction by Taxol. *J Biol Chem.* 2000;275:2251-2254.

[61] Mishra KP, Ganju L, Chanda S, Karan D, Sawhney RC. Aqueous extract of Rhodiola imbricata rhizome stimulates Toll-like receptor 4, granzyme-B and Th1 cytokines in vitro. *Immunobiology.* 2009;214:27-31.

[62] Li D-Q, Zhang L, Pflugfelder SC, de Paiva CS, Zhang X, Zhao G, Zheng X, Su Z, Qu Y. Short ragweed pollen triggers allergic inflammation via TLR4-dependent TSLP/OX40L/OX40 signaling pathways. J Allergy Clin. Immunol. 2011;128: 1318-1325.e2

[63] Tominaga S. A putative protein of a growth specific cDNA from BALB/c-3T3 cells is highly similar to the extracellular portion of mouse interleukin 1 receptor. *FEBS Lett.* 1989;258:301-304.

[64] Kakkar R, Lee RT. The IL-33/ST2 pathway: therapeutic target and novel biomarker. *Nat Rev Drug Discov.* 2008;7:827-840.

[65] Eiwegger T, Akdis CA. IL-33 links tissue cells, dendritic cells and Th2 cell development in a mouse model of asthma. *Eur J Immunol.* 2011;41:1535-1538.

[66] Schmitz J, Owyang A, Oldham E, Song Y, Murphy E, McClanahan TK, Zurawski G, Moshrefi M, Qin J, Li X, Gorman DM, Bazan JF, Kastelein RA. IL-33, an interleukin-

1-like cytokine that signals via the IL-1 receptor-related protein ST2 and induces T helper type 2-associated cytokines. *Immunity.* 2005;23:479-490.

[67] Moussion C, Ortega N, Girard JP. The IL-1-like cytokine IL-33 is constitutively expressed in the nucleus of endothelial cells and epithelial cells in vivo: a novel 'alarmin'? *PLoS One.* 2008;3:e3331.

[68] Smith DE. IL-33: a tissue derived cytokine pathway involved in allergic inflammation and asthma. *Clin Exp Allergy.* 2009.

[69] Allam JP, Bieber T, Novak N. Dendritic cells as potential targets for mucosal immunotherapy. *Curr Opin Allergy Clin Immunol.* 2009;9:554-557.

[70] Zhang L, Lu R, Zhao G, Pflugfelder SC, Li DQ. TLR-mediated induction of pro-allergic cytokine IL-33 in ocular mucosal epithelium. *Int J Biochem Cell Biol.* 2011;43:1385-1391.

[71] Haraldsen G, Balogh J, Pollheimer J, Sponheim J, Kuchler AM. Interleukin-33 - cytokine of dual function or novel alarmin? *Trends Immunol.* 2009;30:227-233.

[72] Hayakawa M, Hayakawa H, Matsuyama Y, Tamemoto H, Okazaki H, Tominaga S. Mature interleukin-33 is produced by calpain-mediated cleavage in vivo. *Biochem Biophys Res Commun.* 2009;387:218-222.

[73] Talabot-Ayer D, Lamacchia C, Gabay C, Palmer G. Interleukin-33 is biologically active independently of caspase-1 cleavage. *J Biol Chem.* 2009;284:19420-19426.

[74] Krishnan J, Selvarajoo K, Tsuchiya M, Lee G, Choi S. Toll-like receptor signal transduction. *Exp Mol Med.* 2007;39:421-438.

[75] Mosmann TR, Coffman RL. TH1 and TH2 cells: different patterns of lymphokine secretion lead to different functional properties. *Annu Rev Immunol.* 1989;7:145-173.

[76] Dong C. Diversification of T-helper-cell lineages: finding the family root of IL-17-producing cells. *Nat Rev Immunol.* 2006;6:329-333.

[77] Komiyama Y, Nakae S, Matsuki T, Nambu A, Ishigame H, Kakuta S, Sudo K, Iwakura Y. IL-17 plays an important role in the development of experimental autoimmune encephalomyelitis. *J Immunol.* 2006;177:566-573.

[78] Hwang SY, Kim HY. Expression of IL-17 homologs and their receptors in the synovial cells of rheumatoid arthritis patients. *Mol Cells.* 2005;19:180-184.

[79] Chang SH, Dong C. A novel heterodimeric cytokine consisting of IL-17 and IL-17F regulates inflammatory responses. *Cell Res.* 2007;17:435-440.

[80] Williams IR. CCR6 and CCL20: partners in intestinal immunity and lymphorganogenesis. *Ann N Y Acad Sci.* 2006;1072:52-61.

[81] Moseley TA, Haudenschild DR, Rose L, Reddi AH. Interleukin-17 family and IL-17 receptors. *Cytokine Growth Factor Rev.* 2003;14:155-174.

[82] Gaffen SL, Kramer JM, Yu JJ, Shen F. The IL-17 cytokine family. *Vitam Horm.* 2006;74:255-282.

[83] Kuestner RE, Taft DW, Haran A, Brandt CS, Brender T, Lum K, Harder B, Okada S, Ostrander CD, Kreindler JL, Aujla SJ, Reardon B, Moore M, Shea P, Schreckhise R, Bukowski TR, Presnell S, Guerra-Lewis P, Parrish-Novak J, Ellsworth JL, Jaspers S, Lewis KE, Appleby M, Kolls JK, Rixon M, West JW, Gao Z, Levin SD. Identification of the IL-17 receptor related molecule IL-17RC as the receptor for IL-17F. *J Immunol.* 2007;179:5462-5473.

[84] Liang SC, Tan XY, Luxenberg DP, Karim R, Dunussi-Joannopoulos K, Collins M, Fouser LA. Interleukin (IL)-22 and IL-17 are coexpressed by Th17 cells and cooperatively enhance expression of antimicrobial peptides. *J Exp Med.* 2006;203:2271-2279.

[85] Zheng Y, Danilenko DM, Valdez P, Kasman I, Eastham-Anderson J, Wu J, Ouyang W. Interleukin-22, a T(H)17 cytokine, mediates IL-23-induced dermal inflammation and acanthosis. *Nature.* 2007;445:648-651.

[86] Hirota K, Yoshitomi H, Hashimoto M, Maeda S, Teradaira S, Sugimoto N, Yamaguchi T, Nomura T, Ito H, Nakamura T, Sakaguchi N, Sakaguchi S. Preferential recruitment of CCR6-expressing Th17 cells to inflamed joints via CCL20 in rheumatoid arthritis and its animal model. *J Exp Med.* 2007;204:2803-2812.

[87] Yang XO, Panopoulos AD, Nurieva R, Chang SH, Wang D, Watowich SS, Dong C. STAT3 regulates cytokine-mediated generation of inflammatory helper T cells. *J Biol Chem.* 2007;282:9358-9363.

[88] Veldhoen M, Hocking RJ, Atkins CJ, Locksley RM, Stockinger B. TGFbeta in the context of an inflammatory cytokine milieu supports de novo differentiation of IL-17-producing T cells. *Immunity.* 2006;24:179-189.

[89] Mangan PR, Harrington LE, O'Quinn DB, Helms WS, Bullard DC, Elson CO, Hatton RD, Wahl SM, Schoeb TR, Weaver CT. Transforming growth factor-beta induces development of the T(H)17 lineage. *Nature.* 2006;441:231-234.

[90] Murphy CA, Langrish CL, Chen Y, Blumenschein W, McClanahan T, Kastelein RA, Sedgwick JD, Cua DJ. Divergent pro- and antiinflammatory roles for IL-23 and IL-12 in joint autoimmune inflammation. *J Exp Med.* 2003;198:1951-1957.

[91] Zhou L, Ivanov II, Spolski R, Min R, Shenderov K, Egawa T, Levy DE, Leonard WJ, Littman DR. IL-6 programs T(H)-17 cell differentiation by promoting sequential engagement of the IL-21 and IL-23 pathways. *Nat Immunol.* 2007;8:967-974.

[92] Langrish CL, Chen Y, Blumenschein WM, Mattson J, Basham B, Sedgwick JD, McClanahan T, Kastelein RA, Cua DJ. IL-23 drives a pathogenic T cell population that induces autoimmune inflammation. *J Exp Med.* 2005;201:233-240.

[93] Leonard WJ, Spolski R. Interleukin-21: a modulator of lymphoid proliferation, apoptosis and differentiation. *Nat Rev Immunol.* 2005;5:688-698.

[94] Korn T, Bettelli E, Gao W, Awasthi A, Jager A, Strom TB, Oukka M, Kuchroo VK. IL-21 initiates an alternative pathway to induce proinflammatory T(H)17 cells. *Nature.* 2007;448:484-487.

[95] Nurieva R, Yang XO, Martinez G, Zhang Y, Panopoulos AD, Ma L, Schluns K, Tian Q, Watowich SS, Jetten AM, Dong C. Essential autocrine regulation by IL-21 in the generation of inflammatory T cells. *Nature.* 2007;448:480-483.

[96] Ivanov II, McKenzie BS, Zhou L, Tadokoro CE, Lepelley A, Lafaille JJ, Cua DJ, Littman DR. The orphan nuclear receptor RORgammat directs the differentiation program of proinflammatory IL-17+ T helper cells. *Cell.* 2006;126:1121-1133.

[97] Zheng X, Bian F, Ma P, de Paiva CS, Stern M, Pflugfelder SC, Li DQ. Induction of Th17 differentiation by corneal epithelial-derived cytokines. *J Cell Physiol.* 2010;222:95-102.

[98] Aujla SJ, Dubin PJ, Kolls JK. Th17 cells and mucosal host defense. *Semin Immunol.* 2007;19:377-382.

[99] Holtta V, Klemetti P, Sipponen T, Westerholm-Ormio M, Kociubinski G, Salo H, Rasanen L, Kolho KL, Farkkila M, Savilahti E, Vaarala O. IL-23/IL-17 immunity as a hallmark of Crohn's disease. *Inflamm Bowel Dis.* 2008;14:1175-1184.

[100] Li D-Q, Luo L, Chen Z, Kim HS, Song XJ, Pflugfelder SC. JNK and ERK MAP kinases mediate induction of IL-1beta, TNF-alpha and IL-8 following hyperosmolar stress in human limbal epithelial cells. *Exp Eye Res.* 2006;82:588-596.

[101] Barton K, Monroy DC, Nava A, Pflugfelder SC. Inflammatory cytokines in the tears of patients with ocular rosacea. *Ophthalmology.* 1997;104:1868-1874.

[102] Corrales RM, Villarreal A, Farley W, Stern ME, Li DQ, Pflugfelder SC. Strain-related cytokine profiles on the murine ocular surface in response to desiccating stress. *Cornea.* 2007;26:579-584.

[103] Turner K, Pflugfelder SC, Ji Z, Feuer WJ, Stern M, Reis BL. Interleukin-6 levels in the conjunctival epithelium of patients with dry eye disease treated with cyclosporine ophthalmic emulsion. *Cornea.* 2000;19:492-496.

[104] Solomon A, Dursun D, Liu Z, Xie Y, Macri A, Pflugfelder SC. Pro- and anti-inflammatory forms of interleukin-1 in the tear fluid and conjunctiva of patients with dry-eye disease. *Invest Ophthalmol Vis Sci.* 2001;42:2283-2292.

[105] Pflugfelder SC, de Paiva CS, Li DQ, Stern ME. Epithelial-immune cell interaction in dry eye. *Cornea.* 2008;27 Suppl 1:S9-11.

[106] Nguyen CQ, Hu MH, Li Y, Stewart C, Peck AB. Salivary gland tissue expression of interleukin-23 and interleukin-17 in Sjogren's syndrome: findings in humans and mice. *Arthritis Rheum.* 2008;58:734-743.

[107] Chotikavanich S, de Paiva CS, Li DQ, Chen JJ, Bian F, Farley WJ, Pflugfelder SC. Production and Activity of Matrix Metalloproteinase-9 on the Ocular Surface Increase in Dysfunctional Tear Syndrome. *Invest Ophthalmol Vis Sci.* 2009; 50:3203-3209.

[108] de Paiva CS, Chotikavanich S, Pangelinan SB, Pitcher JD, III, Fang B, Zheng X, Ma P, Farley WJ, Siemasko KF, Niederkorn JY, Stern ME, Li DQ, Pflugfelder SC. IL-17 disrupts corneal barrier following desiccating stress. *Mucosal Immunol.* 2009;2:243-253.

[109] Chauhan SK, El AJ, Ecoiffier T, Goyal S, Zhang Q, Saban DR, Dana R. Autoimmunity in dry eye is due to resistance of Th17 to Treg suppression. *J Immunol.* 2009;182:1247-1252.

[110] de Paiva CS, Villarreal AL, Corrales RM, Rahman HT, Chang VY, Farley WJ, Stern ME, Niederkorn JY, Li DQ, Pflugfelder SC. Dry eye-induced conjunctival epithelial squamous metaplasia is modulated by interferon-gamma. *Invest Ophthalmol Vis Sci.* 2007;48:2553-2560.

[111] Stern ME, Siemasko KF, Gao J, Calonge M, Niederkorn JY, Pflugfelder SC. Evaluation of ocular surface inflammation in the presence of dry eye and allergic conjunctival disease. *Ocul Surf.* 2005;3:S161-S164.

[112] Zheng X, de Paiva CS, Li DQ, Farley WJ, Pflugfelder SC. Desiccating stress promotion of Th17 differentiation by ocular surface tissues through a dendritic cell-mediated pathway. *Invest Ophthalmol Vis Sci.* 2010;51:3083-3091.

[113] Shainheit MG, Smith PM, Bazzone LE, Wang AC, Rutitzky LI, Stadecker MJ. Dendritic cell IL-23 and IL-1 production in response to schistosome eggs induces Th17 cells in a mouse strain prone to severe immunopathology. *J Immunol.* 2008;181:8559-8567.

[114] Molesworth-Kenyon SJ, Yin R, Oakes JE, Lausch RN. IL-17 receptor signaling influences virus-induced corneal inflammation. *J Leukoc Biol.* 2008;83:401-408.

[115] Bian F, Qi H, Ma P, Zhang L, Yoon KC, Pflugfelder SC, Li DQ. An immunoprotective privilege of corneal epithelial stem cells against Th17 inflammatory stress by producing glial cell-derived neurotrophic factor. *Stem Cells.* 2010;28:2172-2181.

7

Keratoconus Layer by Layer –
Pathology and Matrix Metalloproteinases

Dasha Nelidova and Trevor Sherwin
Department of Ophthalmology, Faculty of Medical and Health Sciences,
University of Auckland, Auckland
New Zealand

1. Introduction

Keratoconus is an ectatic disease in which the cornea develops a conical shape due to thinning of the collagenous corneal stroma. Characteristic morphological features seen on slit lamp examination are well described. This overview describes the recent advances in our understanding of keratoconic pathology, focussing particularly on the matrix metalloproteinase hypothesis of keratoconus disease progression.

2. The diversity and complexity of keratoconus

Keratoconus is a corneal ectatic disease where the cornea assumes a conical shape due to thinning of the corneal stroma, inducing irregular astigmatism and myopia and leading to marked impairment of vision[1]. Keratoconus typically starts at puberty and progresses until the third or fourth decade of life; alternatively it may commence later and arrest at any age. This disease is associated with several conditions, particularly those which encourage eye rubbing.

The mechanism of disease progression has long been the subject of intense research; however, research is complicated by the large degree of variation in clinical features between patients. *Forme fruste* or sub-clinical forms of the disease, likely contribute to the differences in reported incidence are estimated to occur between 50 and 230 per 100,000 of the general population[1]. There are also significant geographical variations. New Zealand, for example, has an unusually high prevalence of keratoconus. 50% of corneal transplants performed in New Zealand are due to this debilitating disease, compared with 30% in Australia[2] and 20% in the UK[3].

3. Clinical signs of keratoconus

The first adequate description of keratoconus, setting it aside from other ectatic conditions, was advanced by Nottingham in 1854 in his treatise 'Practical observations on conical cornea: and on the short sight, and other defects of vision connected with it'[4].

In 1943 Berliner[5] listed the seven distinct features of keratoconus as classified by Von der Heydt and Appelbaum:

1. Thinning of the cornea at the apex of the cone
2. Reflex from the endothelial cup
3. Striae
4. Irregular superficial opacities or scars
5. Ruptures in Descemet's membrane
6. Increased visibility of the nerve fibres and
7. Fleischer's ring.

These morphological features became incorporated by Duke-Elder[6] into the 1965 text 'System of Ophthalmology', which went on to describe keratoconus as a disease which can be recognised by:

1. A thinning of the cornea at the apex of the cone from one half to one fifth of its normal dimensions
2. An endothelial reflex in the central portion of the cornea at the peak of the cone
3. Vertical lines in the deeper layers of the stroma
4. An increased visibility of the nerve fibres which form a network of grey lines interspersed with small dots
5. Fleischer's ring, a line running round the base of the cone
6. Ruptures of Descemet's membrane of characteristic appearance
7. Ruptures in Bowman's membrane in advanced cases producing superficial linear scars.

Rabinowitz[1] lists the following clinical signs which may be present individually or in combination in moderate to advanced keratoconus:

'Stromal thinning (centrally or paracentrally, most commonly inferiorly or inferotemporally); conical protrusion; an iron line partially or completely surrounding the cone (Fleischer's ring); and fine vertical lines in the deep stroma and Descemet's membrane (Vogt's striae)... Other accompanying signs might include epithelial nebulae, anterior stromal scars, enlarged corneal nerves and increased intensity of the corneal endothelial reflex and subepithelial fibrillary lines.'

Since then advances in corneal topographical assessment have greatly aided the diagnosis of early disease. Prior to topography, forme fruste keratoconus was harder to recognise as patients do not necessarily have symptoms or observable clinical signs in these early stages.

4. Antero-posterior review of morphological changes in keratoconus

Pathological and histopathological abnormalities have been documented in every layer of the keratoconic cornea and this has previously been reviewed by our laboratory[7]. The following represents a layer by layer summary of keratoconic morphological variations reported.

4.1 Epithelium

Ex vivo histological analysis of keratoconic corneas has demonstrated significant thinning of the central epithelium[8]. Central epithelial thinning was significantly greater in those corneas which also had breaks in the Bowman's layer, however, the authors thought it likely that differences in the integrity of Bowman's layer could nevertheless be considered to be manifestations of the same disease process. Subsequent studies report thickened epithelia in keratoconus[9,10] or else no difference in epithelial thickness between keratoconus and normal controls[11].

In vivo confocal microscopy studies of the epithelium demonstrate morphological alterations in the area of the keratoconic corneal apex. Elongated superficial epithelial cells, arranged in a whorl-like fashion, can be observed. Near Bowman's membrane highly reflective changes and fold-like structures are visible[12]. These *in vivo* pathological features may well reflect the oedematous disruptions of basal epithelial integrity in keratoconus.

Apoptotic changes have also been detected in epithelia of keratoconic samples. TUNEL positive epithelial cells were confined to the superficial epithelium of normal corneas while extending further down in keratoconic corneas[9].This is supported by the work which reported that intense TUNEL labelling was present in the basal epithelia of fifteen out of sixteen keratoconic corneas examined[13].

The keratoconic basement membrane assumes an irregular appearance and breaks in places[14]. It also undergoes a change in composition[15,16] that cannot be explained by scarring alone. Laminin-1 and laminin-5 staining was shown to be irregular and thickened at defect sites, however monoclonal antibodies against the $\alpha2$ and $\beta2$ chains did not react[15]. Type IV collagen $\alpha1$ and $\alpha2$ reactivity was also only found in the defect regions of keratoconic or scarred corneas[15]. Immunostaining for type VII collagen was patchily localised to the basement membrane defects[15]. Integrin $\beta4$ staining which was positive in the basement membrane and the lateral and apical cell membranes of the epithelial cells, was found to be discontinuous in keratoconic corneas[15]. It has been suggested that a process similar to wound healing might account for such differences in structure. Basement membrane alterations may affect critical interactions of the corneal epithelium with the underlying basement membrane, as well as cell-matrix interactions and matrix organization in the stroma[16].

4.2 Nerve fibres

Increased visibility of nerve fibres by slit lamp biomicroscopy has been demonstrated in keratoconus. Corneal nerves pass between the stroma and epithelium at sites of early degradative change[17]. Keratocytes wrap around the nerves as they pass through an otherwise acellular Bowman's layer[17]. Localised nerve thickenings develop in the epithelium and stress epithelial architecture[17].

4.3 Bowman's layer

Scanning electron microscopy has found defects and ruptures in Bowman's layer to varying degrees in all keratoconic corneas examined[18]. Discontinuities in Bowman's layer are sometimes accompanied by distortion of the stroma beneath the defect[15] or alternatively, direct contact between epithelial and stromal cells[19]. Rather than being seen throughout the affected cornea, such abnormalities of the extracellular matrix are usually confined to several loci, suggesting a localised focus of disease progression.

4.4 Stroma – Collagen lamellae and keratocytes

The thickness of collagen lamellae in keratoconus is unaltered, but the number of lamellae appears to be significantly reduced compared to normal tissue[20]. There is no difference in interfibrillar spacing between keratoconus and control corneas, conclusively demonstrating that stromal thinning in keratoconus is not due to closer packing of the fibrils in the stroma.

There is some evidence for a progressive loss of lamellae from the stroma, for example, a reduction in the volume of proteoglycan along the collagen fibrils has been found in keratoconus[21]. Low angle x-ray scattering has shown that the orientation of collagen fibrils within lamellae is also altered in the disease[22]. It is likely that these changes reflect the presence of a degradative process or alternatively, insufficient repair mechanisms. Biochemical analyses of stromal matrix components are inconclusive: Critchfield and co-workers[23] described decreased collagen and total protein levels in keratoconic tissue by western blotting. Radda et al.[24] found a 5% increase in type I collagen in keratoconus; while Zimmermann et al.[25] found no differences in collagen composition.

Keratoconus is also associated with changes in keratocyte morphology as well as loss of keratocyte density[11, 12]. Keratocytes may be lost though apoptosis[9,13], however, as apoptosis was not seen in all keratoconic samples analysed it was proposed that such cells might not be detected if at the time of analysis the tissue was in a period of keratoconic remission. An alternative explanation suggests that because keratoconus is diagnosed on the basis of clinical findings, there may be several diseases with differing pathophysiological mechanisms that produce the phenotypic change that is referred to as keratoconus.

Keratocyte density was lowest in the anterior-most part of the stroma[12]. Whilst there may be a significant decrease in the density of keratocytes in the stroma immediately underneath Bowmans' membrane, the remaining keratocytes are far from quiet. Such keratocytes and their pseudopodia are oriented apically towards the overlying epithelium and their activated state is reflected by the abundance of rough endoplasmic reticulum within the cells[26].

Studies of the peripheral keratoconic cornea also show discrete incursions of fine keratocytic processes into Bowman's membrane[10]. These processes were often observed in conjunction with posterior collapse of epithelial cells into the Bowman's layer[10].

4.5 Descemet's membrane

Ruptures and folds in Descemet's membrane are common in keratoconus[14]. The origin of these ruptures is unclear as several studies of extracellular matrix proteins have revealed no differences in the levels of collagens, laminin, entactin or perlecan between keratoconus and normal tissue[19,25.] The appearance of the defects in Descemet's membrane may well be associated with environmental factors such as eye rubbing and may lead to the development of hydrops[1].

4.6 Endothelium

The endothelium may be normal in keratoconus or may demonstrate intracellular dark structures, pleomorphisms or elongation of cells[1]. Scanning slit confocal microscopy and ultrasound biomicroscopy in living patients with keratoconus revealed central detachment of Descemet's membrane and endothelium from the posterior part of the stroma[27]. Ruptures in Descemet's membrane may directly lead to endothelial cell loss by triggering cell membrane perforation, loss of cell contents and edema[28]. Alternatively apoptosis may account for decreased endothelial cell density[13].

4.7 Evidence from recurrence of keratoconus

The recurrences of keratoconus in patients after penetrating keratoplasty[29] suggest either a recurrence of the host disease in the graft or else represent transmission of undiagnosed keratoconus from the donor cornea[30]. Histological examination of corneal buttons from patients undergoing repeated penetrating keratoplasty revealed structural changes compatible with a diagnosis of keratoconus in all the examined corneas[31]. Recurrence of keratoconus characteristics may be attributed to graft repopulation by the recipient cells, ageing of the grafted tissue, or both. However a recent study from our own laboratory failed to find evidence of recurrence of keratoconus in patients undergoing regraft surgery[32].

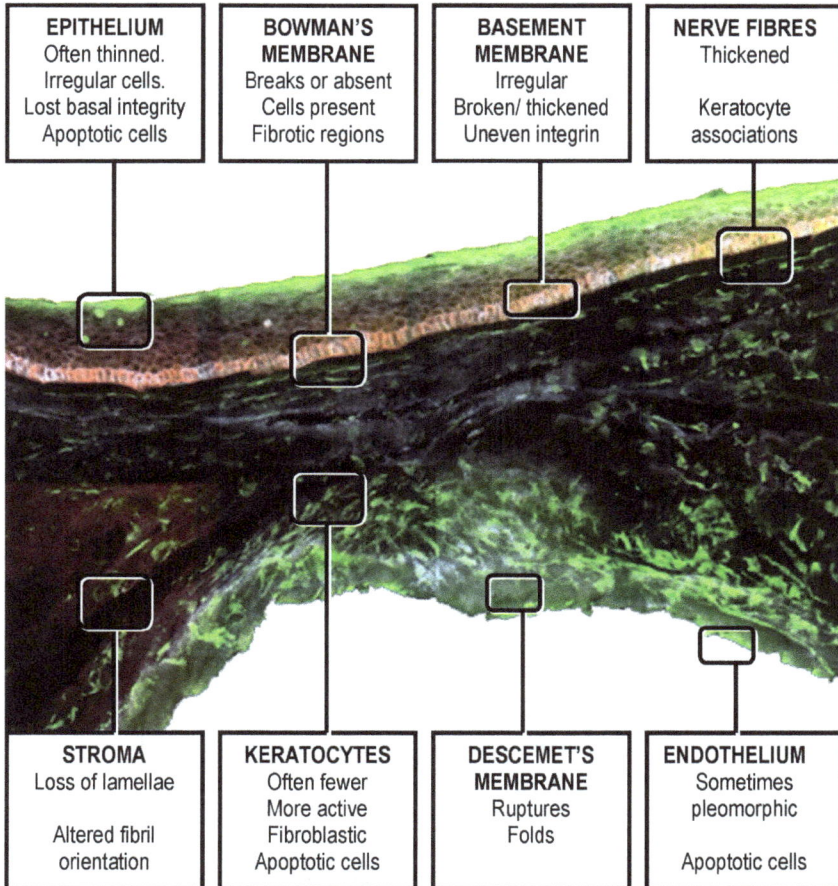

Fig. 1. A diverse range of morphological changes have been described in every layer of the keratoconic cornea. An antero-posterior section of a keratoconic cornea labelled with CellTracker green to highlight cellular morphology and integrin α3β1 labelling the basal epithelium in red helps to summarise characteristic histopathological abnormalities by corneal layer.
Figure reproduced by permission from Wiley-Blackwells[7]

5. Pathology to pathogenesis

The diversity of pathologies described for keratoconus are likely to represent temporal differences in the progression of the disease, positional differences relative to the apical centre of maximum damage and reflect a variety of pathophysiological diseases which make up the clinical pigeonhole of keratoconus.

Matrix metalloproteinases (MMPs) have long been suspected of mediating the pathological progression of keratoconus. The cornea is 70% collagen by weight and the reduced collagen content of the keratoconic cornea suggests a degraded extracellular matrix[23]. Extracellular matrix breakdown is, however, only a small component of the MMP repertoire of activity. Nevertheless, this function is essential for normal remodeling, leading to the constitutive expression of MMPs in healthy tissues.

Various models emphasise the role of MMPs in disease, for example, as mediators of connective tissue destruction in arthritis[33]. Consistent with such an involvement is the MMP hypothesis of keratoconus which proposes that MMPs are over-expressed in the disease while MMP inhibitors may be down-regulated, shifting the balance towards excessive tissue destruction. Over the last decade many studies have set out to measure the levels of MMPs and their inhibitors by a variety of techniques yet over-expression of MMPs or presence of active forms has not been found consistently[34].

It is important to consider that the relative balance between various MMPs could be more significant than absolute concentrations. This is relevant given that MMPs often undergo intermolecular interactions with each other to achieve activation from the latent form or to target MMP action to a particular site such as the cell surface. Paradoxically, tissue inhibitors of matrix metalloproteinases (TIMPs) can associate with pro form MMPs to trigger proteolytic activity[33]. Tissue degradation in thinning disorders, such as keratoconus, also involves the expression of inflammatory mediators, including proinflammatory cytokines and cell adhesion molecules[35], which modulate MMP activity and are themselves modulated by it.

The MMP family includes more than 25 members that make up five families based on their substrate preference: collagenases (MMP-1, MMP-8, and MMP-13), stromelysins (MMP-3, MMP-10), matrilysins (MMP-7, MMP-26), gelatinases (MMP-2, MMP-9), membrane type MMPs (MPP-14 to MMP-17, MMP-24) and others[36]. Most are synthesised by resident cells, some are brought in by invading leukocytes. Specific MMPs appear in specific locations within the cornea[36], likely due to cellular and soluble factors particular to the layer.

MMP changes have been described in every layer of the cornea in keratoconus. The following is a layer by layer summary of MMP changes reported within the last 15 years.

5.1 Tear film and increased MMP-9

Tear film composition reflects ocular surface events and tears may therefore be considered a vehicle for some of the pathogenic protagonists of keratoconus. Unfortunately, the cellular origin of any such molecules cannot be determined conclusively as both corneal and non-corneal secretions will be represented in the tear fluid.

In 2000 the presence of collagen degradation products was reported in the tears of patients with keratoconus[37]. The detected telopeptides were presumed to be of corneal origin but the authors conceded that serum and conjunctiva were also potential sources. The conjunctival epithelium is indeed altered in keratoconus. Elevation of lysosomal enzyme levels has been found in corneal and conjunctival epithelium[38] though such enzymes are mostly involved with lipid metabolism, rather than turnover of proteins or connective tissues. Lipids, however, are crucial to the integrity of the tear film and indeed, chronic ocular desiccation and aqueous tear deficiency can produce inferior corneal steepening and high astigmatism resembling keratoconus[39].

More recently, the levels of interleukin-6 (IL-6), tumour nectosis factor-α (TNF-α), and MMP-9 in the tear fluid of keratoconic patients were measured by enzyme linked immunoadsorbent assay and were found to be significantly higher than in normal subjects[40]. Increases in the levels of these molecules may be intermittent, but sufficient to provoke slowly progressive ectasia[40]. No significant differences in the concentrations of adhesion molecules inter cellular adhesion molecule-1 (ICAM-1) and vascular cell adhesion protein-1 (VCAM-1) were detected and other proteinases were not measured[40].

In most cases, keratoconus initially affects only one eye and later the ectasia may progress to include both eyes. Lema et al. followed up their initial work by measuring the concentrations of IL-6, TNF-α and MMP-9 in thirty patients with unilateral keratoconus - one eye diagnosed with keratoconus and the other eye having subclinical disease. IL-6 and TNF-α levels were found to be raised in both eyes in patients with asymmetric keratoconus, however, only TNF-α was significantly higher in the keratoconic eye, with respect to the subclinical one. Increased MMP-9 levels were found in keratoconic eyes only[35].

TNF-α has been shown to upregulate MMP-9 expression in human corneal epithelial cells[41] and such proinflammatory cytokines are present at the ocular surface even in the absence of inflammation[42]. Interestingly, increased concentrations of cytokines are found in tears from various ocular allergic disease states[43]. While atopy is associated with keratoconus[44], multivariate analysis has shown that the contribution to pathogenesis likely occurs from the eye rubbing encouraged by the itch of atopy rather than from chemical mediators associated with atopy itself[45].

The keratoconic ocular surface is characterised by a disorder of tear quality, decreased corneal sensitivity, conjunctival squamous metaplasia and higher fluorescein and rose bengal staining scores, all of which seem to relate to the extent of keratoconus progression[46]. In that respect the ocular surface is not unlike that of dry eye. It has been shown that inflammation plays an important role in both of these conditions and MMP-9 is found in the tears of both[40,47].

In fact MMP-9 accumulation has been demonstrated in several other disorders with an inflammatory basis, for example, in tears of patients with peripheral ulcerative keratitis, herpetic keratitis and Sjogren's syndrome[48].

Among the MMPs, MMP-9 is of central importance in cleaving epithelial basement membrane components and tight junction proteins that maintain corneal epithelial barrier function[47]. MMP-9 belongs to the gelatinase group of metalloproteinases that degrade denatured collagen; native collagens type IV, V, and VII; and elastin[47]. Expression of MMP-9 by ocular surface epithelia in normal healthy eyes is low. Indeed, MMP-9 knockout mice show significantly less alteration of epithelial barrier function in response to experimental desiccating stress than do wild-type mice, an effect abrogated by topical application of MMP-9 to the ocular surface[49].

5.2 Whole cornea studies and decreased TIMP-1

Studies have also assessed levels of various degradative enzymes in whole processed keratoconic corneas. This research was triggered by observations that cultured human dermal fibroblasts exposed to reactive oxygen species go on to upregulate MMP-1 and MMP-2 mRNA while downregulating TIMP-2 mRNA[50,51]. Thus oxidative stress was thought to be a contributing factor to the pathogenesis of keratoconus by promoting, amongst others, degradative activity.

Kenney et al. measured RNA levels by semi-quantitative reverse transcription-polymerase chain reaction (RT-PCR) and Southern blot. MMP-1, -2, -7, -9, -14, TIMP-2 and TIMP-3 mRNA levels did not differ between normal and keratoconic corneas[52]. There was, however, a 1.8 fold decrease in TIMP-1 mRNA and 2.8 fold decrease in TIMP-1 protein in keratoconus[52].

Decreased TIMP-1 may account for the high gelatinase activity and increased apoptosis of keratoconus. It has been proposed that TIMP-1 curtails the activity of MMP-2, the major protease of the corneal stroma. Unlike the constitutively expressed TIMP-2, TIMP-1 is an inducible inhibitor generally confined to the corneal epithelium[53]. Its synthesis seems to be upregulated in stromal cell cultures from scarred keratoconic corneas[53]. Apart from its anti-proteinase role TIMP-1 prevents TIMP-3 mediated stromal cell apoptosis[53]. Dysequilibrium in the TIMP-1/TIMP-3 system can thus, at least partially, account for the keratoconic condition.

It is likely that changes in MMP and TIMP systems are also present in several other eye diseases. For example, diabetic retinopathy corneas contain higher levels of MMP-3 and MMP-10 mRNA as measured by RT-PCR compared with keratoconic corneas[54]. This is thought to account for the various basement membrane and extracellular matrix alterations in the cornea of diabetic retinopathy.

5.3 Epithelium and increased MMP-1

Collier et al. performed peroxidase immunohistochemistry and determined that MMP-14 (MT1-MMP) was significantly elevated in the epithelium of keratoconic corneas compared to eye bank controls, while MMP-2 was not[55]. This was surprising given that MMP-14 was previously shown to activate latent MMP-2 as well as being able to degrade matrix molecules directly. MMP-14 forms a tri-molecular complex on the cell surface with MMP-2 and TIMP-2 in a complex sequence[55]. The timing of this interaction and concentrations of component molecules determine whether the MMP-14 active site is exposed and available for MMP-2 activation and matrix degradation[55].

It was also noted that the expression of MMP-14 in control corneas varied considerably from virtually none to pronounced levels, raising the possibility that the enzyme is expressed in response to any minor inflammatory or other pathological event.

Subsequent work failed to detect a significant difference in either MMP-2 or MMP-14 between keratoconic and normal epithelium[56], instead reporting higher levels of MMP-13 in the keratoconic epithelium compared to healthy specimens[56]. TNF-α and IL-1β increase corneal epithelial MMP-13 synthesis[57] while MMP-13 has been shown to activate MMP-9 *in vitro*[58]. The temporal and spatial correlation between MMP-13, MMP-9 and corneal re-epithelialisation suggests that MMP-13 plays a role in corneal reepithelialisation after injury[59]. MMP-13 activation seems to be much more prominent in bullous keratopathy than keratoconus[60].

Several studies report increased MMP-1 expression in keratoconus. The epithelia of healthy corneas and corneas with post LASIK keratectasia display nearly absent immunolabelling for MMP-1, whereas strong labelling occurs in the epithelium and stroma of keratoconic specimens[56,61,62]. MMP-1 is able to degrade many non-collagenous components of the extracellular matrix, including fibronectin, laminin, and basement membrane glycoproteins, but first and foremost, it cleaves native interstitial collagens types I and III[62].

MMP-1 can be effectively induced by the extracellular matrix metalloproteinase inducer (EMMPRIN), which is a member of the immunoglobulin superfamily of adhesion molecules[62]. In keratoconus, EMMPRIN expression was found in all layers of the cornea, especially in histopathologically altered areas, however, the distribution of MMP-1 did not totally overlap with histologically apparent corneal damage and EMMPRIN expression[62]. This may be because EMMPRIN upregulates other MMPs (MMP-2, MMP-3) in stromal fibroblasts. In areas of destruction EMMPRIN-inducible MMPs, other than MMP-1, may be participating in the local pathological process.

MMP-8 seems to be down-regulated in keratoconic epithelium compared to normal controls[56]. MMP-8 plays a paradoxical role in tissues, on the one hand being able to cleave collagens despite the presence of TIMPs and on the other controlling the inflammatory load in tissues by downregulating the polymorphonuclear (PMN) burden[63]. Unlike other MMPs epithelial MMP-8 is not upregulated by TNF-α and IL-1β[57]. Such MMPs may contribute to the pathogenesis of keratoconus by proteolytic modulation of proinflammatory cytokines or chemokines or the generation of apoptotic signals for inflammatory and corneal cells.

5.4 Stroma

Despite much research, contradictory reports preclude any conclusive statement on the contribution of specific MMPs to histopathological hallmarks found in the keratoconic corneal stroma.

In one study MMP-1, -2 and -13 immunolabelling was noted to be greater in keratoconic samples compared to normal controls while no difference in MMP-8 or MMP-14 immunolabelling was observed[56]. In another study, keratoconic immunolabelling for MMP-1, -2 and -3 resembled that of the normal cornea and post LASIK keratectasia[61] while peroxidase immunohistochemistry performed by Collier's group showed that MMP-14 was significantly elevated in the keratoconic stroma[55].

Stromal tissue layer supernatant showed no significant difference in MMP-2, MMP-9, pro MMP-13 and TIMP-1 concentrations between bullous keratopathy and keratoconus[60]. Keratocyte cultures from normal and keratoconic corneas also showed no significant changes in mRNA levels for MMP-1, -2, -3, TIMP-1, or TIMP-2[64]. Only TIMP-1 protein was decreased, prompting a three-fold increase in the MMP-2/TIMP-1 ratio in keratoconus[64].

Yet stromal cell cultures performed by Smith et al. found MMP-2 to be over-expressed in clear keratoconic and scarred keratoconic corneas[65]. The quantities of TIMP-1 and TIMP-2 in normal and clear keratoconic cultures were similar. Scarred keratoconic cultures over-expressed TIMP-1[65]. In these cultures the cells remained healthy and the extent of stress induced MMP-2 activation was low[65]. For this reason, in addition to inhibiting MMP activity, upregulated TIMP-1 production may be a feature of corneal scar tissue cells that are refractory to dying. Alternatively, TIMP-1 may prevent cell death that is conceivably initiated by upregulated TIMP-3 production and sequestration in the extracellular matrix[65].

5.5 Endothelium with Descemet's

There are only a few studies assessing MMP changes specific to Descemet's membrane and endothelium. The endothelial monolayer often gets damaged or lost as the result of tissue handling making studies technically difficult. It was noted that endothelial cells and Descemet's membrane were pathologically altered in keratoconus and EMMPRIN was expressed next to areas of histological damage without, however, any evidence of MMP-1 expression in the area[62]. Mackiewicz et al. did not detect a difference in MMP-1, -13 and -14 between keratoconus and healthy controls but did report more MMP-2 in the endothelium and Descemet's of keratoconus and less MMP-8 in the same layers compared to normal controls[56]. Endothelial tissue supernatant showed no significant difference in MMP-2, MMP-9, pro MMP-13 and TIMP-1 concentrations between bullous keratopathy and keratoconus[60].

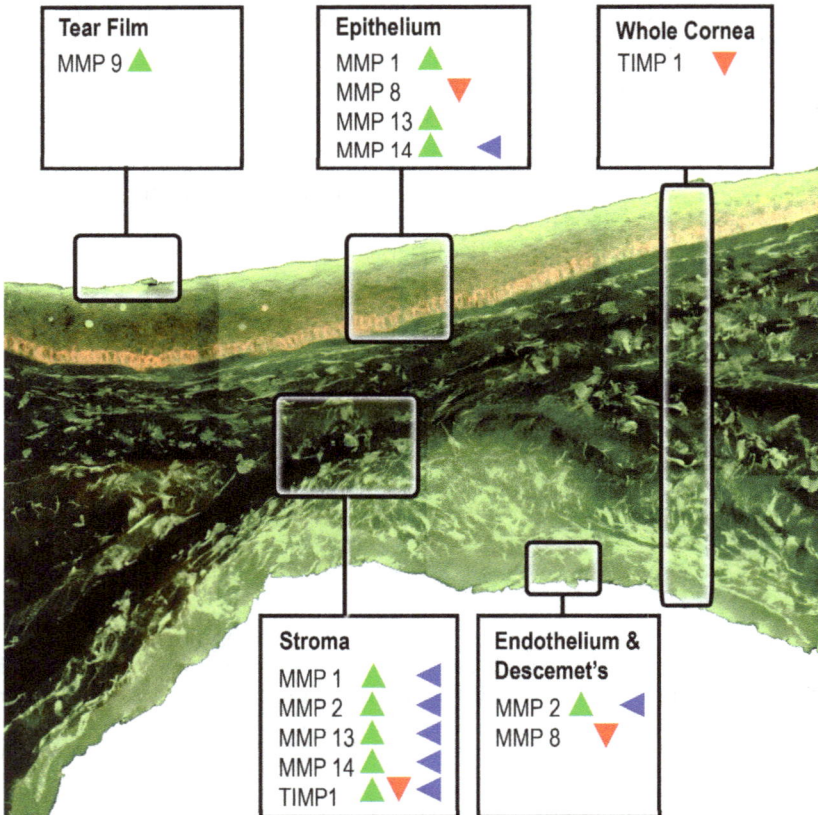

Fig. 2. Matrix metalloproteinase (MMP) and tissue inhibitor of matrix metalloproteinase (TIMP) changes have been described in every layer of the keratoconic cornea. Again, an antero-posterior section of a keratoconic cornea illustrated the MMP and TIMP molecules whose expression have been reported as altered in keratoconus. Green arrows represent increased expression, whilst red represents reported decreased expression and blue no change. It is evident in several cases that reported expression profiles are cotradictory.

6. Conclusion

MMPs are a group of proteolytic enzymes that are able to degrade the main components of the extracellular matrix and corneal membranes. Owing to these activities, MMPs are widely assumed to have a central role in the pathogenesis of keratoconus. However, studies have shown that MMPs can also handle substrates distinct from extracellular matrix proteins, influencing cell processes such as apoptosis. Proteolytic modulation of proinflammatory cytokines or chemokines or the generation of apoptotic signals for resident and inflammatory cells may prove to be as important in mediating keratoconus progression as purported extracellular matrix degradation.

The involvement of proteases in keratoconus has been the subject of much research; however, the exact nature of proteolytic phenomena that contribute to keratoconus progression remains unclear. Studies have described upregulation of MMP-1, MMP-2, MMP-9, MMP-13 and MMP-14 in keratoconus, yet this has not been seen consistently. Other authors report no change in MMP levels or else a downregulation of MMP-8 or TIMP-1. Increased activity of other proteinases such as cathepsins[66] likely contributes to the structural deterioration seen in keratoconus.

For MMP inhibition or TIMP upregulation to be considered a valid therapeutic target for amelioration of the disease process it is important to know exactly which MMPs are culpable. However, due to complex inter-molecular interactions between individual members of the MMP family, the ratios between various MMPs may turn out to be more significant to keratoconus pathogenesis than absolute concentrations of specific MMPs. The ability to measure multiple MMPs in a single corneal specimen is therefore necessary in order to understand the interplay of proteinases within the cornea. Tear fluid analysis affords the opportunity to investigate keratoconus protagonists in the earlier stages of the disease, a significant advantage over end-stage corneal tissue analysis. MMP changes are seen in many other corneal diseases, suggesting that MMP activation may be a nonspecific response to corneal insult. Indeed, the observed changes in inflammatory mediators or MMP levels within the cornea can in fact be epiphenomena of changes in corneal structure[35]. It is also possible that several diseases, with differing pathophysiology produce the phenotypic changes that are called keratoconus, accounting for the difference in proteinase profiles of examined keratoconic samples.

7. References

[1] Rabinowitz YS. Keratoconus. Surv Opthalmol. 1998; 42:297-319.
[2] Williams KA, Muehlberg SM, Lewis RF, Coster DJ. How succesful is corneal transplantation? A report from the Australian corneal graft register. Eye (Lond). 1995; 9:219-227.
[3] Vail A, Gore SM, Bradley BA, Easty DL, Rogers CA. Corneal transplantation in the United Kingdom and Northern Ireland. Brit J Ophthalmol. 1993; 77:650-6.
[4] Nottingham J. Practical observations on conical cornea: and on the short sight, and other defects of vision connected with it. 1854; London, John Churchill.
[5] Berliner ML. Biomicroscopy of the eye. 1943; New York, Paul B Hoeber Inc.
[6] Duke-Elder S. System of Ophthalmology. Vol VIII Diseases of the outer eye. 1965; London, Henry Kimpton.
[7] Sherwin T, Brookes NH. Morphological changes in keratoconus: pathology or pathogenesis. Clin Experiment Ophthalmol. 2004; 32(2):211-7.

[8] Scroggs MW, Proia AD. Histopathological variation in keratoconic corneas. Cornea. 1992; 11:553-559.

[9] Kim W-J, Rabinowitz YS, Meisler DM, Wilson SE. Keratocyte apoptosis associated with keratoconus. Exp Eye Res. 1999; 69:475-481.

[10] Sherwin T, Brookes NH, Loh I-P, Poole CA, Clover GM. Cellular incursion into Bowman's membrane in the peripheral cone of the keratoconic cornea. Exp Eye Res. 2002; 74:473-482.

[11] Erie JC, Patel SV, McLaren JW, Nau CB, Hodge DO, Bourne WM. Keratocyte density in keratoconus: A confocal microscopy study. Am J Ophth. 2002; 134:689-695.

[12] Somodi S, Hahnel C, Slowik C, Richter A, Weiss DG, Guthoff R. Confocal in vivo microscopy and confocal laser scanning fluorescence microscopy in keratoconus. Ger J Ophthalmol. 1997; 5:518-525.

[13] Kaldawy RM, Wagner J, Ching S, Seigel GM. Evidence of apoptotic cell death in keratoconus. Cornea. 2002; 21:206-209.

[14] Teng CC. Electron microscope study of the pathology of keratoconus: Part I. Am J Ophthalmol. 1963; 55:19-47.

[15] Tuori AJ, Virtanen I, Aine E, Kalluri R, Miner JH, Uusitalo HM. The immunohistochemical composition of corneal basement membrane in keratoconus. Curr Eye Res. 1997; 16:792-801.

[16] Cheng EL, Maruyama I, SundarRaj N, Sugar J, Feder RS, Yue BY. Expression of type XII collagen and hemidesmosome-associated proteins in keratoconus corneas. Curr Eye Res. 2001; 22:333-340.

[17] Brookes NH, Loh I-P, Clover GM, Poole CA, Sherwin T. Involvement of corneal nerves in the progression of keratoconus. Exp Eye Res. 2003; 77:515-524.

[18] Sawaguchi S, Fukuchi T, Abe H, Kaiya T, Sugar J, Yue, BT. Three dimensional scanning electron microscopic study of keratoconus corneas. Arch Ophthalmol. 1998; 116:62-68.

[19] Kenney MC, Nesburn AB, Burgeson RE, Butkowski RJ, Ljubimov AV. Abnormalities of the extracellular matrix in keratoconus corneas. Cornea. 1997; 16:345-51.

[20] Takahashi A, Nakayasu K, Okisaka S, Kanai A. Quantitative analysis of collagen fibres in keratoconus. Acta Soc Ophthalmol Jap. 1990; 90:1068-73.

[21] Fullwood NJ, Tuft SJ, Malik NS, Meek KM, Ridgway AEA, Harrison RJ. Synchrotron X-ray diffraction studies of keratoconus corneal stroma. Invest Ophthalmol Vis Sci. 1992; 33:1734-41.

[22] Daxer A, Fratzl P. Collagen fibril orientation in the human corneal stroma and its implication in keratoconus. Invest Ophthalmol Vis Sci. 1997; 38:1289-90.

[23] Critchfield JW, Calandra AJ, Nesburn AB, Kenney MCR. Keratoconus I. Biochemical Studies. Exp Eye Res. 1988; 46:953-64.

[24] Radda TM, Menzel EJ, Freyler H, Gnad HD. Collagen types in keratoconus. Graefes Arch Clin Exp Ophthalmol. 1982; 218:262-6.

[25] Zimmermann DR, Fischer RW, Winterhalter KH, Witmer R, Vaughan L. Comparative studies of collagens in normal and keratoconus corneas. Exp Eye Res. 1988; 46:431-42.

[26] Rock ME, Moore MN, Anderson JA, Binder PS. 3-D computer models of human keratocytes. CLAO J. 1995; 21:57-60.

[27] Wygledowska-Promienska D, Rokita-Wala I, Gierek-Ciaciura S, Piatek-Koronowska G. The alterations in corneal structure at III/IV stage of keratoconus by means of confocal microscopy and ultrasound biomicroscopy before penetrating keratoplasty. Klinika Oczna. 1999; 101:427-432.

[28] Jongebloed WL, Dijk F, Worst JG. Keratoconus morphology and cell dystrophy: a SEM study. Documenta Ophthalmologica. 1989; 72:403-409.

[29] Bechrakis N, Blom ML, Stark WJ, Green WR. Recurrent keratoconus. Cornea. 1994; 13:73-77.

[30] Krivoy D, McCormick S, Zaidman GW. Postkeratoplasty keratoconus in a nonkeratoconus patient. Am J Ophthalmol. 2001; 131:653-654.

[31] Bourges J-L, Salvoldelli M, Dighiero P, Assouline M, Pouliquen Y, BenEzra D, Renard G, Behar-Cohen F. A clinical and histologic follow up analysis of donor grafts. Ophthalmol. 2003; 110:1920-1925.

[32] Brookes NH, Niederer RL, Hickey DG, McGhee CNJ, Sherwin T. Recurrence of keratoconic pathology in penetrating keratoplasty buttons originally transplanted for keratoconus. Cornea. 2009; 28: 688-693.

[33] Brinckerhoff CE, Matrisian LM. Matrix metalloproteinases: a tail of a frog that became a prince. Nat Rev Mol Cell Biol. 2002; 3(3):207-14.

[34] Collier SA. Is the corneal degradation in keratoconus caused by matrix-metalloproteinases? Clin Experiment Ophthalmol. 2001; 29(6):340-4.

[35] Lema I, Sobrino T, Durán JA, Brea D, Díez-Feijoo E. Subclinical keratoconus and inflammatory molecules from tears. Br J Ophthalmol. 2009; 93(6):820-4.

[36] Fournié PR, Gordon GM, Dawson DG, Edelhauser HF, Fini ME. Correlations of long-term matrix metalloproteinase localization in human corneas after successful laser-assisted in situ keratomileusis with minor complications at the flap margin. Arch Ophthalmol. 2008; 126(2):162-70.

[37] Abalain JH, Dossou H, Colin J, Floch HH. Levels of collagen degradation products (telopeptides) in the tear film of patients with keratoconus. Cornea. 2000; 19:474–6.

[38] Fukuchi T, Yue BY, Sugar J, Lam S. Lysosomal enzyme activities in conjunctival tissues of patients with keratoconus. Arch Ophthalmol. 1994; 112(10):1368-74.

[39] De Paiva CS, Harris LD, Pflugfelder SC. Keratoconus-like topographic changes in keratoconjunctivitis sicca. Cornea. 2003; 22(1):22-4.

[40] Lema I, Durán JA. Inflammatory molecules in the tears of patients with keratoconus. Ophthalmology. 2005; 112(4):654-9.

[41] Li DQ, Lokeshwar BL, Solomon A, Monroy D, Ji Z, Pflugfelder SC. Regulation of MMP-9 production by human corneal epithelial cells. Exp Eye Res. 2001; 73:449–59.

[42] Sonoda S, Uchino E, Nakao K, Sakamoto T. Inflammatory cytokine of basal and reflex tears analysed by multicytokine assay. Br J Ophthalmol. 2006; 90(1):120-2.

[43] Cook EB. Tear cytokines in acute and chronic ocular allergic inflammation. Curr Opin Allergy Clin Immunol. 2004; 4(5):441-5.

[44] Jacq PL, Sale Y, Cochener B, Lozach P, Colin J. Keratoconus, changes in corneal topography and allergy. Study of 3 groups of patients. J Fr Ophtalmol. 1997; 20(2):97-102.

[45] Bawazeer AM, Hodge WG, Lorimer B. Atopy and keratoconus: a multivariate analysis. Br J Ophthalmol. 2000; 84(8):834-6.

[46] Dogru M, Karakaya H, Özçetin H, Ertürk H, Yücel A, Ozmen A, Baykara M, Tsubota K. Tear function and ocular surface changes in keratoconus. Ophthalmology. 2003; 110:1110–8.

[47] Chotikavanich S, de Paiva CS, Li de Q, Chen JJ, Bian F, Farley WJ, Pflugfelder SC. Production and activity of matrix metalloproteinase-9 on the ocular surface increase in dysfunctional tear syndrome. Invest Ophthalmol Vis Sci. 2009; 50(7):3203-9.

[48] Smith VA, Rishmawi H, Hussein H, Easty DL. Tear film MMP accumulation and corneal disease. Br J Ophthalmol 2001; 85:147–53.

[49] Pflugfelder SC, Farley W, Luo L, Chen LZ, de Paiva CS, Olmos LC, Li DQ, Fini ME. Matrix metalloproteinase-9 knockout confers resistance to corneal epithelial barrier disruption in experimental dry eye. Am J Pathol. 2005; 166(1):61-71.

[50] Brenneisen P, Briviba K, Wlaschek M, Wenk J, Scharffetter-Kochanek K. Hydrogen peroxide (H2O2) increases the steady-state mRNA levels of collagenase/MMP-1 in human dermal fibroblasts. Free Radic Biol Med. 1997; 22(3):515-24.

[51] Kawaguchi Y, Tanaka H, Okada T, Konishi H, Takahashi M, Ito M, Asai J. The effects of ultraviolet A and reactive oxygen species on the mRNA expression of 72-kDa type IV collagenase and its tissue inhibitor in cultured human dermal fibroblasts. Arch Dermatol Res. 1996; 288(1):39-44.

[52] Kenney MC, Chwa M, Atilano SR, Tran A, Carballo M, Saghizadeh M, Vasiliou V, Adachi W, Brown DJ. Increased levels of catalase and cathepsin V/L2 but decreased TIMP-1 in keratoconus corneas: evidence that oxidative stress plays a role in this disorder. Invest Ophthalmol Vis Sci. 2005; 46(3):823-32.

[53] Matthews FJ, Cook SD, Majid MA, Dick AD, Smith VA. Changes in the balance of the tissue inhibitor of matrix metalloproteinases (TIMPs)-1 and -3 may promote keratocyte apoptosis in keratoconus. Exp Eye Res. 2007 Jun; 84(6):1125-34.

[54] Saghizadeh M, Brown DJ, Castellon R, Chwa M, Huang GH, Ljubimova JY, Rosenberg S, Spirin KS, Stolitenko RB, Adachi W, Kinoshita S, Murphy G, Windsor LJ, Kenney MC, Ljubimov AV. Overexpression of matrix metalloproteinase-10 and matrix metalloproteinase-3 in human diabetic corneas: a possible mechanism of basement membrane and integrin alterations. Am J Pathol. 2001; 158(2):723-34.

[55] Collier SA, Madigan MC, Penfold PL. Expression of membrane-type 1 matrix metalloproteinase (MT1-MMP) and MMP-2 in normal and keratoconus corneas. Curr Eye Res. 2000; 21(2):662-8.

[56] Mackiewicz Z, Määttä M, Stenman M, Konttinen L, Tervo T, Konttinen YT. Collagenolytic proteinases in keratoconus. Cornea. 2006; 25(5):603-10.

[57] Li DQ, Shang TY, Kim HS, Solomon A, Lokeshwar BL, Pflugfelder SC. Regulated expression of collagenases MMP-1, -8, and -13 and stromelysins MMP-3, -10, and -11 by human corneal epithelial cells. Invest Ophthalmol Vis Sci. 2003; 44(7):2928-36.

[58] Knäuper V, Smith B, López-Otin C, Murphy G. Activation of progelatinase B (proMMP-9) by active collagenase-3 (MMP-13). Eur J Biochem. 1997; 248(2):369-73.

[59] Ye HQ, Maeda M, Yu FS, Azar DT. Differential expression of MT1-MMP (MMP-14) and collagenase III (MMP-13) genes in normal and wounded rat corneas. Invest Ophthalmol Vis Sci. 2000; 41(10):2894-9.

[60] Predović J, Balog T, Marotti T, Gabrić N, Bohac M, Romac I, Dekaris I. The expression of human corneal MMP-2, MMP-9, proMMP-13 and TIMP-1 in bullous keratopathy and keratoconus. Coll Antropol. 2008; 32 Suppl 2:15-9.

[61] Meghpara B, Nakamura H, Macsai M, Sugar J, Hidayat A, Yue BY, Edward DP. Keratectasia after laser in situ keratomileusis: a histopathologic and immunohistochemical study. Arch Ophthalmol. 2008; 126(12):1655-63.

[62] Seppälä HP, Määttä M, Rautia M, Mackiewicz Z, Tuisku I, Tervo T, Konttinen YT. EMMPRIN and MMP-1 in keratoconus. Cornea. 2006; 25(3):325-30.

[63] Owen CA, Hu Z, Lopez-Otin C, Shapiro SD. Membrane-bound matrix metalloproteinase-8 on activated polymorphonuclear cells is a potent, tissue inhibitor of metalloproteinase-resistant collagenase and serpinase. J Immunol. 2004; 172(12):7791-803.

[64] Kenney MC, Chwa M, Opbroek AJ, Brown DJ. Increased gelatinolytic activity in keratoconus keratocyte cultures. A correlation to an altered matrix metalloproteinase-2/tissue inhibitor of metalloproteinase ratio. Cornea. 1994; 13(2):114-24. '

[65] Smith VA, Matthews FJ, Majid MA, Cook SD. Keratoconus: matrix metalloproteinase-2 activation and TIMP modulation. Biochim Biophys Acta. 2006; 1762(4):431-9.

[66] Zhou L, Sawaguchi S, Twining SS, Sugar J, Feder RS, Yue BY. Expression of degradative enzymes and protease inhibitors in corneas with keratoconus. Invest Ophthalmol Vis Sci. 1998; 39(7):1117-24.

Part 3

Refraction and Refractive Correction

8

Incidence of Refractive Error and Amblyopia Among Young Adults – A Hospital Based Study

Ashok Kumar Narsani[1], Shafi Muhammad Jatoi[1],
Mohan Perkash Maheshwari[2] and Khairuddin Shah[1]
[1]Department of Ophthalmology,
Liaquat University Eye Hospital, Hyderabad Sindh,
[2]Department of Pharmacology,
Baqai Medical University, Karachi Sindh,
Pakistan

1. Introduction

Visual impairment remains a major public health problem world wide, with an estimated 161 million people with visual impairment, of whom 37 million are blind.[1] Uncorrected or inadequately corrected refractive errors have been shown to be a major cause of visual impairment in population-based studies[2-6]. While amblyopia is a significant cause of unilateral reduced visual acuity in a population aged 40 years and older.[7]

Genetic factors are thought to play a role in development of refractive errors. It has been established that myopia clusters within families, and familial high myopia (refraction of -6 diopter {D} or less) has been linked to long arm regions on chromosomes 7, 12 and 18[8,9]. Environmental risk factors have also been associated with refractive errors, myopia or hypermetropia. Education[10,11] and near-work[12] are both strongly associated with increasing severity of myopia.

In different parts of Asia such as in India, the Andhra Pradesh Eye Disease Study shows 15.2%[13] prevalence rate of myopia (spherical equivalent {SE} at least -1.0D). While study in a 15,068 Singapore military recruits aged 16 to 25 years, the prevalence rates of myopia (SE at least -0.5 D) were much higher with some racial variation, 82.2% in Chinese, 68.8% in Indians, and 65.0% in Malays[14]. Similar high rates of myopia (SE at least -0.25 D; 84%) were present in 16 to 18 years old Chinese children in Taiwan[15]. In Pakistan the prevalence rates of myopia, hypermetropia, astigmatism (with SE worse than –0.5 D, greater than +0.5D, and greater than 0.75D respectively) was 36.5%, 27.1%, and 37%, respectively in adults aged 30 years or more in the National Blindness and Visual Impairment Survey.[16]

In United states, the Baltimore eye survey[17] and Beaver Dam study[18] showed the prevalence rates of myopia (SE at least -0.5 D) were 28.1% in white adults aged 40 years or more and 26.2% in adults aged 43 to 84 years respectively.

Amblyopia is a frequent cause of unilateral or bilateral blindness. The prevalence of amblyopia ranges from 0.73% to 3.06%[7] in previous studies. However, the epidemiology of amblyopia among this region of Asia is not well described and may be different from other because of difference in distribution of refractive error or strabismus.

AIM: To assess the incidence of refractive error and associated amblyopia among young adult.

2. Methodology

2.1 Subjects

This six months study was conducted from June 2008 to November 2008 at tertiary referral center Liaquat University Eye Hospital, Hyderabad Sindh, Pakistan. Three thousand four hundred fifty two patients were included and examined in out patients department with age ranged from 20-40 years. The proportion of men and women was 1:0.54. Both rural and urban residents were evaluated. After taking written consent all subjects underwent a comprehensive ophthalmic examination, and a standardized form was used to extract the data, including the following variables: demographic information, best corrected visual acuity, types of refractive error including myopia, hypermetropia, astigmatism and amblyopia.

2.2 Methods

Monocular visual acuity was determined with current spectacle prescription if any. Pinhole acuity was assessed in eyes with presenting visual acuity <20/20. Non-cycloplegic auto-refraction followed by subjective refinements was performed in all subjects. The best corrected visual acuity was recorded. Refraction data was based on subjective refraction. Only the right phakic eye of each subject was considered for refractive error evaluation and amblyopia evaluated bilaterally.

Amblyopia was defined as best-corrected visual acuity of 20/40 or worse in the absence of any pathological cause. Hypermetropia was defined as a SE greater than +0.5 diopter sphere (DS)[17-21]. Emetropia was defined as a SE between -0.50 and +0.50 DS[20]. Myopia was defined as a SE worse than -0.50 DS[17-21] and a SE or worse than -5.00 DS[19] was classified as high myopia. Astigmatism correction was prescribed in minus cylinder format, and astigmatism was defined as cylindrical error worse than -0.50 diopter cylinder (DC) in any axis. The axis of any cylinder component was classified as with the rule (WTR) if the minus cylinder axis was within 15o of 180o, against the rule (ATR) for minus cylinder axis within 15o of 90o, or oblique (other than WTR or ATR)[22].

3. Results

Of the 3452 patients, 847 (24.54 %) patients had best corrected visual acuity 20/40 or better and remaining 2605 (75.46%) had less than 20/40 due to different anterior and posterior segment eye pathologies, or amblyopia.

Out of the 847 patients 525 (15.20 %) were phakic in right eye, and remaining 322 (9.32%) were pseudophakic. For refractive error the result was analyzed for only 15.20%

phakic ametropic patients. While for amblyopia all patients who met the criteria were evaluated.

There were 341 (64.95% of phakic ametropic patients) male and 184 (35.05%) were female. The age range from 20 to 40 years **(Table 1),** mean age being 26±3.9 years. The mean age of men and women was 28±3.9 and 24±6.3 years respectively (statistically significant at P<0.001). The mean refractive error was 0.75D.

Hypermetropia was found in 185 (35.24% of phakic ametropic) patients (Table 1). The mean age of hypermetropia was 26.31±4.51 years. Which was not significantly different from that of entire population (P=0.5476). There were 121 men (23.04% of total ametropic) and 64 women (12.19%). Man had significantly higher prevalence of hypermetropia than women (P<0.001).

Three hundred and fifteen (60% of phakic ametropic) patients had myopia (Table 1). The mean age of myopes was 23.69±3.98 years. Which was significantly lower than the entire population (P<0.001). There were 205 (39.05%) men and 110 (20.95%) women. The man had a significantly higher prevalence of myopia than did the women (P<0.001)

Twenty five (4.76%) patients of the study population were high myopes (Table 1). Among which 15 patients were males and 10 were females. The mean age among high myopes was 22. 50±3.25 years. Which was also significantly lower than the entire population (P<0.0002). However there was no significant different between the mean age of myopes and high myopes (P=0.1632).

Two hundred and fifteen (25.38 % of phakic ametropic) patients had astigmatism worse than –0.5 DC. The males were 134 (62.32%) of total astigmatic patients and remaining were females. The man had a significantly higher prevalence of astigmatism than women (P<0.001). One hundred and forty two (66.04%) patients had ATR astigmatism, 52 (24.18%) had WTR astigmatism and 21 (9.76%) had oblique astigmatism. The prevalence of against the rule astigmatism increased significantly with age (P=0.007).

The incidence of associated unilateral amblyopia was in 19 (3.62%) of phakic ametropic patients (Table 2). Ten (52.63%) patients were male and 09 (47.37%) were females. Amblyopia was not found to be significantly different by age (p=0.1312) group and gender (p=0.1211). Anisometropia was more common in amblyopic cases (41.75%) compared to the normal population (5.91%), and 69% of amblyopic eyes had visual acuity worse than 20/60. However, two amblyopic patients had strabismus in addition to anisometropia, but the prime reason of both conditions was anisometropia. While none of the case of bilateral amblyopia were seen in this study.

Age (yrs)	Hypermetropia		Myopia		High myopia		Total (%)
	M	F	M	F	M	F	
21-25	38	21	48	25	7	4	143 (27.23)
26-30	29	17	65	27	5	4	147 (28.00)
31-35	27	10	49	32	0	1	119 (22.68)
36-40	27	16	43	26	3	1	116 (22.09)
Total	121	64	205	110	15	10	525 (100)

Table 1. Age and type of refractive error

Age (yrs)	Frequency of amblyopia		Total (%)
	Male	Female	
21 -25	2	2	4 (21.04)
26 -30	3	2	5 (26.32)
31 -35	2	3	5 (26.32)
36 -40	3	2	5 (26.32)
Total	10	9	19 (100)

Table 2. Demography of amblyopia

4. Discussion

The incidence of hypermetropia in this study was 35.24% of total 525 phakic ametropic patients. In contrast to Andhra Paeye disease study (APEDS)[13], Barbados eye study[20], and several other studies[17,18] hypermetropia decrease with increasing age in our study

The incidence of myopia and high myopia in this study was 60% and 4.76% of the phakic ametropic patients and decreased with age. The Attebok et al[18], Wang et al[11], Katz et al[17] reported a significant trends of decreasing myopia with age. However the Chennai glaucoma study[3], Barbodos[20] study reported increase of myopia with age and also have an association of nuclear sclerosis with myopia. Saw[22], Guggenheim et al[23] and Dan et al[24] reported environmental influence such as near work, night lighting and ultraviolet exposure may be responsible for ageing of the crystalline lens and associated myopia. In contrast to population based studies from Australia[18], Singapore[19], and Indonesia[25], the incidence of myopia was more in males than females in our study.

The incidence of astigmatism in this study was 25.38% and increased significantly with age. The same has been reported from Chenni[3], Australia[18], Singapore[19], and Indonesia[25]. ATR astigmatism in this study was predominant that made the 66.04% of the total ametropic patients. In relation to the Chennai[3] study the incidence of ATR astigmatism significantly increased with age and WTR astigmatism decreased with age in our study. Gudmundsdottir et al[26], Pensyl et al[22] and Goss et al[28] reported same and the reason for this could be increased lid laxity with age causing flattening of vertical corneal meridian thereby decreasing WTR astigmatism and increased ATR astigmatism.

In this study the incidence, of associated amblyopia was 3.62% of phakic ametropic patients, which was less than Goel B.S[29] study in which amblyopia was reported 5.97%. One thing common in both were higher rate of amblyopia in ametropic then general population. In contrast to Karki JKD[30] study amblyopia was not found significantly different by age and gender in this study.

In conclusion, 15.20% of people had refractive error and 3.62% has the amblyopia. The prevalence of myopia was 60% and decreased with age. Hypermetropia was more common among men. The prevalence of astigmatism was 25.38%. It was interesting to note that against the rule astigmatism in contrast to other studies was observed more often (66.04%) in this study. Though the above study represent the regional population of limited age (20-40 years), but the differences in the pattern of refractive error in this study leads us to believe that genetic, racial, environmental and occupational influences may play an important role.

5. References

[1] Resnikoff S, Pascolini D, Etya'ale D, et al. Global data onvisual impairment in the year 2002. *Bull World Health Organ*.2004;82:844 –51.

[2] Munoz B, West SK, Rubin GS, Schein OD, Quigley HA, Bressler SB, Bandeen-Roche K. Causes of blindness and visual impairment in a population of older Americans. The Salisbury Eye Evaluation Study. *Arch Ophthalmol*. 2002;118:819–825.

[3] Foran S, Wang JJ, Mitchell P. Causes of incident visual impairment. *Arch Ophthalmol*. 2002;120:613–619.

[4] Weih LM, VanNewkirk MR, McCarty CA, Taylor HR. Age-specific causes of bilateral vision impairment. *Arch Ophthalmol*. 2000;118:264–269.

[5] VanNewkirk MR, Weih L, McCarty CA, Taylor HR. Cause-specific prevalence of bilateral visual impairment in Victoria, Australia. The Visual Impairment Project. *Ophthalmology*. 2001;108:960–967.

[6] Munoz B, West SK, Rodriguez J, Sanchez R, Broman AT, Snyder R, Klein R. Blindness, visual impairment and the problem of uncorrected refractive error in a Mexican-American population: Proyecto VER. *Invest Ophthalmol Vis Sci*. 2002;43:608–614.

[7] Brown SA, Weih LM, Fu CL, Dimitrov P, Taylor HR, McCarty CA. Prevalence of amblyopia and associated refractive errors in an adult population in Victoria, Australia. *Ophthalmic Epdimol* .2000;7:249-58.

[8] Naiglin L, Gazagne C, Dallongeville F, Thalamas C, Idder A, Rascol O, Malecaze F, Calvas P. A genome wide scanfor familial high myopia suggests a novel locus on chromosome7q36. *J Med Genet*. 2002;39:118–124.

[9] Young TL, Ronan SM, Drahozal LA, Wildenberg SC, Alvear AB, Oetting WS, Atwood LD, Wilkin DJ, King RA. Evidence that a locus for familial high myopia maps to chromosome 18p. *Am J Hum Genet*.1998;63:109–119.

[10] The Framingham Offspring Eye Study Group. Familial aggregation and prevalence of myopia in the Framingham Offspring Eye Study. *Arch Ophthalmol*. 1996;114:326–332.

[11] Wang Q, Klein BE, Klein R, Moss SE. Refractive status in the Beaver Dam Eye Study. *Invest Ophthalmol Vis Sci*. 1994;35:4344–4347.

[12] Midelfart A, Aamo B, Sjohaug KA, Dysthe BE. Myopia among medical students in Norway. *Acta Ophthalmol*. 1992;70:317-322.

[13] Dandona R, Dandona L, Naduvilath TJ, Srinivas M, McCarty CA, Rao GN. Refractive errors in an urban population in Southern India: the Andhra Pradesh Eye Disease Study. *Invest Ophthalmol Vis Sci*. 1999;40:2810–2818.

[14] Wu HM, Seet B, Yap EPH, Saw SM, Lim TH, Chia KS. Does education explain ethnic differences in myopia prevalence? A population-based study of young adult males in Singapore. *Optom Vis Sci*. 2001;78:234–239.

[15] Luke LK L, Yung-Feng S, Chong-Bin T, Chien-Jen C, Loung-An L, Port-Tying H, Ping-Kang H. Epidemiologic study of ocular refraction among schoolchildren in Taiwan in 1995. *Optom Vis Sci*. 1999;76:275–281.

[16] Jadoon MZ, Dineen B, Bourne RRA, Shah SP, Khan MA,. Johnson GJ, Gilbert CE, Khan MD. Refractive Errors in the Adult Pakistani Population: The National Blindness and Visual Impairment Survey. *Ophthalmic Epidemiol* 2008;15:183-190.

[17] Katz J, Tielsch JM, Sommer A. Prevalence and risk factors forrefractive error in an adult inner city population. *Invest Ophthalmol Vis Sci*. 1997;38:334–340.

[18]   Attebo K, Ivers RQ, Mitchell P. Refractive errors in an older population: The Blue Mountains eye study. *Ophthalmology*. 1999;106:1066–1072.

[19]   Wong TY, Foster PJ, Hee J, Pin Ng T, Tielsch JM, Chew SJ, Johnson GJ and Seah SKL. Prevalence and risk factors of refractive errors in adult Chinese in Singapore. *Invest Ophthalmol Vis Sci.* 2000;41:2486–2494.

[20]   Wu SY, Nemesure B, Leske MC. Refractive errors in a black adult population: The Barbados Eye Study. *Invest Ophthalmol Vis Sci.* 1999;40:2179–2184.

[21]   Gwiazda J, Scheiman M, Mohindra I, Held R. Astigmatism in children: changes in axis and amount from birth to six years. *Invest Ophthalmol Vis Sci.* 1984;25:88–92.

[22]   Saw SM. A synopsis of the prevalence rates and enviromental risk factors for myopia. *Clin Exp Optom.* 2003;86:289-294.

[23]   Guggenheim JA, Hill C, Yam TF. Myopia, genetics and ambient lighting at night in a UK sample. *Br J Ophthalmol.* 2003;87:580-582.

[24]   Dong X, Dong, Ayala M, Lofgren S, Soderberg PG. Ultraviolet radiation induced catract: age and maximum acceptable dosage. *Invest Ophthalmol Vis Sci.* 2003;44:1150-1154.

[25]   Saw SM, Gazzard G,Koh D, Farook M, Widjaja D, Lee J, Donald T. H. Tan DTH . Prevalence rates of refractive errors in Sumarta, Indonesia. *Invest Ophthalmol Vis Sci.* 2002;43:3174-3180.

[26]   Gudmundsdottir E, Jonasson F, Jonsson V, Stefansson E, Sasaki H, Sasaki K. "With the rule" astigmatism is not the rule in the elderly. *Acta Ophthalmol.* 2000;78:642-646.

[27]   Pensyl CD, Harrson RA, Simpson P, Waterbor JW. Distribution of astigmatism among sioux Indians in South Dakota. *J Am Optom Assoc.* 1997;68:425-431.

[28]   Goss DA. Meridonial Analysis of with the rule astigmatism in Oklahoma *Indians. Optom Vis Sci.* 1989;66:281-287.

[29]   Goel.B.S, Amblyopia: modern concept and management. In current topics in ophthalmology. I Gupta, A.K (ED), B.I Churchil Livingstone New Dehli, 1993, p 145.

[30]   Karki KJD Prevalence of Amblyopia in ametropia in clinical set up. *Katmandu University Medical Journal.* 2006;4;470-73.

9

Amblyopia and Foveal Thickness

Elina Landa[1], Shimon Rumelt[1],
Claudia Yahalom[2], Elaine Wong[3] and Lionel Kowal[3]
[1]Department of Ophthalmology, Western Galilee – Nahariya Medical Center, Nahariya,
[2]Department of Ophthalmology, Hadassah University Hospital, Jerusalem,
[3]Department of Ophthalmology, Eye and Ear Institute, The University of Melbourne, Melbourne,
[1,2]Israel
[3]Australia

1. Introduction

1.1 Definition

Amblyopia in Greek is dullness of vision. It is defined as poor unilateral or bilateral visual acuity due to poor perception in the presence of normal appearing globe.[1] It is caused by poor visual perception during the critical postnatal period required for maturation of the visual pathways and cortex. Clear and corresponding image is required for visual system development in animals including primates.

1.2 Epidemiology

The prevalence of amblyopia in the general population is probably between 2 and 2.5%. The wider range of 1-4% reflects differences in the degree of amblyopia, the studied population and the location. These figures represent the average of the prevalence in the different studies. The frequency of disorder has a socioeconomic impact. These patients have a greater risk for legal blindness if the fellow eye develops a blinding condition or sustain trauma. Indeed, patients with amblyopia as monocular patients are at a greater risk for trauma in the fellow eye although their visual field may be full.

1.3 Development of the visual system

The postnatal visual system development differs in different animals. In humans, the visual acuity improves usually until the age of 5 and this reflects the maturation of both the retina and the visual pathways.[2] The most critical period for amblyopia is the first 2 to 3 years of life.[1] The sensitivity of the visual system to abnormal perception is decreasing gradually afterwards. One should distinguish between the period when amblyopia may develop, which is until 9 years of age (although in most patients, it appears by the age of 5) and the period in which it is treatable, probably until the age of 17.[3]

1.4 Classification

Amblyopia is a result of three mechanisms: deprivation (obscuration of the image on its way to the retina (i.e., ptosis and media opacities), strabismus and refractive (anisometropic or isoamteropic) all causing blurred or non-corresponding images on the fovea.[1] The pathophysiology common to all of these is abnormal binocular interaction and/ or vision deprivation. Strabismic amblyopia occurs in the non-fixating eye and is always unilateral. It occurs in tropia and is more common in esotropia than in exotropia and indeed esotropia is neonatal while exotropia may be neonatal or acquired later in life. It is caused by signaling inhibition of the deviating eye to avoid confusion because of different foveal images between the eyes. Strabismic amblyopia is applied only to cases where the amblyopia is a result of strabismus and not vice versa. In refractive amblyopia, signaling inhibition of the blurred image occurs and in deprivation, there is usually no image. Anisometropia of +2.00, -3.00 and astigmatism of 1.5D or more are associated with amblyopia. The presence of astigmatism causes amblyopia in the astigmatic meridian called meridional amblyopia. Isoametropia of +4.00, -8.00 and astigmatism of 2D or more are associated with bilateral amblyopia. Lesser amount of hypermetropia than myopia is associated with amblyopia because the inability to focus images on the fovea at any distance. While strabismic amblyopia and most of the anisometropic amblyopia are unilateral, isoametropic and some of the deprivative amblyopia are bilateral. Deprivative amblyopia is usually the most profound and most resistant to treatment of all three forms of amblyopia. If it is present in the first 3 months, irreversible nystagmus develops. The unilateral cases are usually the worst.

2. Clinical manifestations

The visual acuity is poorer in the amblyopic eye than in the fellow eye or than in normal eyes and cannot be corrected to full with spectacles or contact lenses. A poorer visual acuity is considered if the visual acuity is less in two Snellen lines or more. Differences in one line may just be fluctuation and within the normal deviation and this is true not only for amblyopia but for all other instances as well. The subject uses the fellow better eye for fixation. The patient sees single signs on the Snellen chart better than several signs in a row (crowding phenomenon or abnormal contour interaction). This is caused by larger receptive fields (larger group of photoreceptors working as a single unit) and lateral inhibition by adjacent fields on the fixating field. Under dim light, the visual acuity decreases in both eyes but the visual acuity of amblyopic eye becomes similar to the normal eye. Thus the decrease in visual acuity is slower in the amblyopic eye than in a normal eye. The use of neutral density filters decreases the visual acuity in the amblyopic eye in much lesser extent compared with eyes with other diseases. In addition, amblyopic eyes have decreased contrast sensitivity, perception of brightness and have longer reaction time.

Other parameters are normal and similar to normal eyes including light perception (visual threshold) and visual field. An afferent pupillary defect is not supposed to occur but is a variable finding.

3. Treatment

Bilateral amblyopia is treated by eliminating the cause of blurred image (removal of the deprivation cause, strabismus surgery or refractive error correction). Unilateral amblyopia is treated similarly along with periodical patching or other penalization of the fellow sound eye. Penalization of the sound eye is usually performed by instilling once drop of atropine sulfate 1% one a day at bedtime. This causes cycloplegia and blurred image in the sound eye and forces the visual system of the amblyopic eye to act. Treatment should be initiated immediately when the condition is diagnosed. The elimination of the deprivative obstacle should be performed as early as possible (usually 2-3 weeks after birth). In strabismic amblyopia, anti-amblyopic treatment is initiated when the condition is diagnosed long before the surgery for strabismus. The reasons for this are improving the possibility to gain binocular vision if visual acuity is improved, easiness to determine the fixation patters, and the strabismus serves as a reminder to the parents on the importance of treatment. Surgery is performed only after achieving alternating fixation and equal visual acuity.

The length of patching or other penalization depends on the severity of the amblyopia. It is increased in direct proportion with the degree of the amblyopia. The follow-up frequency is also increased as the length of patching increases. Amblyopia is more easily reversible if it occurs later (ages 6-9) than earlier in life. Improvement of visual acuity should be both in single and multiple signs on Snellen chart and should be permanent. However, regression may occur and requires re-treatment.

Occlusion may be for full-time (all the day) for several days with one day off, or part time (several hours per day). Full-time occlusion is preserved for severe amblyopia with no binocular vision such as deprivative amblyopia. Full-time occlusion should not exceed one week per one year of age. Part-time treatment is preferred according to the Pediatric Eye Disease Investigator Group (PEDIG) studies because it has a similar outcome as full-time occlusion with less risk for development of amblyopia in the normal fellow eye, especially in the presence of binocular vision and mild amblyopia. Six hours per day of occlusion are sufficient for severe amblyopia of less than 20/100 and 2-3 hours per day for moderate one (better than 20/100). Contact lenses may be employed in anisometropia of more than 3.00D to prevent aniseikonia. However, this is more demanding treatment. Bilateral amblyopia in isoammteropia is usually not treated with occlusion and improves slowly spontaneously once refractive correction has been applied. In all cases, it is essential to rule out the development of amblyopia in the sound eye during treatment.

Obtaining compliance is difficult especially at the beginning of the treatment. The compliance becomes better as visual acuity of the amblyopic eye improves. Children try to remove or pick through the occluder. Therefore, it is better to use eye drops as penalization or a skin sticker rather than a sticker to the eyeglass. A full cooperation is required from the parents. They should be insisting on meticulous treatment for the full period. It is best to occlude when the child is at home under supervision of the parents and to occlude when the child is performing near tasks such as reading or doing homework. A close follow-up is required to ascertain improvement in visual acuity of the amblyopic eye and prevention of developing amblyopia in the fellow eye. In general, the follow-up intervals are one week per each year of life (e.g., a 2-year-old child is followed every 2 weeks). The follow-up includes visual acuity in each eye with full cycloplegic correction after refraction. If the visual acuity decreases, the reason for it should be disclosed. If the correction is not sufficient, it should be adjusted accordingly. If it is sufficient, an adjustment of the anti-amblyopic treatment should be performed. The length of occlusion is gradually decreased if the visual acuity improves to the desired level and no regression is observed in follow-up visits. Occlusion is gradually tapered according to the patient's response. Gradual decrease in occlusion time has been demonstrated to be associated with less recurrence rate than abrupt determination. If regression is noted, the treatment is re-initiated and continued over the vulnerable period (up to the age of 17). Follow-up until the age of 17 is necessary even if the optimal results have been achieved. Recurrence occurs in up to 75% of the patients usually within the first 13 months.[4] If treatment has not been successful after several (usually 6) months, it may be abandoned and visual function will not improve thereafter.

In animal models, L-dopa and bicuculline have been demonstrated to reverse amblyopia.

However, they have not been used in humans because the first one showed only a temporary effect and the second can cause seizures.

4. Prevention

Prevention of amblyopia is of outmost importance. Screening of red reflex at birth should be done to all neonates. Screening programs at preschool and school children are also important.

5. Background

To date, no changes in gross anatomy of the eye were found in the human amblyopic eye. When optical coherence tomography (OCT) was employed to evaluate the overall macular thickness, volume and the retinal nerve fiber layer (RNFL) thickness, it was found that all were similar in one study between strabismic amblyopic and the fellow eyes in 14 patients.[5] Another study did report thicker RNFL in amblyopic eyes than in normal fellow eyes.[6] When the differences in RNFL thickness were compared between amblyopic eyes and normal eyes of other subjects, they were found to be statistically insignificant.[7] In this study, the foveal thickness in the amblyopic eyes was similar to normal control eyes (p=0.551), but the authors did not compare it with the normal fellow eye. It would be expected that any differences in the anatomy in vivo between amblyopic and normal eyes would be microscopic. One should also consider the reproducibility of the OCT and the normal variations between normal eyes at different ages. Therefore, to show differences, a comparison should be made first with the fellow normal eye in unilateral amblyopia.

We compared the foveal thickness of amblyopic eyes with the fellow normal eye by OCT. Furthermore, we compared the foveal thickness of amblyopic eyes that underwent successful occlusion therapy with amblyopic eyes refractory to treatment. Such a study has not been previously reported according to Medline® search. The rationale for the current study was that even if the gross anatomy is normal, subtle structural variations such as foveal hypoplasia might exist.

6. Methods

In a prospective study, we compared the foveal thickness of amblyopic eyes with the fellow normal eyes in unilateral strabismic and anisometropic amblyopia by OCT (spectral OCT/SLO, OTI, Ophthalmic Technologies, Toronto, Canada). The inclusion criteria included best-corrected visual acuity (BCVA) of 20/80 or less in the involved eye, BCVA of 20/25 or better of the fellow eye, normal eye exam of each eye and no explanation for the low visual acuity except for amblyopia, presence of one of the causes for amblyopia (anisometropia of more than −3.00D or more than +1.00D, or strabismus), no other ocular, neurologic or systemic disorders, and children between 4 and 10 years of age who can undergo OCT and be treated for amblyopia and that followed the treatment orders. All other patients were excluded from the study. Ocular and general medical history were obtained and the patients underwent a complete ophthalmic examination of each eye including visual acuity by Snellen charts, pupil reactions, slit lamp examination, dilated funduscopic examination with a slit lamp biomicroscopy and indirect ophthalmoscopy.

All eyes were analyzed by OCT. Measurement was performed at the thinnest point of the macular center, representing the fovea. Several topographic 3D, linear and radial scans were obtained. The acceptance criteria of OCT included a central reflex, signal strength of at least 4 and standard deviation of the foveal thickness of less than 10% of the mean for each individual.

Amblyopic patients with refractive errors were treated by refractive full cycloplegic correction. Amblyopic patients with strabismus underwent strabismus surgery. All patients underwent occlusion (patching) therapy of the sound eye at least 6 for months and were followed according to previous recommendations.[3,8-10] Successful treatment was defined as an improvement in visual acuity in the amblyopic eye in at least 2 Snellen lines. The follow-up time ranged between 12 and 54 months.

Statistical analysis was performed with SPSS version 11.5 program (SPSS Inc., Chicago, IL, USA). Paired sample T-test was used for samples larger than 15 and Wilcoxon signed rank test was employed for smaller samples. Two-tailed $p<0.05$ was considered as statistically significant. Approval by the IRB/Ethics Committee was obtained and the patients' parents received a full explanation about the exam.

7. Patients

Nineteen children aged 4-10 with unilateral amblyopia were included. Ten patients had anisometropic (refractive) and 9 had strabismic amblyopia. Eight patients had successful occlusion therapy, while the other 11 had unsuccessful treatment.

8. Results

The foveal thickness in amblyopic eyes was 201±42 µm (average±SD) and in the normal fellow eyes 174±27 µm. The fovea was statistically thicker in the amblyopic eyes of whatever cause than in the normal fellow eye (p=0.011, paired sample T-test). The foveal thickness in eyes with anisometropic amblyopia (n=10) was 194±45 µm and in the fellow eyes of the same patients 167±23 µm (p=0.059, Wilcoxon signed rank test). The foveal thickness in eyes with strabismic amblyopia (n=9) was 210±39 µm and in the fellow eyes of the same patients 181± 30 µm (p=0.070, Wilcoxon signed rank test).

Eight (42%) of the 19 patients experienced improvement in BCVA after occlusion therapy. Six of the 8 had anisometropic and 2 had strabismic amblyopia. From the group of 11 (58%) patients that did not show improvement in BCVA, 4 had anisometropic and 7 had strabismic amblyopia (p=1.000). The foveal thickness in the patients who showed no improvement in BCVA after treatment was 216±41 µm and in their fellow eyes 176±31 µm (p=0.016, Wilcoxon signed rank test) (Table 1). In those who showed improvement, the foveal thickness in the amblyopic eyes was 181±36 µm and in their fellow eyes 171±21 µm (p=0.297, Wilcoxon signed rank test). Examples of the topographic 3-dimensional OCT maps of an amblyopic and normal fellow eye are seen in figures 1 and 2.

Parameter	Amblyopic eye	Fellow eye	P-value
Total (n=19)	201±42	174±27	0.011
Refractive (n=10)	194±45	167±23	0.059
Strabismic (n=9)	210±39	181±30	0.070
VA improvement (n=8)	216±41	176±31	0.016
No VA improvement (n=11)	181±36	171±21	0.297

Mean±SD in µm

Table 1. The foveal thickness in µm as measured by optical coherence tomography in amblyopic versus the normal fellow eye.

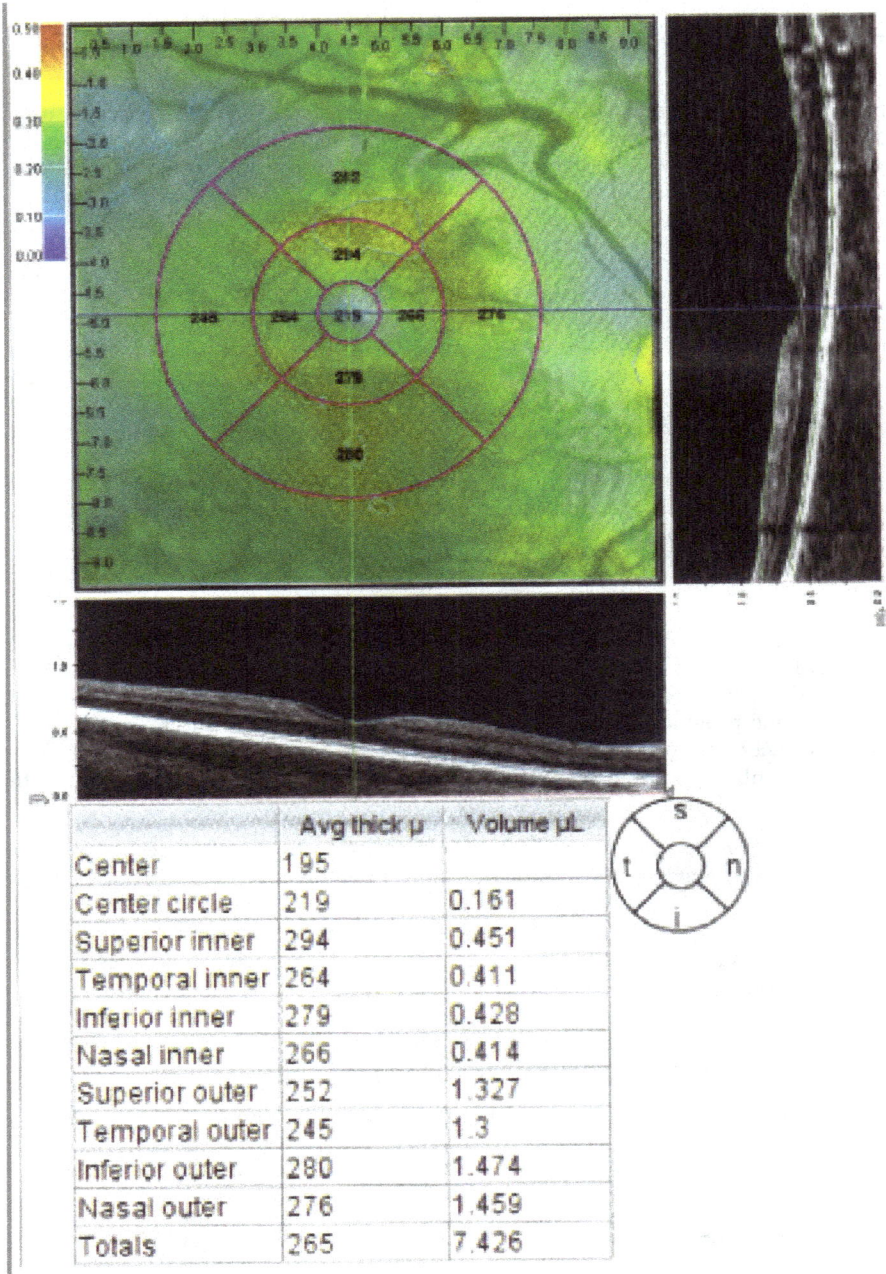

	Avg thick μ	Volume μL
Center	195	
Center circle	219	0.161
Superior inner	294	0.451
Temporal inner	264	0.411
Inferior inner	279	0.428
Nasal inner	266	0.414
Superior outer	252	1.327
Temporal outer	245	1.3
Inferior outer	280	1.474
Nasal outer	276	1.459
Totals	265	7.426

Fig. 1. A topographic 3-dimensional OCT image of the right amblyopic eye of a 10-year-old boy that was refractory to treatment measured a foveal thickness of 195 μm.

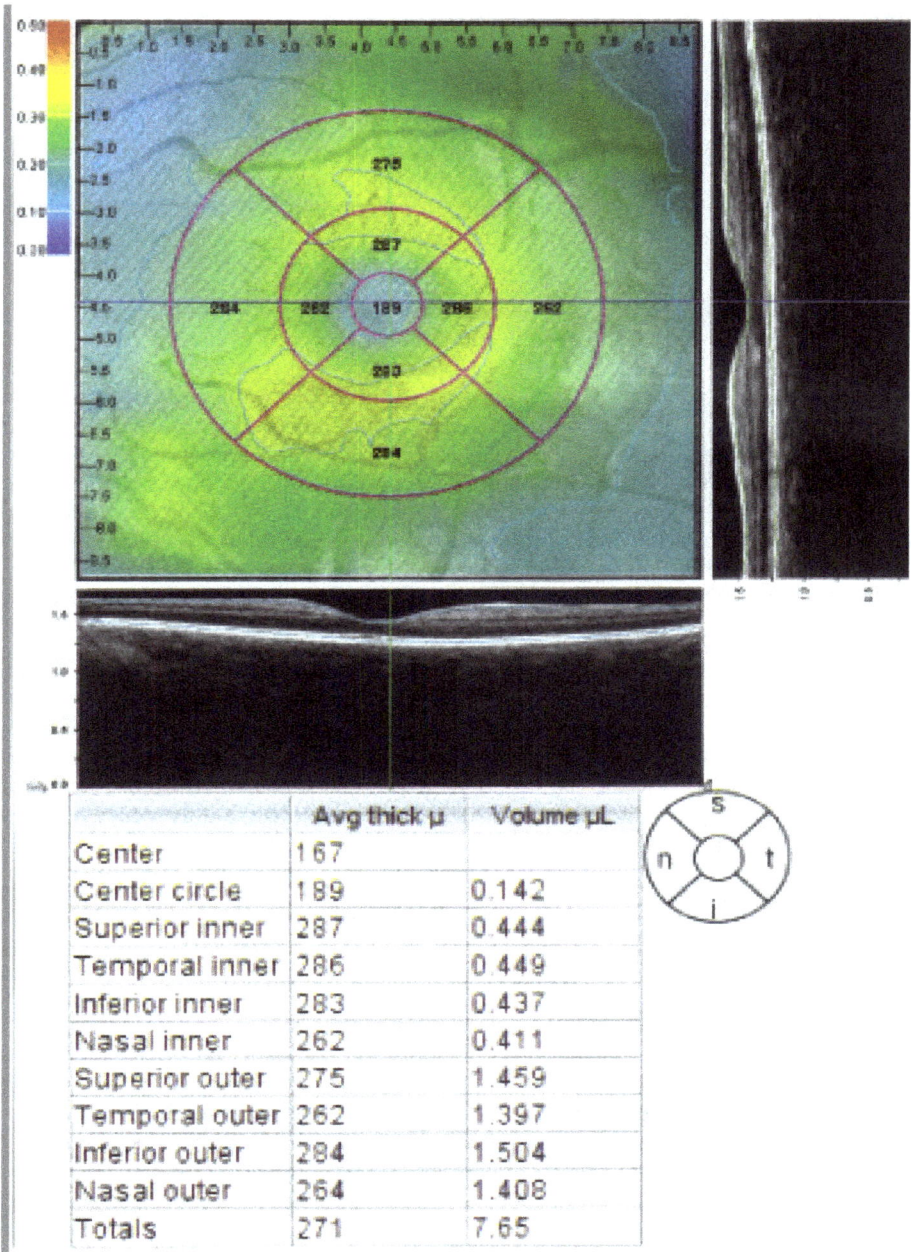

	Avg thick µ	Volume µL
Center	167	
Center circle	189	0.142
Superior inner	287	0.444
Temporal inner	286	0.449
Inferior inner	283	0.437
Nasal inner	262	0.411
Superior outer	275	1.459
Temporal outer	262	1.397
Inferior outer	284	1.504
Nasal outer	264	1.408
Totals	271	7.65

Fig. 2. A topographic 3-dimensional OCT image of the left normal eye of the same patient as in figure 1 measured a foveal thickness of 167 µm. The fovea was thinner in this normal eye than the amblyopic eye.

9. Discussion

Amblyopic eyes are classically considered as having a normal structure.[1] The only changes that have been found were smaller parvocellular cells in layers II, III and V in the ipsilateral lateral geniculate body, layers I, IV and VI of the contralateral lateral geniculate body and reduction in the number of cells in the primary (striate) visual cortex V1 receiving input from the affected eye.[11,12] Reduction was noted in the number of cells receiving binocular input. An increase in the number of cortical cells responding to a contour orientation also occurs. Positron emission tomography demonstrated a reduced cortical activity under visual stimulation of the amblyopic eye.[13]

We found that in the amblyopic eyes the fovea was thicker than in the normal fellow eyes. This was common both for anisometropic and strabismic eyes. Our finding is supported by a recent study in 3,529 children aged 6-12 years that found thicker fovea in amblyopic eyes than in the normal fellow eyes by 5μm.[14] These and our results differ from a recent evaluation of the foveal thickness that did not show statistically significant differences (p=0.551) of the foveae in patients with unilateral anisometropic and strabismic amblyopia compared with normal subjects.[7] Nonetheless, the authors did not compare the amblyopic eye with the normal fellow eyes and therefore, did not have an internal control. The differences between our study and the previous one probably relate to variability of foveal thickness in different individuals and indeed such differences were found between different individuals in our study and therefore the standard deviation between different individual was quite high.

Careful review of the OCT images indicated that the foveal thickening was due to either thicker outer retinal layers or immature retinal tissue. The structural feature of the foveae in amblyopic eyes is hypoplasia similar to albinotic and nanophthalmic eyes.[15-18] The fovea is thicker and flatter in these eyes. Since there are no histologic preparations of the retina in amblyopic eyes, it is impossible to determine the exact composition of the foveal area. However, in oculocutaneous albinism the retinal tissue was intact and the Bruch's layer was thickened in one specimen.[19]

We found that amblyopic eyes refractory to occlusion therapy had thicker fovea than those of the normal fellow eyes, while the differences in thickness between amblyopic eyes that responded to treatment and the fellow eyes were insignificant. This finding could have been different if patients and their parents would not be cooperative. No previous study addressed this issue and therefore we cannot compare our data with previous ones.

In our study, patients with anisometropic amblyopia had not statistical significant success of the occlusion therapy compared with patients with strabismic amblyopia. The differences in foveal thickness in the amblyopic and the sound fellow eyes in each group were not statistically significant although they were marginal in the amblyopic eyes of the anisometropic group. The higher number of anisometropic patients that underwent successful occlusion therapy might explain this tendency. A larger population will be required to confirm if the foveal thickness differs in these two groups and if the type of the amblyopia is the cause for different foveal thickness rather than treatment success. The higher success of occlusion therapy in anisometropic amblyopia than in strabismic amblyopia might be related to the thinner foveae in anisometropic patients. Thicker foveae were found in strabismic than in anisometropic amblyopia in another study as well (p=0.046).[7]

In our sample, the foveae of the amblyopic eyes were thicker than in the fellow normal eyes except for one in which the thickness was the same and another 3 with thicker normal fovea. Two of these patients experienced an improvement in BCVA after occlusion therapy. If in all future patients, the fovea of the amblyopic eye will be thicker than in the fellow normal eye, the foveal thickness may serve as a prognostic factor for improvement after proper therapy. To validate this, more patients should be recruited and a scale should be established for the measures that may predict improvement or non-improvement. It is possible that there will be patients in whom the fovea in the amblyopic eye would be thinner than in the normal fellow eye and would not experience an improvement in BCVA after treatment. In such event, it may not be possible to predict the success of a treatment based on the foveal thickness at least in those patients.

In patients with bilateral amblyopia, measurements of each fovea and a comparison with normal foveae will be needed. In such cases, the differences might be subtle as after comparing unilateral amblyopic eyes with normal controls and prediction of successful treatment may be difficult. According to our findings, it might be worthwhile to create a database for foveal thickness in the normal population according to age, since the foveal thickness may change with age.[20] In addition, a correlation between BCVA and foveal thickness might be established as well.

OCT measurements in children are demanding because of inattention, especially in children under age 4. In addition, amblyopic eyes tend to fixate less and if nystagmus is present, clear images may not be possible to obtain, unless the eye is mechanically fixated. We should also consider the accuracy and reproducibility of the OCT. When assessing thin layers as in the fovea, if the accuracy and reproducibility are not perfect, subtle differences may not be measured accurately, even if the image resolution is of 2μm. For macular thickness, OCT was found accurate and reproducible[21] and it is expected that with better technologies including high-resolution Fourier-domain OCT, this problem will be solved.

It will be interesting to verify our results in amblyopic adults and to find what is the foveal thickness in children that had regression after treatment. The last and the most intriguing issue is whether treatment influences the foveal thickness. Since the fovea, as well as other structures such as the lateral geniculate body and visual cortex, continue to develop after birth (the "critical" period), it is tempting to hypothesize that in successful treatment, the foveal thickness might also change.

10. Acknowledgments

We thank Orly Yakir, MA for the statistical analysis.

11. References

[1] von Noorden GK. Binocular Vision and Ocular Motility: Theory and Management. 5th Ed. St. Louis: Mosby-Year book Inc. 1996;216-54.
[2] Daw NW. Critical periods and amblyopia. Arch Opthalmol 1998;116:502-5.
[3] Scheiman MN, Hertle RW, Beck RW et at. Randomized trial of treatment of amblyopia in children aged 7 to 17 years. Arch Ophthalmol 2005;123:437-47.

[4] Levartovsky S, Oliver M, Gottesman N, Shimshoni M. Factors affecting long term results of successfully treated amblyopia: initial visual acuity and type of amblyopia. Br J Ophthalmol 1995;79:225-8.

[5] Altintas O, Yüksel N, Ozkan B, Caglar Y. Thickness of the retinal nerve fiber layer, macular thickness, and macular volume in patients with strabismic amblyopia. J Pediatr Ophthalmol Strabismus 2005;42:216-21.

[6] Yen M, Cheng C, Wang A. Retinal nerve fiber layer thickness in unilateral amblyopia. Invest Ophthalmol Vis Sci 2004;45:2224-30.

[7] Kee SY, Lee SY, Lee YC. Thicknesses of the fovea and retinal nerve fiber layer in amblyopic and normal eyes in children. Korean J Ophthalmol 2006;20:177-81.

[8] Park KH, Hwang JM, Ahn JK. Efficacy of amblyopia therapy initiated after 9 years of age. Eye 2004;18:571-4.

[9] Repka MX, Wallace DK, Beck RW et al. Two-year follow-up of a 6-month randomized trial of atropine vs patching for treatment of moderate amblyopia in children. Arch Ophthalmol 2005;123:149-57.

[10] Scheiman MN, Hertle RW, Kraker RT et at. Patching vs atropine to treat amblyopia in children aged 7 to 12 years: a randomiz. Arch Ophthalmol 126;1634-42.

[11] von Noorden GK, Crawford ML, Levacy RA. The lateral geniculate nucleus in human anisometropic amblyopia. Invest Ophthalmol Vis Sci 1983;24:788-90.

[12] Grigg J, Thomas R, Billson F. Neuronal basis of amblyopia: a review. Indian J Ophthalmol 1996;44:69-76.

[13] Demer JL, von Noorden GK, Volkow ND, Gould KL. Imaging of cerebral blood flow and metabolism in amblyopia by positron emission tomography. Am J Ophthalmol 1988;105:337-347.

[14] Huynh SC, Samarawichkama C, Wang XY et al. Macular and nerve fiber layer thickness in amblyopia. The Sydney Childhood Eye Study. Ophthalmology 2009;116:1604-9.

[15] Meyer CH, Lapolice DJ, Freedman SF. Foveal hypoplasia in oculocutaneous albinism demonstrated by optical coherence tomography. Am J Ophthalmol 2002;133:409-10.

[16] Harvey PS, King RA, SummeCG. Spectrum of foveal development in albinism detected with optical coherence tomography. J AAPOS 2006;10:237-42.

[17] Izquierdo NJ, Emanuelli A, Izquierdo JC et al. Foveal thickness and macular volume in patients with oculocutaneous albinism. Retina 2007;27:1227-30.

[18] Bijlsma WR, van Schooneveld MJ, Van der Lelij A. Optical coherence tomography findings for nanophthalmic eyes. Retina 2008;28:1002-7.

[19] Mietz H, Green WR, Wolff SM, Abundo GP. Foveal hypoplasia in complete oculocutaneous albinism. A histopathologic study. Retina 1992;12:254-60.

[20] Neuville JM, Bronson-Castain K, Bears MA Jr et al. OCT reveals regional differences in macular thickness with age. Optom Vis Sci 2009;86:E810-6.

[21] Muscat S, Parks S, Kemp E, Keating D. Repeatability and reproducibility of macular thickness measurements with the Humphrey OCT system. Invest Ophthalmol Vis Sci 2002;43:490-5.

10

Myopia, Light and Circadian Rhythms

John R. Phillips, Simon Backhouse and Andrew V. Collins
Department of Optometry and Vision Science, The University of Auckland
New Zealand

1. Introduction

Myopia has been investigated scientifically for over a century but the search for an effective remedy has been manifestly unsuccessful. The prevalence of myopia in developed societies has now risen to about 30% in USA (Vitale, Sperduto et al. 2009) and up to 70% in some Asian centres (Lin, Shih et al. 2004). In addition to the socio-economic burden of providing optical corrections for myopia, common myopia limits career choice and increases the risk of glaucoma and cataract. High myopia also increases the risk of retinal detachment, chorio-retinal degeneration and subsequent visual impairment (Saw, Gazzard et al. 2005). Both genetic and environmental factors have been implicated in the aetiology of myopia. Children with myopic parents have a higher than normal risk of developing myopia (Mutti, Mitchell et al. 2002) and twin studies show a higher level of concordance of common myopia in monozygotic compared to dizygotic twins (Dirani, Chamberlain et al. 2006). However, the rapid rise in myopia prevalence over recent decades argues strongly that changing environmental factors also play an important role in the aetiology of myopia.

In the early 1900s Fuchs asserted *'The following means are advised to put a stop to the extension of myopia in schools. First, the excess of work which many scholars have at present to struggle with should be reduced'*…. *'Instruction ought not to begin too early (if possible not before the completion of the sixth year) and more time should be allotted to bodily exercise, especially in the open air, than has hitherto been the case.'* (Duane 1919). Although the long-held view that myopia primarily results from too much near-work is now regarded as an over-simplification, several recent studies support Fuchs's idea that outdoor activity may have an important role in protecting against myopia.

There have been many attempts to inhibit the progression of myopia in children. More recently, these have included treatment with antimuscarinic agents such as atropine eye-drops (Chua, Balakrishnan et al. 2006) and optical devices including multifocal spectacle lenses (Gwiazda, Hyman et al. 2003), dual-focus contact lenses (Anstice and Phillips 2011) and orthokeratology (Kakita, Hiraoka et al. 2011). However, none of these approaches entirely arrests myopia progression in the long term and the vast majority of myopia is managed by optical correction alone. Although conventional optical corrections including refractive surgery restore acuity, they do not prevent the abnormal enlargement of the myopic eye, so children with myopia remain at increased risk of ocular disease later in life.

In this review we examine evidence from human and animal studies that one aspect of outdoor activity, namely exposure to natural light, may reduce the prevalence and progression of myopia. We focus on the timing of light exposure in relation to the circadian cycle and on the potential roles of dopamine and melatonin in control of ocular growth and refractive development.

2. Human myopia and light

2.1 Outdoor activity

Current epidemiological research, as quantified by validated surveys, supports the idea that time spent in outdoor activities has a beneficial effect in reducing myopia prevalence in children and young adults (Jones, Sinnott et al. 2007; Rose, Morgan et al. 2008a; Rose, Morgan et al. 2008b). Whether the effect derives predominantly from increased natural light exposure or increased activity (e.g. sport) or from greater viewing distances outdoors has yet to be ascertained. An association between greater physical activity and reduced myopia progression has been reported in university students (Jacobsen, Jensen et al. 2008) although this association may have been confounded by other factors in the outdoor environment where much of the activity took place. Other studies have found an association between increased outdoor hours and lower myopia even when time spent playing sport outdoors was excluded (Rose, Morgan et al. 2008a). Moreover, indoor sport appears to have no beneficial effect (Rose, Morgan et al. 2008a; Dirani, Tong et al. 2009) suggesting that physical activity alone cannot account for the effect of outdoor activity. Whether the increased viewing distance typically associated with being outdoors has a positive effect in reducing myopia is unknown. The idea that time spent outdoors may act beneficially by substituting for time spent in near and mid-working distance activities seems not to be the case (Rose, Morgan et al. 2008a). In relation to distance viewing outdoors, the accommodative demand for viewing beyond about 6 metres is minimal. Indoor environments, particularly in city apartments, inevitably restrict viewing distance and typically include low dioptric stimuli for accommodation over the peripheral visual field (Charman 2011). However, the most obvious difference between spending time outdoors and time indoors is in light exposure. The spectral composition of light outdoors includes large amounts of ultraviolet (UV) and infrared (IR) in addition to light in the visible spectrum. Indoors, the UV portion of the spectrum is largely absent and if incandescent lighting is used the composition of the light is often biased towards the red end of the spectrum. Light intensity indoors is rarely more than 800 lux, whereas outdoor light intensity is around 50,000 lux on a sunny, blue-sky day and is rarely less than 5,000 lux, even when overcast. The cumulative light exposure for one hour spent outdoors is thus very much greater than for one hour spent indoors (Backhouse, Ng et al. 2011). This increased light exposure during the day is generally believed to be the most likely basis for the beneficial effect of outdoor activity in reducing myopia prevalence (Rose, Morgan et al. 2008a).

2.2 Light at night

Between birth and 2 years of age, the normal eye grows very rapidly, with axial length increasing at a rate of about 2 mm/year before slowing to about 0.1 mm/year until the eye reaches adult size (Larsen 1971). It has been suggested that environmental influences acting in this early period of rapid eye growth may potentially affect refractive development later in life. Quinn et al. (Quinn, Shin et al. 1999) investigated the effects of light exposure early in life on refractive status later in childhood. Their study, which was based on a questionnaire completed by parents of children aged 2-16 years (median 8 years) on their child's night-time light-exposure, reported a strong, dose-dependent association between the prevalence of myopia at the time of the study and night-time lighting conditions experienced by the children before the age of 2 years. Remarkably, 55% of children who slept with the room lights on developed myopia whereas 34% of children who slept with night-lights, and 10% of children who slept in darkness, had developed myopia at the time of the study. On the statistical strength of their findings, the authors suggested that the absence of a daily period of darkness could be a precipitating factor in the later development of myopia. A similar study (Czepita, Goslawski et al. 2004) also reported increased prevalence of myopia in children who had experienced ambient light at night before the age of 2 years. However, several studies in different parts of the world, also based on parental questionnaires, have reported no difference in prevalence of myopia in children sleeping in darkness or with ambient light at night before the age of 2 years (USA (Gwiazda, Ong et al. 2000; Zadnik, Jones et al. 2000), Asia (Saw, Zhang et al. 2002), UK (Guggenheim, Hill et al. 2003)). Both studies from the USA found associations between the number of myopic parents in the family and nursery lighting experienced by the child before the age of 2 years, suggesting that the results obtained by Quinn et al. may have been confounded by the uncontrolled effect of parental myopia. However, exposure to light at night may also affect the refractive development of young adults. A study of law students (Loman, Quinn et al. 2002) reported an association between increased myopia progression during law school with less daily exposure to darkness (i.e. more artificial light at night).

2.3 Season of birth

Further evidence for the influence of light exposure early in life on later refractive error comes from studies on the effect of season of birth (and by implication perinatal photoperiod) on adult refractive status. In a study population of 276,911 adolescents born in Israel (Mandel, Grotto et al. 2008), moderate and severe myopia prevalence varied by birth month, with the summer months (June/July) being associated with a higher myopia prevalence than the winter months (December/January). Moreover, increasing photoperiod was associated with increasing myopia prevalence in a dose-dependent pattern. Mild myopia was not associated with either season of birth or photoperiod. Birth during the summer was also found to be significantly associated with high myopia in a UK study (McMahon, Zayats et al. 2009) but no association was found between postnatal photoperiod and prevalence of myopia in adulthood. Seasonal variations in photoperiod are particularly extreme above the Arctic Circle. However, in a study of Finnish military conscripts (Vannas, Ying et al. 2003) no associations between myopia prevalence and birth month, global irradiance at birth month or daily hours of darkness during the birth month were found, although there was a trend towards higher prevalence of myopia among conscripts living above the Arctic Circle.

The human data on light exposure and refractive development suggest that increased day-time outdoor light exposure is associated with reduced myopia prevalence whereas increased night-time exposure to artificial light may be associated with increased myopia development – a case of day-light good, night-light bad. The remainder of this review examines the underlying processes which could explain why perturbations in the daily light-dark cycle may affect eye growth and refractive development.

3. Light and animal models of myopia

Animal studies have shown that a diurnal light:dark photoperiod is required for the normal refractive development of the eye in chicks (Li, Troilo et al. 1995; Stone, Lin et al. 1995), tree shrews (Norton, Amedo et al. 2006) and Rhesus monkeys (Smith, Bradley et al. 2001). In normal chick eyes there is a diurnal growth rhythm in which greatest eye elongation occurs during the day with reduced growth rates at night (Weiss and Schaeffel 1993; Nickla, Wildsoet et al. 1998). The choroid also demonstrates a similar diurnal rhythm in which the choroid thins during the day and thickens at night (Papastergiou, Schmid et al. 1998). In eyes deprived of form vision in order to induce myopia, a phase shift occurs in the relationship between the axial length and choroidal rhythms such that peak axial growth occurs earlier than in normal eyes (Nickla, Wildsoet et al. 1998).

3.1 Effect of constant light

Rearing chicks under constant light with open eyes produces hyperopia, due to corneal flattening resulting in shallow anterior chambers (Li, Troilo et al. 1995; Stone, Lin et al. 1995). While the anterior chamber becomes shallower, the vitreous chamber lengthens, resulting in no net change in axial length at 2 weeks of age. Continued rearing of chicks in constant light beyond 2 weeks produces macrophthalmos (Oishi, Lauber et al. 1987). The final refractive state may be hyperopic despite the development of significantly deeper vitreous chambers (Li, Troilo et al. 1995). In form-deprived eyes, constant light also produces hyperopia despite overall longer axial lengths and enlarged vitreous chambers in both axial and equatorial directions; (Stone, Lin et al. 1995).

While rearing chicks under continuous light produces hyperopia, the effect is dependent on the level of ambient illumination. Thus, higher light intensities are correlated with higher degrees of hyperopia, lower corneal power and increased vitreous chamber depth. Cohen et al. (Cohen, Belkin et al. 2008) reported that chicks raised under continuous illumination at 10,000 lux for 90 days developed a hyperopic mean refraction of +11.97D, while those raised under 50 lux resulted in an emmetropic mean refraction of +0.63D. An illumination level of 500 lux also produced a relatively high hyperopic outcome of +7.90D. While vitreous chamber depth was positively correlated with light intensity, overall axial length did not vary significantly between groups due to the corneal flattening associated with increasing light intensity, resulting in an overall hyperopic refraction at the moderate and high illumination levels (Cohen, Belkin et al. 2008).

Monkeys raised under continuous light conditions (Smith, Bradley et al. 2001) do not exhibit the increase in ocular growth typically found in the chick. Rhesus monkeys raised under continuous light for 6 months developed hyperopic refractions similar in magnitude to animals raised under normal diurnal light cycles. However, the refractions were more variable in outcome, with some animals developing axial anisometropia and low myopia (Smith, Bradley et al. 2001). The authors cautioned that the animals may have been able to re-establish at least a partial diurnal cycle by shielding their eyes during sleep with their arms, although no significant difference in behaviour was observed (Smith, Bradley et al. 2001).

3.2 Effect of constant darkness

Rearing chicks in complete darkness also produces hyperopia irrespective of whether a diffusing goggle is worn (Gottlieb, Fugate-Wentzek et al. 1987). The degree of hyperopia produced is approximately double that of normal chicks by 42 days. In contrast, tree shrews placed in continuous darkness eventually exhibit a myopic shift in refraction (Norton, Amedo et al. 2006). Although the animals initially stabilise at a low degree of hyperopia following 16 days of normal visual experience after eye opening, a subsequent period of 10 days of continuous darkness results in vitreous elongation and a myopic refraction (Norton, Amedo et al. 2006). While both chicks and tree shrews exhibit ocular growth under constant darkness, the significant corneal flattening which produces hyperopia in chicks does not occur in the tree shrew. Conversely, raising rhesus monkeys in continuous darkness appears to interfere with the emmetropisation process such that they retain their relatively high hyperopic neonatal refractions (Guyton, Greene et al. 1989).

Gottlieb et al. (Gottlieb, Fugate-Wentzek et al. 1987) proposed that two mechanisms may combine under dark-rearing in chicks to produce the hyperopic outcome: a visual deprivation mechanism which triggers enlargement of the eye, as occurs in form-deprivation myopia, and a second photoperiod-related mechanism which results in corneal flattening.

A phase advance in the cycle of eye growth is found in chicks raised under constant darkness which is associated with an overall increase in axial growth and choroidal thinning (Nickla, Wildsoet et al. 2001). As the rhythms in choroidal thinning and axial growth persist under constant darkness, they must be circadian in origin, rather than simply diurnal in response to external light-dark cycles (Nickla, Wildsoet et al. 2001). Nickla (Nickla 2006) provides further evidence for the role of a phase shift in the temporal relationship between axial length and choroidal thickness cycles in the control of ocular growth in a study comparing recovery from form-deprivation, myopic defocus and hyperopic defocus in chicks. It appears that where the treatment requires a decrease in ocular growth (such as recovery from form-deprivation) the axial length and choroidal rhythms shift into phase. The mechanism by which such a phase shift might influence ocular growth is not certain, although it has been proposed that the variation in thickness of the choroid may regulate diffusion of a signal molecule from the retina to the sclera, or may act as a mechanical scaffolding against the influence of diurnal intra-ocular pressure changes on the sclera (Nickla 2006).

3.3 Diurnal modulation of illumination

In order to determine the minimum period of darkness within the diurnal light:dark cycle that is required for normal eye growth, Li et al. (Li, Howland et al. 2000) investigated the effect of various periods of darkness from zero (constant light) to a standard 12:12 h light:dark cycle in chicks. They found that at least 4 hours darkness per diurnal cycle produced a normal emmetropisation response in the chick (Li, Howland et al. 2000). Further investigations demonstrated that the 4 hours of darkness was most effective in blocking the effects of excess light exposure when presented in a single period at the same time of day, rather than at random times or as multiple periods totalling 4 hours (Li, Howland et al. 2000). Li et al. (Li, Howland et al. 2000) concluded that this period of darkness may be sufficient to entrain the intrinsic circadian clock of the avian retina (Morgan and Boelen 1996). The requirement for periods of darkness during a diurnal cycle in order to produce normal eye growth in chicks has a potential corollary in humans. As noted earlier, the use of night lights in children's bedrooms under the age of 2 years has been associated with the development of myopia in later life (Quinn, Shin et al. 1999).

Diurnal modulation of ambient illumination rather than the need for periods of total darkness may be the significant requirement for normal emmetropisation in chicks. Liu et al. (Liu, Pendrak et al. 2004) reared chicks under light:dark, light:dim and constant light cycles with the aim of investigating the effect of ambient lighting at night on emmetropisation. The irradiance of the light phase was 1500 $\mu W/cm^2$, while the dim phase varied between 0.01 and 500 $\mu W/cm^2$. The eyes of chicks raised under light:dark and light:dim cycles had comparable ocular refractions and dimensions. Conversely, rearing under constant light levels from 1 $\mu W/cm^2$ (~0.3 lux) to 1500 $\mu W/cm^2$ (~500 lux) produced the typical shallow anterior chamber and hyperopic shift in refraction as found previously in chicks. These results imply that the modulation of light levels during a diurnal cycle may be of more importance in the maintenance of the normal emmetropisation response than the absolute light (or dark) levels. Consequently, the use of light:dim diurnal cycles may be a more pertinent paradigm for study as it more closely approximates the typical urban environment with artificial lighting at night (Liu, Pendrak et al. 2004).

3.4 Amplitude modulation of illumination

Recent animal investigations support the fundamental hypothesis that light exposure is the mediator of the antimyopiagenic effect of outdoor activity (Rose, Morgan et al. 2008a). Experiments in chicks have shown that exposure to high ambient light levels, either artificial or natural, modifies the development of experimental myopia due to either visual form deprivation using translucent occluders, or induced defocus using spectacle lenses (Ashby, Ohlendorf et al. 2009; Ashby and Schaeffel 2010). While exposure to high illumination levels of 15,000 lux for 5 hours per day significantly reduced form-deprivation myopia by around 60%, in lens-induced myopia the rate of compensation for the induced defocus was modified, but not the final degree of refractive error produced (Ashby and Schaeffel 2010). The normal emmetropisation process in chicks can also be directly influenced by ambient light levels: raising animals under low light levels (50 lux) produced myopic refractive outcomes on average, while high light levels (10,000 lux) produced hyperopic refractive outcomes (Cohen, Belkin et al. 2011).

In form-deprivation experiments in chicks, exposure to high artificial light (15,000 lux) indoors or natural light (30,000 lux) outdoors for 15 minutes per day with occluders removed was sufficient to produce a statistically significant decrease in axial myopia beyond that produced by the removal of the occluders under normal laboratory light levels (500 lux) (Ashby, Ohlendorf et al. 2009). The antimyopiagenic effect of high illumination levels was also demonstrated under constant occluder wear conditions where a significant decrease in axial myopia development was also demonstrated in chicks raised under 15,000 lux for 6 hours per day when compared to animals raised under 50 or 500 lux (Ashby, Ohlendorf et al. 2009). As the antimyopiagenic effect occurred during continuous occluder wear the authors conclude that the effect cannot be due to a reduction in image blur resulting from pupil constriction as these animals did not receive clear form vision at any time in the occluded eye. It has been suggested that high ambient illumination levels may affect the diurnal variation in retinal dopamine, which is disrupted in form-deprivation in chicks (Weiss and Schaeffel 1993), with the proposal that the chick retina has a graded release of dopamine under high illumination levels which results in a retardation of myopia development (Ashby, Ohlendorf et al. 2009). The intra-vitreal administration of a dopamine antagonist (spiperone) blocked the protective effect of high illumination levels against form-deprivation myopia in chicks (Ashby and Schaeffel 2010) further supporting the hypothesis that this neurotransmitter is intrinsically involved in the control of the emmetropisation mechanism (Ashby and Schaeffel 2010; Mao, Liu et al. 2010; Nickla, Totonelly et al. 2010).

3.5 Chromaticity and refractive development

The contribution of the chromatic component of light to refractive development has been investigated in a number of animal models including chicks (Rucker and Wallman 2009), fish (Kroger and Wagner 1996) and guinea pigs (Long, Chen et al. 2009). Guinea pigs raised under long-wavelength light (peak at 760 nm) reportedly develop a significant degree of myopia, associated with a significant increase in vitreous chamber depth, over a period of 4 weeks when compared to animals raised under mixed-wavelength light (unfiltered halogen lamps) (Long, Chen et al. 2009). The myopiagenic effect of long-wavelength light was reversed by allowing the animals to recover under mixed-wavelength light conditions for two weeks, after which there was no significant difference in refraction (Long, Chen et al. 2009).

One possible explanation for the effect of wavelength on refractive outcome is based on the intrinsic chromatic aberration of the vertebrate eye (Mandelman and Sivak 1983) which could provide a sign-of-defocus signal for emmetropisation (Flitcroft 1990) as the long and short wavelength components would produce relative hyperopic and myopic defocus of the retinal image respectively. For example, in a comparison of the effects of raising guinea pigs under equiluminant short wavelength light (430 nm) or middle wavelength light (530 nm), Liu et al. (Liu, Qian et al. 2011) demonstrated that after 12 weeks the 530 nm group was less hyperopic due to faster vitreous elongation, while the 430 nm group was more hyperopic following slower vitreous elongation. The difference in refraction between the groups (4.50 D) exceeded the longitudinal chromatic aberration of the guinea pig eye (approximately 1.5 D) at the selected wavelengths, which was possibly due to additional accommodative effects produced by the monochromatic illumination (Seidemann and Schaeffel 2002), or by wavelength-dependent alteration of retinal or retinal pigment epithelium growth signals (Liu, Qian et al. 2011).

4. Light and circadian rhythms

The role of illumination level and the requirement for periodic light:dark cycles during normal refractive development points to a role for the intrinsic circadian clock and the associated dopamine-melatonin cycle in the control of eye growth (Cahill and Besharse 1995; Witkovsky 2004; Iuvone, Tosini et al. 2005). The presumed role of circadian rhythms, which persist in constant darkness independent of the diurnal light:dark cycle, is to regulate the timing of biological events so as to optimise the metabolic function and energy use of the organism (Roenneberg and Foster 1997; Levi and Schibler 2007).

4.1 The circadian pacemaker

Although the control of the circadian rhythm is a complex, multivariate process, it has been known for some time that light plays a pivotal role (Iuvone, Tosini et al. 2005). The underlying circadian rhythm is controlled by a circadian clock, through the expression of "clock genes" and their products, and entrainment cues known as zeitgebers ("time givers") which influence the timing of these rhythms (Roenneberg and Foster 1997; Iuvone, Tosini et al. 2005). The primary, central time keeping clock in the body is the suprachiasmatic nucleus (SCN) of the hypothalamus (Roenneberg and Foster 1997). The primary input to the SCN is from the retina via the retinohypothalamic tract (RHT) (Simonneaux and Ribelayga 2003), which makes light the primary zeitgeber for entrainment of the circadian rhythm (Roenneberg and Foster 1997). While input via the RHT is not necessary for the generation of a circadian rhythm (evidenced by the free running nature of the SCN rhythm), it is necessary for the entrainment of the circadian rhythm to the normal light:dark cycle (Inouye and Kawamura 1979).

4.2 The light entrainment pathway

The traditional view of the photosensitive retinal organisation is of a dual photoreceptor system comprising both rods and cones. However, circadian entrainment has been found to originate from a small subset of retinal ganglion cells, the intrinsically photosensitive retinal ganglion cells (ipRGCs) (Berson, Dunn et al. 2002; Hattar, Liao et al. 2002). The photopigment melanopsin, first described in melanophores on frog skin and subsequently found in the inner retina of a number of mammals including humans, provides the ipRGCs with this photosensitivity (Provencio, Rodriguez et al. 2000; Hattar, Liao et al. 2002). Melanopsin has an action spectrum that peaks around 480 nm (Berson, Dunn et al. 2002). However, studies in melanopsin-knockout mice showed that melanopsin is not essential for light entrainment of the circadian pacemaker, but improves the magnitude of the response (Ruby, Brennan et al. 2002). It transpires that the melanopsin-containing ipRGCs also receive input from the traditional rod and cone photoreceptors (Perez-Leon, Warren et al. 2006). There is a loss of photo-entrainment, but a persistence of pattern vision, in animals without functional ipRGCs providing definitive support for the role of the ipRGCs in the entrainment of the circadian system by light (Guler, Ecker et al. 2008). The entrainment of the circadian system in mammals is thus mediated by the ipRGCs as a balance between intrinsic photoreception enabled by melanopsin and input from the traditional retinal photoreceptors. In chicks melanopsin is found in both the retina and the pineal gland, indicating light can entrain the circadian pacemaker through both retinal (via ipRGCs) and direct pineal routes (Torii, Kojima et al. 2007; Neumann, Ziegler et al. 2008).

The SCN, working as a central master clock, controls the circadian timing of the organism through a multisynaptic pathway. The SCN projects to neurones in the paraventricular hypothalamic nucleus, which synapse preganglionic sympathetic neurons in the intermediolateral cell column, stimulating postganglionic sympathetic neurons in the superior cervical ganglion, before finally providing sympathetic input to the pineal gland (Larsen, Enquist et al. 1998). The main circadian mediator from the pineal gland is melatonin, a hormone first isolated from bovine pineal glands and named for its ability to lighten the melanocytes in frog skin (Lerner, Case et al. 1958). Melatonin acts through melatonin receptors in a diverse range of tissues, performing a variety of roles in circadian entrainment, endocrine functions, cardiovascular responses, the immune system, and ocular physiology (Alarma-Estrany and Pintor 2007).

4.3 Melatonin precursors

Melatonin (N-acetyl-5-methoxytryptamine) is a circadian hormone produced through a pathway involving four precursor intermediaries (Fig. 1.). All of the components necessary for the production of melatonin are active within the pineal gland, which is the main site of production (Axelrod 1974; Zawilska, Skene et al. 2009). The first step is the conversion of the dietary amino acid tryptophan to 5-hydroxytryptophan by the enzyme tryptophan hydroxylase (TPH); the second step involves the conversion of 5-hydroxytryptophan to serotonin via the enzyme aromatic L-amino acid decarboxylase (AADC); serotonin is converted in the third step to N-acetylserotonin by the enzyme arylalkylamine-N-acetyltransferase (AANAT); the final step is the O-methylation of N-acetylserotonin to melatonin by the enzyme hydroxyindole-O-methyltransferase (HIOMT). The rate limiting enzyme in the production of melatonin is widely thought to be AANAT, although recent work suggests that HIOMT may be the crucial limiting factor (Liu and Borjigin 2005). The precursor components of melatonin synthesis also show inherent circadian rhythms of production (Axelrod 1974). The retina is another significant producer of melatonin in some animals, providing the basis for a peripheral clock in addition to the central clock of the pineal gland (Iuvone, Tosini et al. 2005)

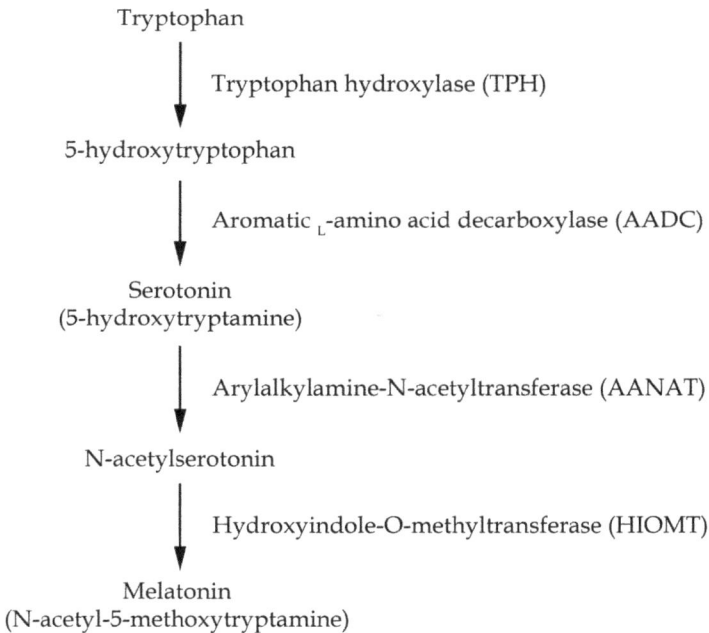

Tryptophan

$\downarrow$ Tryptophan hydroxylase (TPH)

5-hydroxytryptophan

$\downarrow$ Aromatic $_{L}$-amino acid decarboxylase (AADC)

Serotonin
(5-hydroxytryptamine)

$\downarrow$ Arylalkylamine-N-acetyltransferase (AANAT)

N-acetylserotonin

$\downarrow$ Hydroxyindole-O-methyltransferase (HIOMT)

Melatonin
(N-acetyl-5-methoxytryptamine)

Fig. 1. Melatonin production pathway showing the precursor compounds and the enzymes involved.

4.4 Circadian melatonin rhythms

In the majority of species studied to date, whether they are diurnally or nocturnally active, there is a circadian secretion pattern of melatonin with high levels present at night and low levels during the day (Zawilska, Skene et al. 2009). The onset of darkness following a period of light leads to an increase in pineal AANAT and melatonin levels in phase with each other (Wilkinson, Arendt et al. 1977). However, there appears to be a refractory period for dark-induced melatonin rises such that darkness during periods when the organism is expecting it to be light does not induce the rise (Binkley, Macbride et al. 1975). Three distinct patterns of nocturnal melatonin production have been described in mammals: Type A is uncommon and represents a peak in melatonin late in the dark phase (e.g. Syrian hamster and house mouse); Type B is most common and shows peak melatonin expression occurring around midnight (e.g. rat, guinea pig, and human); and Type C which is also common and shows elevated melatonin levels for most of the dark phase (e.g. sheep and cat) (Zawilska, Skene et al. 2009). The human melatonin cycle, like that of animals (Tast, Love et al. 2001), can be entrained to variations in the light:dark cycle. When the light:dark cycle is phase-shifted by 12 hours, the human rhythm in melatonin secretion re-entrains to the new dark phase over a period of 5 to 7 days (Lynch, Jimerson et al. 1978).

4.5 Light and melatonin suppression

Darkness is required for the rise in melatonin, as animals kept in constant light show a reduction or complete loss of melatonin synthesis (Perlow, Reppert et al. 1980). However, the factor mediating the entrainment of the melatonin rhythm appears to be light exposure. Presentation of light during the dark phase, when melatonin levels are elevated, results in a rapid suppression of production and a reduction in serum melatonin concentration (e.g. (Illnerova, Backstrom et al. 1978; Rollag, O'Callaghan et al. 1978)). Human melatonin suppression by light is intensity dependant, with brighter light leading to greater levels of melatonin suppression (McIntyre, Norman et al. 1989; Zeitzer, Dijk et al. 2000). Suppression to near daytime levels (67% suppression) is achieved with 1000 lux (McIntyre, Norman et al. 1989), while a half maximal suppression response can be seen between approximately 50 and 130 lux (Zeitzer, Dijk et al. 2000). This light induced suppression also shows an inverse correlation with duration, such that longer durations of light require lower intensities of light to induce suppression (Aoki, Yamada et al. 1998). However, independent of light level there appears to be an asymptote for melatonin suppression after around 60 minutes of light exposure (Figueiro, Rea et al. 2006). Interestingly the melatonin suppression by light appears to be sensitised/desensitised by the amount of light received during the day prior, such that less light exposure (as experienced during winter months) results in much greater melatonin suppression for a given amount of light at night (Smith, Schoen et al. 2004; Higuchi, Motohashi et al. 2007).

The action spectrum for melatonin suppression shows peak effect between 446 and 477 nm (Brainard, Hanifin et al. 2001; Thapan, Arendt et al. 2001). The light response of the melanopsin containing ipRGCs mirrors that of the melatonin suppression action spectrum, indicating that these cells are the likely mediators of the response (Berson, Dunn et al. 2002). Circadian photo-entrainment also appears to be mediated by a peak action spectrum response from the same blue wavelength portion of the spectrum (Hattar, Lucas et al. 2003). These responses are also seen in humans, although a greater response is seen when polychromatic light is used instead of monochromatic light at peak melanopsin sensitivity, suggesting melanopsin may not be solely responsible and that rod and cone input also play a role (Revell and Skene 2007). Despite uncertainty as to the exact cellular input driving the circadian entrainment, it is clear that the blue end of the spectrum is important. Interestingly, exposure to the blue part of the spectrum also appears to suppress myopia development in guinea pigs (e.g. (Liu, Qian et al. 2011; Wang, Zhou et al. 2011)).

Wang et al. (Wang, Zhou et al. 2011) raised guinea pigs under blue light (480 nm), green light (530 nm) and broadband white light. After 10 days the levels of melatonin in the pineal glands were significantly lower in both the blue light and white light groups when compared to the green light group. This difference existed in both daytime (10 am) and night-time (10 pm) samples. The green-light group were also about 2 D more myopic, had greater axial lengths and greater vitreous depths than the other groups. Furthermore the green-light group exhibited reduced expression of retinal melanopsin mRNA and reduced levels of melanopsin protein. MT1 receptor mRNA expression was higher in both the retina and sclera of the green-light group. Overall this study demonstrated a clear link between wavelength of illumination, refractive error development and modulation of the melatonin pathway in guinea pigs.

4.6 Light as a zeitgeber

Light is the primary zeitgeber for the entrainment of the circadian system (Roenneberg and Foster 1997). Phase response curves have shown that the timing of light exposure is critical to circadian responses to light (Daan and Pittendrigh 1976). When light is presented at the beginning of the subjective night there is a phase delay of the subsequent activity-rest cycle, while light presented at the end of the subjective night leads to a phase advance. Presentation of light during the subjective day has little effect on the phase response curve, suggesting the twilight zones of dusk and dawn are the key times for entrainment (Roenneberg and Foster 1997). The phase shifting effect of light also affects the timing of the dim light melatonin onset (the increase in melatonin levels at night) (Lewy, Sack et al. 1985). Bright light in the evening delays dim light melatonin onset while bright light in the morning advances it. Bright light presented both in the morning and evening gives an intermediate response between delay and advance (Lewy, Sack et al. 1987). Exposure to bright light results in immediate melatonin suppression, but longer exposure of greater intensity is required to entrain the pacemaker (Hashimoto, Nakamura et al. 1996). However, dim light exposure at the appropriate time and for a long enough period has also been shown to entrain the circadian system (Zeitzer, Dijk et al. 2000). The importance of the timing of the signal for entrainment has a parallel in form-deprivation myopia wherein removal of the occluder for 40 minutes in the evening is more effective at reducing the induced myopia than if the occluder is removed in the morning (Ohngemach, Feldkaemper et al. 2001).

4.7 Photoperiodism and photoperiodic history

Photoperiodism, the adaptation of an organism's physiological functions to changes in season, is thought to be determined by both the absolute photoperiod length and by changes (either increasing or decreasing) in photoperiod length (Goldman 2001). Three main hypotheses to explain the influence of melatonin on this phenomenon exist: the duration, coincidence, and amplitude hypotheses.

The duration hypothesis proposes that the duration of night-time melatonin release is used as a signal encoding day length, with a shorter duration melatonin signal indicating long day/short night periods and vice versa (Simonneaux and Ribelayga 2003). In pinealectomised animals, short duration infusion of melatonin replicates a long day reproductive response while long duration infusion replicates a short day response (e.g.

(Bittman and Karsch 1984; Maywood, Buttery et al. 1990)). The coincidence hypothesis proposes that there is a coincidence between a sensitive period for signal detection and the presence of the melatonin signal. Infusion of melatonin at specific circadian time points in pinealectomised individuals suggests a critical period of sensitivity either at the onset of the dark phase (Gunduz and Stetson 2001), or at a specific time after the initial melatonin rise (Pitrosky, Kirsch et al. 1995). More recent work suggests that the coincidence timing effect of melatonin acts through clock gene expression oscillations (for review see (Hazlerigg and Wagner 2006)). While the amplitude hypothesis, which proposes that the peak amplitude of melatonin secretion is the signal for seasonal timing, is often discussed (e.g. (Simonneaux and Ribelayga 2003)), very little experimental data exists to back it up. Thus duration and timing of circadian signals may be more important than signal amplitude for circadian entrainment.

During periods of intermediate day-length between the winter and summer solstices a single day-length signal is insufficient to determine whether the days are becoming longer or shorter, so photoperiodic history, based upon the length of the preceding days, is used. The photoperiodic history appears to rely on the summation of recent photoperiod information over a number of days (Prendergast, Gorman et al. 2000), and the prenatal photoperiod actually appears to modify the postnatal day-length threshold which controls the maximal rate of development (Shaw and Goldman 1995). The ability of the perinatal photoperiodic history to influence future development rates may explain the observed season of birth effect in human refractive development (see Section 2.3).

5. Peripheral clocks

In addition to the master central circadian clock, peripheral systems and indeed individual cells also possess clocks (reviewed by (Balsalobre 2002)). Of these the retina, which also provides the main entrainment cue for the central clock, constitutes the most relevant peripheral clock for refractive development. The retina is a highly circadian tissue, showing rhythms in a variety of functions including visual sensitivity, the electroretinogram response, rod outer segment disc shedding, melanopsin mRNA expression, melatonin synthesis, and dopamine synthesis (for excellent reviews see (Iuvone, Tosini et al. 2005; Tosini, Pozdeyev et al. 2008)).

5.1 Retinal melatonin

Melatonin is synthesised in the retina in a circadian manner, independent of the SCN, in both non-mammalian (Cahill and Besharse 1992; Thomas, Tigges et al. 1993) and mammalian (Tosini and Menaker 1996) vertebrates. The retinal photoreceptors appear to be the source of this retinal melatonin production, with AANAT and HIOMT activity having been localised mainly to these cells, and only minimal activity in the inner nuclear layer and ganglion cells (Guerlotte, Greve et al. 1996; Coon, Del Olmo et al. 2002). Moreover, melatonin continues to be produced despite partial or complete destruction of the inner retina (Cahill and Besharse 1992; Thomas, Tigges et al. 1993). Human and primate retinas appear to be missing activity of the HIOMT enzyme, with expression of HIOMT mRNA in such small quantities that it contributes little to the production of melatonin (Bernard, Donohue et al. 1995; Coon, Del Olmo et al. 2002). However, labelling and activity of HIOMT in human photoreceptors has been demonstrated (Wiechmann and

Hollyfield 1987), although this has not been repeated by other groups. It has been postulated that N-acetylserotonin might take the place of a local melatonin signal in the retina of humans and primates (Iuvone, Tosini et al. 2005), or that the signal is provided by circulating melatonin levels (Osol and Schwartz 1984). Interestingly, human RPE and ciliary body also synthesise melatonin (Martin, Malina et al. 1992; Zmijewski, Sweatman et al. 2009).

5.2 Central and retinal dopamine rhythms

Dopamine is a neurotransmitter that has a multitude of roles, such as in learning and movement (Witkovsky 2004). Plasma dopamine levels in humans show a circadian rhythm in concentration that is phase-shifted relative to melatonin by approximately 180 degrees, peaking in the light phase and reaching lowest levels during the dark phase (Sowers and Vlachakis 1984). Primates (Perlow, Gordon et al. 1977), rats (Schade, Vick et al. 1995), and birds (Kang, Thayananuphat et al. 2007) also show these circadian rhythms in dopamine production; high in light, low in dark, and out of phase with melatonin. In pinealectomised rats the administration of melatonin suppresses dopamine expression in a dose-dependent manner (Khaldy, Leon et al. 2002).

Dopamine also has many roles in the retina, for example in light adaptation and cell death, as well as a potential role in ocular growth (Witkovsky 2004). As in the brain, retinal dopamine shows a diurnal rhythm with peak levels during the day and low levels during the night in non-human vertebrates (Nowak, Zurawska et al. 1989; Megaw, Boelen et al. 2006), and in human retinas (Di Paolo, Harnois et al. 1987). The diurnal variation in dopamine levels persists in constant darkness in mice, indicating that it has a circadian rhythm of release (Doyle, Grace et al. 2002), although others have found no circadian rhythm but a light activated fluctuation in retinal dopamine (Melamed, Frucht et al. 1984).

5.3 Light and dopamine

Dopamine is released from the perfused retina on exposing it to light (Kramer 1971), and light also stimulates retinal dopamine synthesis and turnover (Iuvone, Galli et al. 1978; Cohen, Hadjiconstantinou et al. 1983). Moreover, the light-activated rise in dopamine levels in the retina is much greater than the rise seen with the underlying circadian rhythm in constant darkness (Megaw, Boelen et al. 2006), and the metabolism of dopamine in the light is much greater than in the dark (Parkinson and Rando 1983; Megaw, Boelen et al. 2006). Furthermore, the intensity of light appears to be important for dopamine release and synthesis in the retina, with maximal stimulation and saturation of the response occurring between 32 to 80 lux in rats (Proll, Kamp et al. 1982; Brainard and Morgan 1987).

It transpires that change in light, in the form of flicker, is a more potent stimulus to dopamine release than constant light levels. This effect has been shown in several species, with increasing release rates seen with increasing stimulus presentation rates, and an increase in dopamine release above that seen with constant light alone (Kramer 1971; Weiler, Baldridge et al. 1997). Flickering light appears to increase dopamine release two to three times that of basal release levels. High frequency flicker at 6 Hz has also been shown to inhibit both form-deprivation myopia and lens-induced myopia in the chick (Schwahn and Schaeffel 1997). The degree of suppression is correlated with the length of the dark phase of the flicker duty cycle (Schwahn and Schaeffel 1997). This may be due to increased retinal dopamine levels as 2 hours of exposure to flickering light at 10 Hz was shown to restore the rate of dopamine synthesis under form-deprivation conditions in chicks, possibly due to increased transcription of the tyrosine hydroxylase gene in dopaminergic amacrine cells (Luft, Iuvone et al. 2004).

5.4 Dopamine and melatonin

When light is presented during the dark phase there is a rapid suppression of melatonin and an increase in dopamine to normal daytime levels (Adachi, Nogi et al. 1998). Interestingly, in knockout mice that do not produce melatonin there is a loss of the circadian dopamine rhythm when the animals are maintained in constant darkness, but the rhythm is restored on administering exogenous melatonin (Doyle, Grace et al. 2002). These results are intriguing as they show that in the absence of melatonin a normal dopamine rhythm can be maintained by light exposure in a rhythmic light:dark cycle, but that melatonin can, in the absence of a light driven zeitgeber, also influence dopamine rhythms. Indeed there is a complex interaction between melatonin and dopamine in the retina with mutual inhibitory effects between the two compounds. Intra-vitreal injection of dopamine into the eye at night suppresses melatonin while the injection of melatonin during the day suppresses dopamine (Adachi, Nogi et al. 1998). Melatonin leads to an increase in AANAT activity in the retina and a decrease in dopamine levels (Nowak, Zurawska et al. 1989; Nowak, Kazula et al. 1992), while dopamine inhibits retinal AANAT activity and melatonin release (Iuvone and Besharse 1986; Tosini and Dirden 2000).

As melatonin production has not been demonstrated in the human retina, endogenous melatonin released from the pineal gland potentially acts in the retina. Indeed high levels of melatonin are found in human retinas, and intraperitoneal injection of melatonin in mice leads to an increase in retinal melatonin levels (Osol and Schwartz 1984; Doyle, Grace et al. 2002). In chicks the pineal gland has been shown to have a significant influence over both expression of the dopamine D_2-receptor mRNA and dopamine release in the retina (Ohngemach, Feldkaemper et al. 2001). Dopamine has also been shown to increase the expression of melanopsin mRNA via a D_2-receptor pathway in ipRGCs (Sakamoto, Liu et al. 2005).

6. Dopamine, melatonin and refractive development

6.1 Dopamine

Retinal dopamine levels are reduced during the induction of form-deprivation myopia in the chick (Stone, Lin et al. 1989), rhesus monkey (Iuvone, Tigges et al. 1991) and guinea pig (Mao, Liu et al. 2010). In the chick, this reduction is due to a decreased rate of dopamine synthesis during the light phase of the diurnal light:dark cycle (Stone, Lin et al. 1989). The use of modified translucent occluders demonstrates that retinal dopamine levels inversely correlate with the degree of axial elongation (Stone, Pendrak et al. 2006). Retinal dopamine levels exhibit a bidirectional response to retinal blur in chicks, with lens-induced myopia decreasing and hyperopia increasing the levels respectively (Guo, Sivak et al. 1995) although this effect is not universally reported (Bartmann, Schaeffel et al. 1994). The increase in retinal dopamine associated with the slowing of axial growth in lens-induced hyperopia parallels recovery from form-deprivation myopia in the chick where a similar relationship between dopamine level and axial growth is reported (Pendrak, Nguyen et al. 1997).

The role of dopamine in the control of ocular growth is further supported by the demonstration that ocular administration of dopamine agonists can inhibit the axial growth and myopic refractions produced by form-deprivation in chicks (Rohrer, Spira et al. 1993; Nickla, Totonelly et al. 2010) and primates (Iuvone, Tigges et al. 1991). Also, extraocular administration of the dopamine precursor levodopa by intraperitoneal injection in guinea pigs raises retinal dopamine content and reduces the development of myopia during form-deprivation (Mao, Liu et al. 2010). The relationship between retinal dopamine pathways and lens-induced myopia is less certain. At dosages sufficient to suppress form-deprivation myopia in chicks, development of lens-induced myopia was not suppressed by intra-vitreal injections of 6-hydroxy dopamine, a drug which inhibits dopaminergic pathways (Schaeffel, Hagel et al. 1994). Conversely the non-specific dopaminergic agonist apomorphine has been shown to block negative lens-induced myopia in other chick studies (Schmid and Wildsoet 2004; Nickla, Totonelly et al. 2010).

Investigations using dopamine receptor subtype-specific agonists and antagonists have shown that the antimyopiagenic effect of dopamine is primarily mediated by D_2 receptors. For example, in form-deprivation in chicks, the protective effects of the non-specific dopaminergic agonist apomorphine were blocked by the D_2 specific antagonist spiperone, but not by the D_1 specific antagonist SCH-23390 (Rohrer, Spira et al. 1993).

In lens-induced myopia in chicks, both apomorphine (non-selective) and quinpirole (D_2 specific) agonists prevent the axial elongation and development of myopia associated with hyperopic defocus (Nickla, Totonelly et al. 2010). The effect is associated with an initial period of choroidal thickening, which is implicated in the inhibition of ocular growth either by the action of the choroid as a diffusion barrier to a growth signal or as an additional mechanical resistance to the effects of intraocular pressure (Nickla 2006). The D_2 antagonist spiperone is not as effective in abolishing the protective effect of periodic lens removal as has been previously found for the removal of form-depriving diffusers in chicks (McCarthy, Megaw et al. 2007). This may suggest a partial role for D_1 receptors in the control of ocular growth (Nickla, Totonelly et al. 2010).

6.2 Melatonin

While experimental evidence supports the role of retinal dopamine in the control of ocular growth and in the protective effect of light on myopia development, the role of melatonin, with which it is intrinsically linked in a counterphase cycle, is less certain (Cahill and Besharse 1995; Witkovsky 2004; Iuvone, Tosini et al. 2005).

Evidence for the role of an intrinsic melatonin rhythm in the control of eye growth is provided by Li and Howland (Li and Howland 2003) who demonstrated that the use of an opaque hood preventing light reaching the pineal gland for 12 hours per day is sufficient to significantly reduce the development of constant-light hyperopia in chicks. Covering one eye alone with an opaque occluder for 12 hours also partially prevented hyperopia development in the fellow eye under constant light conditions. The conclusion was that the eyes and pineal gland act as independent photoreceptors able to entrain the melatonin circadian rhythm which is protective against the effects of constant light on eye growth (Li and Howland 2003).

While diurnal retinal melatonin rhythms appear unaffected during form-deprivation (Hoffmann and Schaeffel 1996), the intra-vitreal injection of melatonin at relatively high doses (1000 µg) increases the level of form-deprivation myopia induced in the chick (Schaeffel, Bartmann et al. 1995; Hoffmann and Schaeffel 1996). Although retinal melatonin content was sampled twice a day (day and night) during monocular occlusion, and an expected diurnal variation in melatonin was found, no significant difference was found between the occluded and non-occluded eyes (Hoffmann and Schaeffel 1996). While the authors concluded that melatonin was not a significant component of the ocular growth control mechanism in form-deprivation in chicks a number of factors may have colluded to disguise the role of melatonin in form-deprivation myopia. These include the timing of the intra-vitreal injection of melatonin (between 2:00-3:00 pm) which may have occurred during a refractory period where the system was less sensitive, or that the duration (rather than the amplitude) of the nocturnal melatonin pulse may have been altered under form-deprivation conditions (see Section 4.7).

Rada and Wiechmann (Rada and Wiechmann 2006) demonstrated that the intraperitoneal injection of melatonin in chick at the beginning of each dark phase of the diurnal light cycle during a 5 day period of form-deprivation altered ocular growth patterns in both the form-deprived and control eyes. In form-deprived eyes, melatonin injection resulted in a significant reduction in anterior chamber depth, while vitreous chamber depth only exhibited a non-significant trend towards increased growth. The choroidal thickness was also significantly reduced in this group when compared to the sham-treatment group. The study also demonstrated the presence of melatonin receptors Mel(1A), Mel(1B) and Mel(1C) in the cornea, choroid, sclera, and retina of the chick. A diurnal rhythm in the expression of these receptors was identified where Mel(1C) expression was highest in the early morning around the onset of the light phase, while Mel(1A) and Mel(1B) expression was highest around the onset of the dark phase in the evenings. Rada and Wiechmann (Rada and Wiechmann 2006) concluded that the presence of melatonin receptors and diurnal rhythms of receptor expression, along with the effects of exogenous melatonin, suggests a significant role for melatonin in the control of ocular growth, and by extension, in the control of refractive development.

7. Conclusion

Recent human epidemiological studies propose that light exposure mediates the antimyopiagenic effect of outdoor activity. However, light may also have a causative role in myopia development when it is presented at an inappropriate time. Animal investigations demonstrate that light is a potent modulator of ocular growth and associated rhythms, including the interplay between dopamine and melatonin. One question is whether the effect of light on refractive development primarily acts through modification of circadian rhythms, or through some other intensity or wavelength dependent mechanism.

If the effect is circadian in origin, is there an optimal period for presenting light in order to control ocular growth and prevent myopia? Both constant light and constant dark disrupt ocular growth in animals and result in refractive error development. This can be ameliorated by either pharmacological interventions or controlled light exposure which re-establish more typical circadian rhythms. Light at night disrupts the normal circadian rhythm, rapidly decreasing melatonin and increasing dopamine, which potentially upsets the normal balance in ocular growth. As bright light presented in the middle of the day does not affect the timing of the circadian rhythm, presentation of a light signal during the twilight zones (dawn and dusk) is the most potent circadian zeitgeber. We hypothesise that the phase-advancing properties of morning light would be the most effective means of regulating the dopamine-melatonin circadian rhythm for the purposes of myopia control.

If the effect is not circadian in origin, then does the timing of the light signal matter or is it the nature of the stimulus (intensity and/or wavelength) that is important? Time spent outdoors leads to a significantly greater light dose than that received indoors, resulting in greater melatonin suppression and an increase in retinal dopamine. Additionally, the blue light spectral bias of outdoor light preferentially stimulates the melanopsin-containing ipRGCs, which would also lead to greater melatonin suppression. Both the intensity and wavelength of outdoor light favour increased retinal dopamine levels at the expense of melatonin. We hypothesise that it is this bias towards retinal dopamine production when outdoors that influences human refractive development, because increased dopamine has antimyopiagenic effects in animal experiments.

While the adage 'day-light good, night-light bad' in relation to refractive development is appealing, the true relationship between light and myopia is likely to be far more complex, with intricate interactions between the circadian cycle and the timing, intensity, and wavelength of the light exposure.

8. Acknowledgements

Simon Backhouse was supported by the New Zealand Association of Optometrists Education and Research Fund.

9. References

Adachi, A., T. Nogi, et al. (1998). "Phase-relationship and mutual effects between circadian rhythms of ocular melatonin and dopamine in the pigeon." *Brain Res* 792(2): 361-369.

Alarma-Estrany, P. and J. Pintor (2007). "Melatonin receptors in the eye: location, second messengers and role in ocular physiology." *Pharmacol Ther* 113(3): 507-522.

Anstice, N. S. and J. R. Phillips (2011). "Effect of dual-focus soft contact lens wear on axial myopia progression in children." *Ophthalmology* 118(6): 1152-1161.

Aoki, H., N. Yamada, et al. (1998). "Minimum light intensity required to suppress nocturnal melatonin concentration in human saliva." *Neurosci Lett* 252(2): 91-94.

Ashby, R., A. Ohlendorf, et al. (2009). "The effect of ambient illuminance on the development of deprivation myopia in chicks." *Invest Ophthalmol Vis Sci* 50(11): 5348-5354.

Ashby, R. S. and F. Schaeffel (2010). "The effect of bright light on lens compensation in chicks." *Invest Ophthalmol Vis Sci* 51(10): 5247-5253.

Axelrod, J. (1974). "The pineal gland: a neurochemical transducer." *Science* 184(144): 1341-1348.

Backhouse, S., H. Ng, et al. (2011). Light exposure patterns in children: a pilot study. Proceedings of the 13th International Myopia Conference, Tübingen, Germany, *Optom Vis Sci* 88(3): 395-403.

Balsalobre, A. (2002). "Clock genes in mammalian peripheral tissues." *Cell Tissue Res* 309(1): 193-199.

Bartmann, M., F. Schaeffel, et al. (1994). "Constant light affects retinal dopamine levels and blocks deprivation myopia but not lens-induced refractive errors in chickens." *Vis Neurosci* 11(2): 199-208.

Bernard, M., S. J. Donohue, et al. (1995). "Human hydroxyindole-O-methyltransferase in pineal gland, retina and Y79 retinoblastoma cells." *Brain Res* 696(1-2): 37-48.

Berson, D. M., F. A. Dunn, et al. (2002). "Phototransduction by retinal ganglion cells that set the circadian clock." *Science* 295(5557): 1070-1073.

Binkley, S., S. E. Macbride, et al. (1975). "Regulation of pineal rhythms in chickens: refractory period and nonvisual light perception." *Endocrinology* 96(4): 848-853.

Bittman, E. L. and F. J. Karsch (1984). "Nightly duration of pineal melatonin secretion determines the reproductive response to inhibitory day length in the ewe." *Biol Reprod* 30(3): 585-593.

Brainard, G. C., J. P. Hanifin, et al. (2001). "Action spectrum for melatonin regulation in humans: evidence for a novel circadian photoreceptor." *J Neurosci* 21(16): 6405-6412.

Brainard, G. C. and W. W. Morgan (1987). "Light-induced stimulation of retinal dopamine: a dose-response relationship." *Brain Res* 424(1): 199-203.

Cahill, G. M. and J. C. Besharse (1992). "Light-sensitive melatonin synthesis by Xenopus photoreceptors after destruction of the inner retina." *Vis Neurosci* 8(5): 487-490.

Cahill, G. M. and J. C. Besharse (1995). "Circadian rhythmicity in vertebrate retinas: Regulation by a photoreceptor oscillator." *Prog Retin Eye Res* 14(1): 267-291.

Charman, W. N. (2011). "Myopia, posture and the visual environment." *Ophthalmic Physiol Opt.* 31(5):494-501

Chua, W. H., V. Balakrishnan, et al. (2006). "Atropine for the treatment of childhood myopia." *Ophthalmology* 113(12): 2285-2291.

Cohen, J., M. Hadjiconstantinou, et al. (1983). "Activation of dopamine-containing amacrine cells of retina: light-induced increase of acidic dopamine metabolites." *Brain Res* 260(1): 125-127.

Cohen, Y., M. Belkin, et al. (2008). "Light intensity modulates corneal power and refraction in the chick eye exposed to continuous light." *Vision Res* 48(21): 2329-2335.

Cohen, Y., M. Belkin, et al. (2011). "Dependency between light intensity and refractive development under light-dark cycles." *Exp Eye Res* 92(1):40-46.

Coon, S. L., E. Del Olmo, et al. (2002). "Melatonin synthesis enzymes in Macaca mulatta: focus on arylalkylamine N-acetyltransferase (EC 2.3.1.87)." *J Clin Endocrinol Metab* 87(10): 4699-4706.

Czepita, D., W. Goslawski, et al. (2004). "Role of light emitted by incandescent or fluorescent lamps in the development of myopia and astigmatism." *Med Sci Monit* 10(4): CR168-171.

Daan, S. and C. S. Pittendrigh (1976). "A Functional Analysis of Circadian Pacemakers in Nocturnal Rodents. II. The Variability of Phase Response Curves." *J Comp Physiol* 106(3): 253-266.

Di Paolo, T., C. Harnois, et al. (1987). "Assay of dopamine and its metabolites in human and rat retina." *Neurosci Lett* 74(2): 250-254.

Dirani, M., M. Chamberlain, et al. (2006). "Refractive errors in twin studies." *Twin Res Hum Genet* 9(4): 566-572.

Dirani, M., L. Tong, et al. (2009). "Outdoor activity and myopia in Singapore teenage children." *Br J Ophthalmol* 93(8): 997-1000.

Doyle, S. E., M. S. Grace, et al. (2002). "Circadian rhythms of dopamine in mouse retina: the role of melatonin." *Vis Neurosci* 19(5): 593-601.

Duane, A. (1919). *Fuch's Textbook of Ophthalmology*. Philadelphia, Lippincott.

Figueiro, M. G., M. S. Rea, et al. (2006). "Circadian effectiveness of two polychromatic lights in suppressing human nocturnal melatonin." *Neurosci Lett* 406(3): 293-297.

Flitcroft, D. I. (1990). "A neural and computational model for the chromatic control of accommodation." *Vis Neurosci* 5(6): 547-555.

Goldman, B. D. (2001). "Mammalian photoperiodic system: formal properties and neuroendocrine mechanisms of photoperiodic time measurement." *J Biol Rhythms* 16(4): 283-301.

Gottlieb, M. D., L. A. Fugate-Wentzek, et al. (1987). "Different visual deprivations produce different ametropias and different eye shapes." *Invest Ophthalmol Vis Sci* 28(8): 1225-1235.

Guerlotte, J., P. Greve, et al. (1996). "Hydroxyindole-O-methyltransferase in the chicken retina: immunocytochemical localization and daily rhythm of mRNA." *Eur J Neurosci* 8(4): 710-715.

Guggenheim, J. A., C. Hill, et al. (2003). "Myopia, genetics, and ambient lighting at night in a UK sample." *Br J Ophthalmol* 87(5): 580-582.

Guler, A. D., J. L. Ecker, et al. (2008). "Melanopsin cells are the principal conduits for rod-cone input to non-image-forming vision." *Nature* 453(7191): 102-105.

Gunduz, B. and M. H. Stetson (2001). "A test of the coincidence and duration models of melatonin action in Siberian hamsters: the effects of 1-hr melatonin infusions on testicular development in intact and pinealectomized prepubertal Phodopus sungorus." *J Pineal Res* 30(2): 97-107.

Guo, S. S., J. G. Sivak, et al. (1995). "Retinal dopamine and lens-induced refractive errors in chicks." *Curr Eye Res* 14(5): 385-389.

Guyton, D. L., P. R. Greene, et al. (1989). "Dark-rearing interference with emmetropization in the rhesus monkey." *Invest Ophthalmol Vis Sci* 30(4): 761-764.

Gwiazda, J., L. Hyman, et al. (2003). "A randomized clinical trial of progressive addition lenses versus single vision lenses on the progression of myopia in children." *Invest Ophthalmol Vis Sci* 44(4): 1492-1500.

Gwiazda, J., E. Ong, et al. (2000). "Myopia and ambient night-time lighting." *Nature* 404(6774): 144.

Hashimoto, S., K. Nakamura, et al. (1996). "Melatonin rhythm is not shifted by lights that suppress nocturnal melatonin in humans under entrainment." *Am J Physiol* 270(5 Pt 2): R1073-1077.

Hattar, S., H. W. Liao, et al. (2002). "Melanopsin-containing retinal ganglion cells: architecture, projections, and intrinsic photosensitivity." *Science* 295(5557): 1065-1070.

Hattar, S., R. J. Lucas, et al. (2003). "Melanopsin and rod-cone photoreceptive systems account for all major accessory visual functions in mice." *Nature* 424(6944): 76-81.

Hazlerigg, D. G. and G. C. Wagner (2006). "Seasonal photoperiodism in vertebrates: from coincidence to amplitude." *Trends Endocrinol Metab* 17(3): 83-91.

Higuchi, S., Y. Motohashi, et al. (2007). "Less exposure to daily ambient light in winter increases sensitivity of melatonin to light suppression." *Chronobiol Int* 24(1): 31-43.

Hoffmann, M. and F. Schaeffel (1996). "Melatonin and deprivation myopia in chickens." *Neurochem Int* 28(1): 95-107.

Illnerova, H., M. Backstrom, et al. (1978). "Melatonin in rat pineal gland and serum; rapid parallel decline after light exposure at night." *Neurosci Lett* 9(2-3): 189-193.

Inouye, S. T. and H. Kawamura (1979). "Persistence of circadian rhythmicity in a mammalian hypothalamic "island" containing the suprachiasmatic nucleus." *Proc Natl Acad Sci U S A* 76(11): 5962-5966.

Iuvone, P. M. and J. C. Besharse (1986). "Dopamine receptor-mediated inhibition of serotonin N-acetyltransferase activity in retina." *Brain Res* 369(1-2): 168-176.

Iuvone, P. M., C. L. Galli, et al. (1978). "Light stimulates tyrosine hydroxylase activity and dopamine synthesis in retinal amacrine neurons." *Science* 202(4370): 901-902.

Iuvone, P. M., M. Tigges, et al. (1991). "Effects of apomorphine, a dopamine receptor agonist, on ocular refraction and axial elongation in a primate model of myopia." *Invest Ophthalmol Vis Sci* 32(5): 1674-1677.

Iuvone, P. M., G. Tosini, et al. (2005). "Circadian clocks, clock networks, arylalkylamine N-acetyltransferase, and melatonin in the retina." *Prog Retin Eye Res* 24(4): 433-456.

Jacobsen, N., H. Jensen, et al. (2008). "Does the level of physical activity in university students influence development and progression of myopia? - A 2-year prospective cohort study." *Invest Ophthalmol Vis Sci* 49(4): 1322-1327.

Jones, L. A., L. T. Sinnott, et al. (2007). "Parental history of myopia, sports and outdoor activities, and future myopia." *Invest Ophthalmol Vis Sci* 48(8): 3524-3532.

Kakita, T., T. Hiraoka, et al. (2011). "Influence of overnight orthokeratology on axial elongation in childhood myopia." *Invest Ophthalmol Vis Sci* 52(5): 2170-2174.

Kang, S. W., A. Thayananuphat, et al. (2007). "Dopamine-melatonin neurons in the avian hypothalamus controlling seasonal reproduction." *Neuroscience* 150(1): 223-233.

Khaldy, H., J. Leon, et al. (2002). "Circadian rhythms of dopamine and dihydroxyphenyl acetic acid in the mouse striatum: effects of pinealectomy and of melatonin treatment." *Neuroendocrinology* 75(3): 201-208.

Kramer, S. G. (1971). "Dopamine: A retinal neurotransmitter. I. Retinal uptake, storage, and light-stimulated release of H3-dopamine in vivo." *Invest Ophthalmol* 10(6): 438-452.

Kroger, R. H. and H. J. Wagner (1996). "The eye of the blue acara (Aequidens pulcher, Cichlidae) grows to compensate for defocus due to chromatic aberration." *J Comp Physiol A* 179(6): 837-842.

Larsen, J. S. (1971). "The sagittal growth of the eye. IV. Ultrasonic measurement of the axial length of the eye from birth to puberty." *Acta Ophthalmol* 49(6): 873-886.

Larsen, P. J., L. W. Enquist, et al. (1998). "Characterization of the multisynaptic neuronal control of the rat pineal gland using viral transneuronal tracing." *Eur J Neurosci* 10(1): 128-145.

Lerner, A. B., J. D. Case, et al. (1958). "Isolation of Melatonin, the Pineal Gland Factor That Lightens Melanocytes." *J Am Chem Soc* 80(10): 2587-2587.

Levi, F. and U. Schibler (2007). "Circadian rhythms: mechanisms and therapeutic implications." *Annu Rev Pharmacol Toxicol* 47: 593-628.

Lewy, A. J., R. L. Sack, et al. (1987). "Antidepressant and circadian phase-shifting effects of light." *Science* 235(4786): 352-354.

Lewy, A. J., R. L. Sack, et al. (1985). "Immediate and delayed effects of bright light on human melatonin production: shifting "dawn" and "dusk" shifts the dim light melatonin onset (DLMO)." *Ann N Y Acad Sci* 453: 253-259.

Li, T. and H. C. Howland (2003). "The effects of constant and diurnal illumination of the pineal gland and the eyes on ocular growth in chicks." *Invest Ophthalmol Vis Sci* 44(8): 3692-3697.

Li, T., H. C. Howland, et al. (2000). "Diurnal illumination patterns affect the development of the chick eye." *Vision Res* 40(18): 2387-2393.

Li, T., D. Troilo, et al. (1995). "Constant light produces severe corneal flattening and hyperopia in chickens." *Vision Res* 35(9): 1203-1209.

Lin, L. L., Y. F. Shih, et al. (2004). "Prevalence of myopia in Taiwanese schoolchildren: 1983 to 2000." *Ann Acad Med Singapore* 33(1): 27-33.

Liu, J., K. Pendrak, et al. (2004). "Emmetropisation under continuous but non-constant light in chicks." *Exp Eye Res* 79(5): 719-728.

Liu, R., Y. F. Qian, et al. (2011). "Effects of different monochromatic lights on refractive development and eye growth in guinea pigs." *Exp Eye Res.* 92(6):447-453

Liu, T. and J. Borjigin (2005). "N-acetyltransferase is not the rate-limiting enzyme of melatonin synthesis at night." *J Pineal Res* 39(1): 91-96.

Loman, J., G. E. Quinn, et al. (2002). "Darkness and near work: myopia and its progression in third-year law students." *Ophthalmology* 109(5): 1032-1038.

Long, Q., D. Chen, et al. (2009). "Illumination with monochromatic long-wavelength light promotes myopic shift and ocular elongation in newborn pigmented guinea pigs." *Cutan Ocul Toxicol* 28(4): 176-180.

Luft, W. A., P. M. Iuvone, et al. (2004). "Spatial, temporal, and intensive determinants of dopamine release in the chick retina." *Vis Neurosci* 21(4): 627-635.

Lynch, H. J., D. C. Jimerson, et al. (1978). "Entrainment of rhythmic melatonin secretion in man to a 12-hour phase shift in the light/dark cycle." *Life Sci* 23(15): 1557-1563.

Mandel, Y., I. Grotto, et al. (2008). "Season of birth, natural light, and myopia." *Ophthalmology* 115(4): 686-692.

Mandelman, T. and J. G. Sivak (1983). "Longitudinal chromatic aberration of the vertebrate eye." *Vision Res* 23(12): 1555-1559.

Mao, J., S. Liu, et al. (2010). "Levodopa inhibits the development of form-deprivation myopia in guinea pigs." *Optom Vis Sci* 87(1): 53-60.

Martin, X. D., H. Z. Malina, et al. (1992). "The ciliary body - the third organ found to synthesize indoleamines in humans." *Eur J Ophthalmol* 2(2): 67-72.

Maywood, E. S., R. C. Buttery, et al. (1990). "Gonadal responses of the male Syrian hamster to programmed infusions of melatonin are sensitive to signal duration and frequency but not to signal phase nor to lesions of the suprachiasmatic nuclei." *Biol Reprod* 43(2): 174-182.

McCarthy, C. S., P. Megaw, et al. (2007). "Dopaminergic agents affect the ability of brief periods of normal vision to prevent form-deprivation myopia." *Exp Eye Res* 84(1): 100-107.

McIntyre, I. M., T. R. Norman, et al. (1989). "Human melatonin suppression by light is intensity dependent." *J Pineal Res* 6(2): 149-156.

McMahon, G., T. Zayats, et al. (2009). "Season of Birth, Daylight Hours at Birth, and High Myopia." *Ophthalmology.* 116(3):468-473

Megaw, P. L., M. G. Boelen, et al. (2006). "Diurnal patterns of dopamine release in chicken retina." *Neurochem Int* 48(1): 17-23.

Melamed, E., Y. Frucht, et al. (1984). "Dopamine turnover in rat retina: a 24-hour light-dependent rhythm." *Brain Res* 305(1): 148-151.

Morgan, I. G. and M. K. Boelen (1996). "A retinal dark-light switch: a review of the evidence." *Vis Neurosci* 13(3): 399-409.

Mutti, D. O., G. L. Mitchell, et al. (2002). "Parental myopia, near work, school achievement, and children's refractive error." *Invest Ophthalmol Vis Sci* 43(12): 3633-3640.

Neumann, T., C. Ziegler, et al. (2008). "Multielectrode array recordings reveal physiological diversity of intrinsically photosensitive retinal ganglion cells in the chick embryo." *Brain Res* 1207: 120-127.

Nickla, D. L. (2006). "The phase relationships between the diurnal rhythms in axial length and choroidal thickness and the association with ocular growth rate in chicks." *J Comp Physiol A Neuroethol Sens Neural Behav Physiol* 192(4): 399-407.

Nickla, D. L., K. Totonelly, et al. (2010). "Dopaminergic agonists that result in ocular growth inhibition also elicit transient increases in choroidal thickness in chicks." *Exp Eye Res* 91(5): 715-720.

Nickla, D. L., C. Wildsoet, et al. (1998). "Visual influences on diurnal rhythms in ocular length and choroidal thickness in chick eyes." *Exp Eye Res* 66(2): 163-181.

Nickla, D. L., C. F. Wildsoet, et al. (2001). "Endogenous rhythms in axial length and choroidal thickness in chicks: implications for ocular growth regulation." *Invest Ophthalmol Vis Sci* 42(3): 584-588.

Norton, T. T., A. O. Amedo, et al. (2006). "Darkness causes myopia in visually experienced tree shrews." *Invest Ophthalmol Vis Sci* 47(11): 4700-4707.

Nowak, J. Z., A. Kazula, et al. (1992). "Melatonin increases serotonin N-acetyltransferase activity and decreases dopamine synthesis in light-exposed chick retina: in vivo evidence supporting melatonin-dopamine interaction in retina." *J Neurochem* 59(4): 1499-1505.

Nowak, J. Z., E. Zurawska, et al. (1989). "Melatonin and its generating system in vertebrate retina: circadian rhythm, effect of environmental lighting and interaction with dopamine." *Neurochem Int* 14(4): 397-406.

Ohngemach, S., M. Feldkaemper, et al. (2001). "Pineal control of the dopamine D2-receptor gene and dopamine release in the retina of the chicken and their possible relation to growth rhythms of the eye." *J Pineal Res* 31(2): 145-154.

Oishi, T., J. K. Lauber, et al. (1987). "Experimental myopia and glaucoma in chicks." *Zoolog Sci* 4: 455-464.

Osol, G. and B. Schwartz (1984). "Melatonin in the human retina." *Exp Eye Res* 38(2): 213-215.

Papastergiou, G. I., G. F. Schmid, et al. (1998). "Ocular axial length and choroidal thickness in newly hatched chicks and one-year-old chickens fluctuate in a diurnal pattern that is influenced by visual experience and intraocular pressure changes." *Exp Eye Res* 66(2): 195-205.

Parkinson, D. and R. R. Rando (1983). "Effect of light on dopamine turnover and metabolism in rabbit retina." *Invest Ophthalmol Vis Sci* 24(3): 384-388.

Pendrak, K., T. Nguyen, et al. (1997). "Retinal dopamine in the recovery from experimental myopia." *Curr Eye Res* 16(2): 152-157.

Perez-Leon, J. A., E. J. Warren, et al. (2006). "Synaptic inputs to retinal ganglion cells that set the circadian clock." *Eur J Neurosci* 24(4): 1117-1123.

Perlow, M. J., E. K. Gordon, et al. (1977). "The circadian variation in dopamine metabolism in the subhuman primate." *J Neurochem* 28(6): 1381-1383.

Perlow, M. J., S. M. Reppert, et al. (1980). "Photic regulation of the melatonin rhythm: monkey and man are not the same." *Brain Res* 182(1): 211-216.

Pitrosky, B., R. Kirsch, et al. (1995). "The photoperiodic response in Syrian hamster depends upon a melatonin-driven circadian rhythm of sensitivity to melatonin." *J Neuroendocrinol* 7(11): 889-895.

Prendergast, B. J., M. R. Gorman, et al. (2000). "Establishment and persistence of photoperiodic memory in hamsters." *Proc Natl Acad Sci U S A* 97(10): 5586-5591.

Proll, M. A., C. W. Kamp, et al. (1982). "Use of liquid chromatography with electrochemistry to measure effects of varying intensities of white light on DOPA accumulation in rat retinas." *Life Sci* 30(1): 11-19.

Provencio, I., I. R. Rodriguez, et al. (2000). "A novel human opsin in the inner retina." *J Neurosci* 20(2): 600-605.

Quinn, G. E., C. H. Shin, et al. (1999). "Myopia and ambient lighting at night." *Nature* 399(6732): 113-114.

Rada, J. A. and A. F. Wiechmann (2006). "Melatonin receptors in chick ocular tissues: implications for a role of melatonin in ocular growth regulation." *Invest Ophthalmol Vis Sci* 47(1): 25-33.

Revell, V. L. and D. J. Skene (2007). "Light-induced melatonin suppression in humans with polychromatic and monochromatic light." *Chronobiol Int* 24(6): 1125-1137.

Roenneberg, T. and R. G. Foster (1997). "Twilight times: light and the circadian system." *Photochem Photobiol* 66(5): 549-561.

Rohrer, B., A. W. Spira, et al. (1993). "Apomorphine blocks form-deprivation myopia in chickens by a dopamine D2-receptor mechanism acting in retina or pigmented epithelium." *Vis Neurosci* 10(3): 447-453.

Rollag, M. D., P. L. O'Callaghan, et al. (1978). "Serum melatonin concentrations during different stages of the annual reproductive cycle in ewes." *Biol Reprod* 18(2): 279-285.

Rose, K. A., I. G. Morgan, et al. (2008a). "Outdoor activity reduces the prevalence of myopia in children." *Ophthalmology* 115(8): 1279-1285.

Rose, K. A., I. G. Morgan, et al. (2008b). "Myopia, lifestyle, and schooling in students of Chinese ethnicity in Singapore and Sydney." *Arch Ophthalmol* 126(4): 527-530.

Ruby, N. F., T. J. Brennan, et al. (2002). "Role of melanopsin in circadian responses to light." *Science* 298(5601): 2211-2213.

Rucker, F. J. and J. Wallman (2009). "Chick eyes compensate for chromatic simulations of hyperopic and myopic defocus: evidence that the eye uses longitudinal chromatic aberration to guide eye-growth." *Vision Res* 49(14): 1775-1783.

Sakamoto, K., C. Liu, et al. (2005). "Dopamine regulates melanopsin mRNA expression in intrinsically photosensitive retinal ganglion cells." *Eur J Neurosci* 22(12): 3129-3136.

Saw, S. M., G. Gazzard, et al. (2005). "Myopia and associated pathological complications." *Ophthalmic Physiol Opt* 25(5): 381-391.

Saw, S. M., M. Z. Zhang, et al. (2002). "Near-work activity, night-lights, and myopia in the Singapore-China study." *Arch Ophthalmol* 120(5): 620-627.

Schade, R., K. Vick, et al. (1995). "Circadian rhythms of dopamine and cholecystokinin in nucleus accumbens and striatum of rats - influence on dopaminergic stimulation." *Chronobiol Int* 12(2): 87-99.

Schaeffel, F., M. Bartmann, et al. (1995). "Studies on the role of the retinal dopamine/melatonin system in experimental refractive errors in chickens." *Vision Res* 35(9): 1247-1264.

Schaeffel, F., G. Hagel, et al. (1994). "6-Hydroxy dopamine does not affect lens-induced refractive errors but suppresses deprivation myopia." *Vision Res* 34(2): 143-149.

Schmid, K. L. and C. F. Wildsoet (2004). "Inhibitory effects of apomorphine and atropine and their combination on myopia in chicks." *Optom Vis Sci* 81(2): 137-147.

Schwahn, H. N. and F. Schaeffel (1997). "Flicker parameters are different for suppression of myopia and hyperopia." *Vision Res* 37(19): 2661-2673.

Seidemann, A. and F. Schaeffel (2002). "Effects of longitudinal chromatic aberration on accommodation and emmetropization." *Vision Res* 42(21): 2409-2417.

Shaw, D. and B. D. Goldman (1995). "Influence of prenatal and postnatal photoperiods on postnatal testis development in the Siberian hamster (Phodopus sungorus)." *Biol Reprod* 52(4): 833-838.

Simonneaux, V. and C. Ribelayga (2003). "Generation of the melatonin endocrine message in mammals: a review of the complex regulation of melatonin synthesis by norepinephrine, peptides, and other pineal transmitters." *Pharmacol Rev* 55(2): 325-395.

Smith, E. L., 3rd, D. V. Bradley, et al. (2001). "Continuous ambient lighting and eye growth in primates." *Invest Ophthalmol Vis Sci* 42(6): 1146-1152.

Smith, K. A., M. W. Schoen, et al. (2004). "Adaptation of human pineal melatonin suppression by recent photic history." *J Clin Endocrinol Metab* 89(7): 3610-3614.

Sowers, J. R. and N. Vlachakis (1984). "Circadian variation in plasma dopamine levels in man." *J Endocrinol Invest* 7(4): 341-345.

Stone, R. A., T. Lin, et al. (1995). "Photoperiod, early post-natal eye growth, and visual deprivation." *Vision Res* 35(9): 1195-1202.

Stone, R. A., T. Lin, et al. (1989). "Retinal dopamine and form-deprivation myopia." *Proc Natl Acad Sci U S A* 86(2): 704-706.

Stone, R. A., K. Pendrak, et al. (2006). "Local patterns of image degradation differentially affect refraction and eye shape in chick." *Curr Eye Res* 31(1): 91-105.

Tast, A., R. J. Love, et al. (2001). "The pattern of melatonin secretion is rhythmic in the domestic pig and responds rapidly to changes in daylength." *J Pineal Res* 31(4): 294-300.

Thapan, K., J. Arendt, et al. (2001). "An action spectrum for melatonin suppression: evidence for a novel non-rod, non-cone photoreceptor system in humans." *J Physiol* 535(Pt 1): 261-267.

Thomas, K. B., M. Tigges, et al. (1993). "Melatonin synthesis and circadian tryptophan hydroxylase activity in chicken retina following destruction of serotonin immunoreactive amacrine and bipolar cells by kainic acid." *Brain Res* 601(1-2): 303-307.

Torii, M., D. Kojima, et al. (2007). "Two isoforms of chicken melanopsins show blue light sensitivity." *FEBS Lett* 581(27): 5327-5331.

Tosini, G. and J. C. Dirden (2000). "Dopamine inhibits melatonin release in the mammalian retina: in vitro evidence." *Neurosci Lett* 286(2): 119-122.

Tosini, G. and M. Menaker (1996). "Circadian rhythms in cultured mammalian retina." *Science* 272(5260): 419-421.

Tosini, G., N. Pozdeyev, et al. (2008). "The circadian clock system in the mammalian retina." *Bioessays* 30(7): 624-633.

Vannas, A. E., G. S. Ying, et al. (2003). "Myopia and natural lighting extremes: risk factors in Finnish army conscripts." *Acta Ophthalmol Scand* 81(6): 588-595.

Vitale, S., R. D. Sperduto, et al. (2009). "Increased prevalence of myopia in the United States between 1971-1972 and 1999-2004." *Arch Ophthalmol* 127(12): 1632-1639.

Wang, F., J. Zhou, et al. (2011). "Effects of 530 nm Green Light on Refractive Status, Melatonin, MT1 Receptor, and Melanopsin in the Guinea Pig." *Curr Eye Res* 36(2): 103-111.

Weiler, R., W. H. Baldridge, et al. (1997). "Modulation of endogenous dopamine release in the fish retina by light and prolonged darkness." *Vis Neurosci* 14(2): 351-356.

Weiss, S. and F. Schaeffel (1993). "Diurnal growth rhythms in the chicken eye: relation to myopia development and retinal dopamine levels." *J Comp Physiol A Neuroethol Sens Neural Behav Physiol* 172(3): 263-270.

Wiechmann, A. F. and J. G. Hollyfield (1987). "Localization of hydroxyindole-O-methyltransferase-like immunoreactivity in photoreceptors and cone bipolar cells in the human retina: a light and electron microscope study." *J Comp Neurol* 258(2): 253-266.

Wilkinson, M., J. Arendt, et al. (1977). "Determination of a dark-induced increase of pineal N-acetyl transferase activity and simultaneous radioimmunoassay of melatonin in pineal, serum and pituitary tissue of the male rat." *J Endocrinol* 72(2): 243-244.

Witkovsky, P. (2004). "Dopamine and retinal function." *Doc Ophthalmol* 108(1): 17-39.

Zadnik, K., L. A. Jones, et al. (2000). "Myopia and ambient night-time lighting. CLEERE Study Group. Collaborative Longitudinal Evaluation of Ethnicity and Refractive Error." *Nature* 404(6774): 143-144.

Zawilska, J. B., D. J. Skene, et al. (2009). "Physiology and pharmacology of melatonin in relation to biological rhythms." *Pharmacol Rep* 61(3): 383-410.

Zeitzer, J. M., D. J. Dijk, et al. (2000). "Sensitivity of the human circadian pacemaker to nocturnal light: melatonin phase resetting and suppression." *J Physiol* 526 Pt 3: 695-702.

Zmijewski, M. A., T. W. Sweatman, et al. (2009). "The melatonin-producing system is fully functional in retinal pigment epithelium (ARPE-19)." *Mol Cell Endocrinol* 307(1-2): 211-216.

11

Non-Surgical Treatment of Astigmatism

Luciane B. Moreira

Ophthalmology Department, Federal University of Paraná, Curitiba
Brazil

1. Introduction

People with astigmatism have several options available to regain clear vision. They include eyeglasses, contact lenses, orthokeratology and refractive surgery procedures. In this chapter, we will talk about non-surgical treatment only.

2. Eyeglasses

Eyeglasses are a choice for correction for people with regular astigmatism and it doesn't improve vision for irregular astigmatism. They will contain a cylindrical lens prescription for the astigmatism in a specific meridian of the lens which designates the axis of the lens power. Myopia or hyperopia can be associated to astigmatism. Generally, a single vision lens is prescribed so as to provide clear vision at all distances. However, for patients over the age of 40 who have presbyopia, a bifocal or progressive addition lens may be needed in order to focus effectively for near vision work.

A wide variety of lens-types and frame designs are now available for patients of all ages. Eyeglasses are no longer just a medical device that provides needed vision correction, but also a means of enhancing appearance. However, any astigmatism correction numerically higher than a cylinder +1.50 or -2.50 should warrant special consideration of lenses and frames.[1]

Some consideration must be made with the intention of obtaining the best adaptation of the patient to their eyeglasses. A good frame should be lightweight, strong, fit comfortably and suit the wearer's sense of style. Over-sized lenses or much curved frames need to be avoided because they can induce distortion in the periphery of the lens. Eyeglasses with small scaffoldings have a minor possibility of producing alterations in the periphery of the lens. The lesser the distance-vertex, the less will be the disparity in the magnification of the image as it enters the meridians of the astigmatism. The use of negative cylindrical lenses for this sends information to locate the correction of the astigmatism in the posterior part of the lens and consequently next to the ocular globe.[2]

The design of the lens influences the adaptation of the eyeglasses. The lenses of spectacles for correcting astigmatism should have a toric or cylindrical surface in order to give a single focal point in the retina. The thickness of the lens is not the same across its surface. This difference in thickness is increased due to the strength of the astigmatism.[3]

Aspheric lenses are not like conventional lenses in that they do not have a spherical front curvature but instead have differing degrees of curvature. This allows wearers to see clearly whether they are looking directly ahead or to either side. Aspheric lenses can also be combined with a high index material so as to produce extremely thin lenses which provide the same great vision improvement.[1]

Lens material is also important. In general, lenses are made from three materials: plastic, glass, and polycarbonate.[3] Glass is still used for lenses and it is scratch resistant, but it is also heavy and breakable. Polycarbonate and Trivex lenses are designed for high impact resistance and are ideal for occupational hazards, children and athletes. They provide the best eye protection. Plastic is the most used material for lenses. The ones made of high index resin are thin, lightweight, provide good optical quality and do not magnify the eyes as with the others. The term 'Index of refraction' is used to describe the speed at which light travels through a material: a higher index results in thinner lenses.

The lenses of eye glasses can also be upgraded with scratch protectant, anti-reflective, UV-protectants, colour tints, or photochromics. A scratch protectant coating helps the lenses become more resistant against most abrasions. A UV coating helps to reduce the amount of UV rays that enter the eyes by blocking it through the lens. Anti-reflective lenses diminish glare and reflections, and allow people to see your eyes without any problem. They are designed to lighten up the tint when in the shade and darken the tint when in direct sunlight. Polarised lenses are like sunglasses in that they are tinted with a polarisation filter and they block vertical light from placing stress on the eyes. They are good for outdoor activities where the sun will be glaring down.[3]

Doctors should instruct patients about the best glasses for their needs, checking the history and the eye exam of each one. The ideal method is to prescribe the spectacles after eyeglass trials, giving the patients the opportunity to see how they feel in the situations that are common in their everyday life. Often, the physician will try to give the best monocular correction at the refractor to their patients; however, when the patient uses the eyeglasses, with both eyes open, they will not obtain much comfort and will sometimes feel dizzy and get a headache. Ultimately, one needs to take into consideration the binocular vision, the differences between the eyes, the interpupillary distance and the pantoscopic angle of the scaffolding.[4] (figure 1).

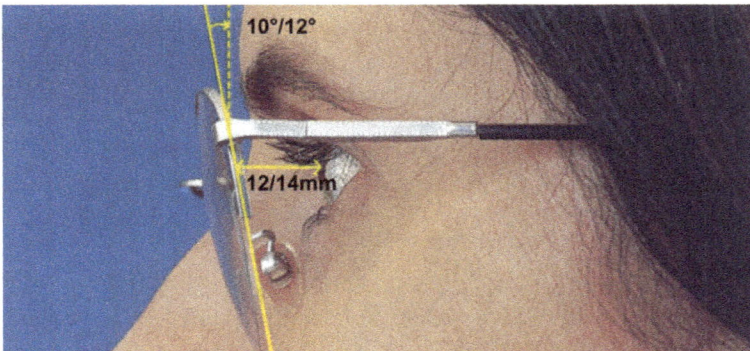

Fig. 1. Pantoscopic angle of glasses.[4]

3. Contact lenses

For some individuals, contact lenses can offer better vision than eyeglasses. They can be used for people with regular and irregular astigmatism, such as keratoconus. They may provide clearer vision and a wider field of view. However, since contact lenses are worn directly on the eyes, they require regular cleaning and care to safeguard eye health[5]

Contact lenses are the first choice for difficult cases such as corneal ecstasies (e.g. keratoconus, keratoglobus and pellucid marginal degeneration). For these cases, there are special lenses with a variety of designs. In this current chapter we will focus only on regular astigmatisms, since to address this kind of adaptation would require a whole chapter to itself.

Almost everybody has the option of using contact lenses. Before initiating any contact lens fitting, it is important to evaluate the patient's motivation, ocular needs, and ocular and medical history. There are four principal indications for contact lens fitting: 1) optical indications (myopia, hyperopia, astigmatism and presbyopia); 2) medical indications (keratoconus, irregular astigmatism, corneal opacification, anisometropia, unilateral aphakia, nystagmus, after refractive surgery or keratoplasty); 3) cosmetic or prosthetic indication to hide imperfections of the eye; 4) therapeutic indications for corneal abrasion.[4]

The contraindications are generally relative, and they will depend upon the criteria of the ophthalmologist's evaluation. Unmotivated patient; poor personal hygiene; inability to follow directions of lens maintenance and handling; inability to understand the risks associated with contact lens use; allergies that affect the eye; immunosuppressed patients, diabetic patients, and alcoholics have a large risk of complications; any effective eye disease affecting the cornea, the conjunctiva and lids as, for example, with inflammations, infections, dry eye, lagophthalmos and glaucoma; moreover, psychological intolerance can be a contraindication for contact lenses use.[4]

Contact lens can be classified by the nature of the material, by their design or by their wearing and replacement schedule, as will seen. A well-made clinical history, along with a complete ophthalmological examination and the patient's needs, determines whether contact lenses are appropriate for each patient[5]

As to the nature of the material of the lens, it can be hard, soft or hybrid. Hard lenses can be non-gas permeable or gas permeable. Polymethylmethacrylate (PMMA) is the polymer from which hard non-gas permeables are made. The disadvantage with this is a lack of gas permeability. The rigid gas permeable lenses (RGP) permit the passage of oxygen and carbon dioxide gas but they contain no water. The general categories of gas permeable polymers are: cellulose acetate butyrate, pure silicone, silicone acrylate and fluorocarbonate. The soft lenses can be hydrogel or silicone hydrogel, both of which have a low water-content (less than 50% water) or high water-content (greater than 50% water). The oxygen transmissibility of a hydrogel lens is directly related to its water-content. For the silicone hydrogel, a higher water-content gives more comfort because it diminishes the roughness of the lens.[6]

There are many designs of lenses. In this chapter, the three basic designs that exist will be addressed: spherical (having anterior and posterior spherical surfaces); aspheric (different radii of curvature in the centre and periphery, simulating the structure of the cornea); and toric (two principal meridians having different radii of curvature; this may be the anterior or posterior surfaces of the lenses or both).[6] Other designs, such as multi-curvature, reverse curve, progressive and bifocal, are related to other refractive errors besides astigmatism and will not be considered here.

The wearing schedule can be: 1) continuous wear (overnight lenses – utilised both during waking and sleeping hours); 2) daily wear (removed daily and not utilised during sleep); 3) flexible wear (removed daily with sporadic sleepers wearing lenses); 4) occasional wear (utilises glasses most of the time and lenses only sometimes, in social activities or sports).[5]

The replacement schedule can be done in three ways: 1) a traditional or conventional way is used when the lens must be replaced annually; 2) the planned replacement way which is nowadays the most used and where the lens needs to be replaced every 15, 30 or 60 days (as defined by the manufacturer's guidelines); 3) disposable lenses, which are probably are the easiest way, because they are immediately discarded after use and do not need maintenance.[5]

Many people ask whether or not RGP lenses are better than hydrogel lenses. The answer to this question depends upon vision accuracy, the comfort and satisfaction of the patient and corneal health. The adaptation of contact lens is different for each person. Generally, to get used to them, the patients need between 1 and 15 days and seem to be easier for those wearing hydrogel lenses than for the ones who wear RGP lenses.

There are many pamphlets to help and teach users how to put on and take off contact lenses, as well as how to store them and keep them clean. However, it is necessary to review these steps at every follow-up visit to the ophthalmologist. The control of contact lens use needs to be done with a specialist every year or else every 6 months, depending on the lens fitting and eye condition.

3.1 Soft contact lenses

Soft contact lenses conform to the shape of the eye. Spherical soft lenses may not be effective in correcting astigmatism;[7] however, toric soft contact lenses can provide a correction for regular astigmatism similar to that of eyeglasses.

A strategy for correcting low degrees of astigmatism with spherical soft lenses is to increase the thickness of the lens. Considering that a thicker or stiffer lens may drape less on the cornea and mask more astigmatism, thicker lenses associated with a special design can give good vision even for irregular astigmatism, such as keratoconus.[5] Another strategy that has been described is the use of lenses with low water-content, since it is not so malleable. However, a low water-content spherical silicone hydrogel material has been shown to have no significant impact on the amount of astigmatism masked.[8]

Visual acuity with a spherical equivalent refraction remained at tolerable limits with the use of spherical contact lenses. Spherical lenses failed to mask corneal toricity during topography, while toric lenses caused central neutralisation and a decrease in corneal cylinder in low and moderate astigmatic eyes.[9]

Soft aspheric contact lenses have been recommended for low astigmatic patients because its design could decrease the level of spherical aberration that is a distortion in image formation. However, clinical studies have reported that non-toric aspheric soft contact lenses did not improve visual acuity significantly when compared to spherical lenses on low astigmats. One reason for why these non-toric lenses do not improve visual acuity is that aspheric soft contact lenses do not correct astigmatism. Additionally, decentration of spherical aberration correction has been shown to induce a coma-like aberration that is another distortion in image formation.[9]

Visual acuity with toric lenses is better than with spherical or aspheric lenses, but initially lens quality and stability was a problem. Nowadays, improved lens designs and the availability of disposable toric contact lenses have resulted in improved health benefits and adaptation[10] Well-fitted hydrogel toric lenses can provide visual acuity and visual performance equivalent to that of spherical RGP lenses.[9]

All the literature agrees that the best way to fit a soft lens is by considering the response to the trial lens fitting. By slit lamp, the physician observes centralisation, the movement of the lens and the lens-cornea relationship. After this, over-refraction has to be done.[5] However, the fitting without trial lens has proven to be an efficient way to prescribe it. 50% to 80% of patients are being fitted successfully with this method for soft toric contact lenses.[11] To fit a soft contact lens, keratometry needs to be done. The base curve of the lens should be approximately 0.6 to 0.8 mm flatter than the average corneal curvature measurement. The lens diameter should be approximately 2.0 mm larger than the horizontal visible iris diameter. The dioptric power of the contact lens should consider the total eye refraction and, if it is greater than 4.00 D, a table for the correction of the vertex distance should be used.[6] It can also be calculated using the following formula:[5]

$$DL = \frac{DA}{1 - d \cdot DA}$$

DL= dioptric power of contact lens.
DA= dioptric power of glasses.
d= vertex distance (which has an average of 12mm).

There remains some disagreement as to when to fit soft toric lenses or else spherical lenses. In practice, high myopia associated with low astigmatism has good acuity with spherical contact lenses; however, low myopes with higher astigmatism had significantly better acuity with toric lenses than with the spherical equivalent.[5]

3.2 Rigid gas permeable lenses

Rigid gas permeable contact lenses maintain their regular shape while on the cornea, and they offer an effective way to compensate for the cornea's irregular shape and improve the vision of persons with astigmatism and other refractive errors.

Gas permeable (GP) lenses could be very acceptable as a viable option for the correction of moderate to severe astigmatism. Patients preferred RGP lenses for visual acuity, especially at near and intermediate distances.[12]

Spherical lenses can compensate for corneal astigmatism up to 3.00 D, although it is known that using them on corneas showing more than 2.00 D of toricity may be inappropriate. Because of this, it is recommended that spherical fittings should be done where the base curve of the lens is equal to the cornea's flattest meridian. The limits of this approach are reached on highly toric corneas where the lens may alter the tear film flow, leading to peripheral desiccation of the cornea (known as 3–9 o'clock staining). This is why a spherical GP lens should be used with extreme caution on a cornea presenting toricity greater than 2.00 D. At present, it is recommended that reliance should be placed on a topographic map of the cornea so as to determine the optimal parameters.[13]

Many methods can be used to find the base curve. That most frequently used by practitioners involves adding 1/3 to 1/4 of the astigmatism measure to K (the flattest meridian of the topographic corneal map).[12] The diameter of the lenses is dependent to the base curve. A great diameter needs a flatter adaptation (table 1). Another tip is to remember is that steeper corneas require lenses with a smaller diameter, and that flatter corneas require lenses with a greater diameter (table 2).[5]

The selected trial lens is placed on the cornea and then, for the evaluation, it is necessary to take into account its comfort, position, movement and stability. The slit lamp evaluates the relationship between the lens and cornea with fluorescein. After the fitting is complete, the over-refraction should be done.

Corneal cylinder	8.6 mm diameter lens	9.2 mm diameter lens	10.2 mm diameter lens
0,00 to 0,50 D	0.25 D STK	On K	0.25 D FTK
0,75 to 1,25 D	0.50 D STK	0,25 D STK	On K
1,50 to 2,00 D	0.75 D STK	0.50 D STK	0.25 D STK
2,25 to 2,75 D	1.00 D STK	0.75 D STK	0.50 D STK
3,00 to 3,50 D	1.25 D STK	1.00 D STK	0.75 D STK

STK = steeper than K / FTK = flatter then K.

Table 1. Base curve lens determination in dependence of lens diameter and topographic corneal cylinder.

Corneal curvature (K)	Lens diameter
38.00 to 42.00 D	9.8 mm or bigger
42.25 to 44.25 D	9.1 to 9.7 mm
44.50 to 50.00 D	9.0 mm or smaller

Table 2. Correlation between corneal curvature flattest meridian of the topographic corneal map (K) and contact lens diameter

Aspheric lenses will always move in the direction of least resistance: this implies that a lens that is restricted along the vertical meridian and which is free along the horizontal meridian will move freely up and down. Conversely, if there is a restriction along the horizontal meridian, the lens will decentre on the nasal or temporal side.[13]

For those wearing RGP contact lenses, only 18% to 22% wear toric correction, suggesting that many practitioners tend to mask astigmatism using spherical equivalence with contact lenses. One reason for this behaviour is that toric gas permeable lenses are more complex to fit and have variable results.[13] Some practitioners will consider toric lenses only if the patient reports unsatisfactory vision in spherical contact lenses or else when the corneal toricity is too great and the fitting has become unstable. Toric lens designs can have different radii of curvature on the front surface, back surface or both of what are known as bitoric lenses.

Back-toric design implies that the back surface of the lens is toric and that its front surface is spherical. This design is most successful when the corneal toricity represents more than two thirds of the refractive astigmatism. Back-toric gas permeable lenses are not designed with prism ballasts; their stabilisation is mainly achieved by the correspondence between the back curves and the corneal toricity. This type of lens is designed with only 66% corneal toricity so as to provide more comfort. However, because of this, the lens will quite certainly rotate in the eye. Clinically, this translates as induced astigmatism that can disturb the visual outcome where it exceeds 0.75 D.[5]

Front-toric designs are designed with the astigmatic correction on the front surface of the lens, leaving the back surface spherical. They are stabilised with a base-down prism and represent the best choice for correcting residual astigmatism, in which the cornea is spherical.[5] Residual astigmatism results from causes other than the shape of the anterior corneal surface and can refer to astigmatism of the posterior cornea surface, lens, and retina.

A bitoric lens offers both surfaces as toric. The back toric surface curves are designed to be aligned with the corneal toricity. Optically speaking, this generates an over-correction of the refractive astigmatism. This is why a front toric surface is needed to compensate the power of the lens. Bi-toric designs are the most popular toric design in RGP contact lens practice, and represent the best choice if corneal toricity is less than or exceeds refractive astigmatism.[5]

For RGP toric lenses, I believe that the most appropriate fitting method is a 4-step approach, known as the two-thirds rule, as seen below.[14]

Step 1. Calculation of corneal toricity: calculate the difference between the two principal meridians of the cornea.

Step 2. Calculation of Base curve 1 (BC-1): the base curve 1 of the lens is determined by dividing the corneal toricity (found in Step 1) into two-thirds and then adding it to the flattest meridian of the cornea.

Step 3. Calculation of base curve 2 (BC-2): the base curve 2 of the lens is determined by flattening the steepest meridian of the cornea according to Remba's rule (Table 3).

Step 4. Calculation of lachrymal lens power and induced astigmatism: this type of astigmatism is induced by the relationship of the back surface of the lens to the cornea, and can be seen doing the over-refraction. If this value is less than 1.00 D, a back-toric design should be ordered because the induced astigmatism is not considered to be a contributing factor affecting visual acuity. At this point, a spherical equivalence is made in order to determine the final power of the back-toric lens. However, if the induced astigmatism value exceeds 1.00 D, a bitoric design should then be selected because the induced astigmatism should be corrected by the addition of the cylinder power to the front-surface of the lens.

Cornea toricity	Flattening of the steepest meridian
2.0 D	0.25 D
3.0 D	0.50 D
4.0 D or more	0.75 D

Table 3. Usable values according to Remba's rule

3.3 Orthokeratology

Orthokeratology (ortho-k) involves the fitting of specially designed rigid contact lenses to reshape the cornea so as to temporarily reduce or eliminate refractive error. The contact lenses are worn for limited periods, such as overnight, and then removed. Persons with mild to moderate myopia and mild astigmatism may be able to temporarily obtain clear vision without lenses for most of their daily activities. Ortho-k does not permanently improve vision, and if the person stops wearing the retainer lenses, the cornea may return to its original condition and vision will be bad again. Ortho-k is a good option for people who need RGP contact lenses to improve vision but who cannot wear common lenses for many reasons.[5] The main reasons for using this kind of lens are: workers in polluted environments or who use chemical products; boxers or water-sports athletes; people who feel discomfort with regular lenses and cannot have refractive surgery; people who have problems with blinking, dry eye, giant papillary conjunctivitis or nystagmus.

Ortho-k makes many changes to the shape of the cornea, as can be seen by topography maps, wave front measurements and pachymetry. The corneal changes induced by reverse-geometry – because of the relatively flat-fitting base curve – create a central flattened zone called the treatment zone, corresponding approximately to the lens back optic zone. Successful ortho-k treatment produces a well-centred regular treatment zone which encompasses the pupil diameter, as revealed by inspection of the difference map on the corneal topographer's data display (figure 2).[15]

The induction of higher-order aberrations with the use of reverse-geometry lenses for overnight ortho-k has been reported.[16] The significant increase in spherical aberrations is seen by the annular zone of mid-peripheral corneal steepening induced by the reverse-geometry lens, and the consequent change in corneal shape from prolate[1] towards oblate[2] asphericity.[16] However, the patients do not complain about these kinds of visual problems. A higher-order aberration is a distortion acquired when light passes through an eye with irregularities. Everyone's eyes have it, but the quantity of it is what determines whether it will affect quality of vision, by giving symptoms as glare, halos, starburst effects and ghost images.

Most of the studies concern ortho-k for myopia of 4.0D and with-the-rule corneal astigmatism of less than 1.50D showing rapid results, with most change after the first night of lens wear and most stability in refractive change after 4 weeks.[17] However, a few studies show good results for irregular astigmatism, such as keratoconus.[15]

Spherical reverse-geometry lenses can be used on toric corneas in order to reduce astigmatism. In a retrospective analysis, Mountford and Pesudovs[18] demonstrated that up

---

[1] The normal cornea is a prolate surface - steeper in the centre and flatter in the periphery.
[2] The oblate surface is a surface after myopic laser photorefractive keratectomy – flatter in the centre and steeper in the periphery.

to 50% of corneal astigmatism could be reduced with standard reverse-geometry ortho-k lenses, provided that the toricity was with-the-rule and restricted to the central region of the cornea. Corneal toricity reaching from limbus to limbus on the topographic map was less amenable to modification by ortho-k lenses.

Toric ortho-k lenses were created for an oval treatment zone and different meridional topographic changes, with more corneal flattening in the meridian requiring more myopic refractive error correction. Details of corneal topographic changes induced by these different ortho-k lens designs over longer periods of wear are yet to be published.[19]

There is slight regression of effect (about 0.25 to 0.75 D) during the day, and lenses must be periodically worn overnight (from every night to every three to four nights) to retain the effect. No serious adverse events have been reported from published clinical studies, although overnight lens adherence and clinically significant corneal staining in the morning after lens removal appear to be relatively common and have caused some clinical concerns in some studies.[20]

Patient satisfaction with overnight ortho-k has been reported as similar to or better than other popular modalities of contact lens wear. Unlike refractive surgery, if patients fail to achieve a subjectively successful outcome, they can cease lens wear and return to other corrective options, such as spectacles or conventional contact lenses. The corneal changes induced by overnight ortho-k are fully reversible on cessation of lens wear.[20]

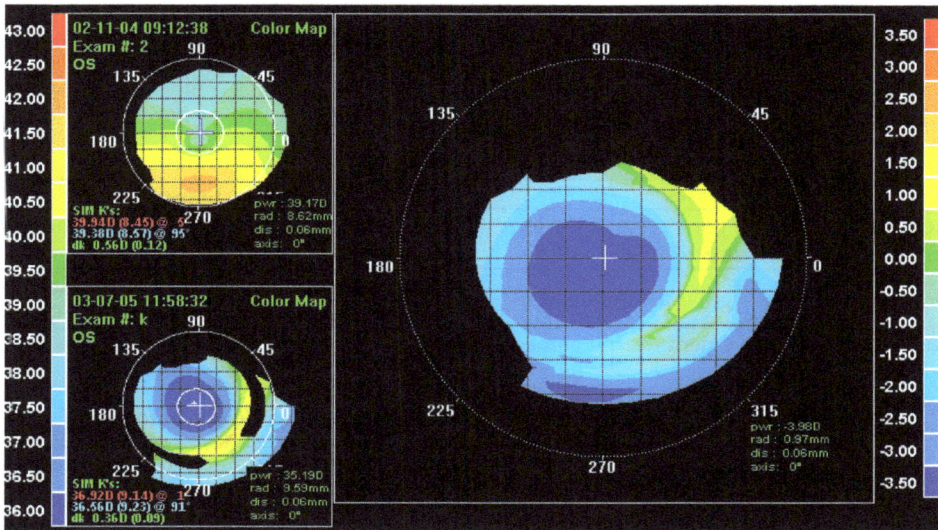

Fig. 2. Topography before and after orthokeratology in a case of irregular astigmatism (keratoconus).[15]

4. Visual stimulation

Brain plasticity in the visual functions of adults has been shown to improve with repetitive practice on specific controlled visual tasks. Through these repetitive practices are initiated neural modifications that lead to an improvement in neuronal efficiency. These neural modifications can enhance image quality by compensating for blurred retinal images due to optical defocus for all the refract errors.[21] It is indicated by those who have good Snellen visual acuity but still have symptoms of ghost images. This commonly happens to people with low astigmatism.

RevitalVision by NeuroVision (NeuroVision Inc., Singapore), based on visual stimulation, have developed a computer programme for amblyopia, post lasik (laser assisted in situ keratomileusis) and post cataract. However, it can be extended for others refractive errors. During training sessions, the user is presented with a series of precise visual tasks consisting of Gabor patches with subtle differences in orientation, size and contrast. Through repetitive practice, the brain is trained to be more efficient and to improve visual processing by improving contrast sensitivity and visual acuity.[22]

Studies showed mean improvements of visual acuity of about 2.0 LogMar, and the contrast sensitivity function also improved at all spatial frequencies. However, the mean refractive error remained unchanged after treatment. Follow-up data for up to 12 months post-treatment showed that the gains were retained.[23] This method has never been proven. The effect is probably related to the memory of the patients, and this would be the reason that the refractive error remains unchanged.

Besides this, it requires more evaluation to see the real value of this kind of stimulation for the treatment of astigmatism.[21-23]

5. Advantages and disadvantages for each correcting method

There are many differences between contact lens and glasses, as can be seen in the chart below, but both need an eye doctor's prescription and periodic evaluation.

Eyeglasses	Contact Lenses
The distance between your eye and the lens sometimes creates distortion.	When worn right on the eye it sometimes can blur because of tears.
Glasses correct only regular astigmatism.	Contact lenses can also correct irregular cornea shape that distorts vision.
Glasses can be inconvenient during games and sports.	Contact lenses are a favourite among athletes.
Poor peripheral vision (visual field) because of the frame.	Your entire field of view is in focus.
Eyeglasses can get dirty and decrease vision.	Contact lenses can form deposits on the lens and blur the vision acuity.
Glasses must be sprayed and wiped several times a day.	Contact lenses should be cleaned, disinfected and stored properly after each use.
Periodic need for tightening or other adjustment.	Maintenance and handling of the lens every day.
Sometimes an uncomfortable weight on your face and ears.	Sometimes uncomfortable in the eye as a strange body, dry eye or allergy.
Glasses are fashionable, functional and complement your outfit.	Cosmetic lens may alter the colour of the eye.

Also, there are advantages and disadvantages associated with various types of contact lens, as seen below. All of the contact lenses require visits to the ophthalmologist for follow-up care.

Lens Types	Advantages	Disadvantages
Soft lenses	Very short adaptation period. More comfortable and more difficult to dislodge than RGP lenses.	Maintenance and handling every day. Do not last long comparing to RGP lenses. Vision may not be as sharp as RGP lenses.
Daily wear disposable lenses	Thinner lenses. Require no cleaning. Minimal risk of eye infection if the wearing instructions are followed.	Do not correct all vision problems.
Extended ware disposable lenses	Can usually be worn up to several days without removal (the wearing period is defined by the manufacturer's guidelines). Require no cleaning.	Do not correct all vision problems. Increases risk of complication with night and day wear. Requires regular monitoring and professional care.
Planned replacement lenses	Require simplified cleaning and disinfection. Good for eye health. Available in most prescriptions.	Vision may not be as sharp as RGP lenses. Maintenance and handling every day.
Rigid gas permeable lenses (RGP)	Excellent vision. Easier than the soft lens for maintenance and handling. Correct most vision problems. Durable, with a relatively long life.	Require consistent wear to maintain good vision. Can slip off the centre of the eye more easily than other types. Debris can easily get under the lenses. Longer period to get used to compared to soft lenses.
Ortoceratologia	Worn only at times of sleeping. Eliminates the use of the lens on walking hour. Short adaptation period. Comfortable to wear. Less friction with the lid. Durable, with a long life.	Correct only low astigmatism and low to moderate myopia. Vision may not be as sharp as with other lenses.

6. Conclusion

Individuals with astigmatism have a wide range of options to correct their vision problems and, together with an eye exam, the selection of the best treatment that meets vision and lifestyle needs must be done.

7. References

[1] Guyton DL. Prescribing cylinders: the problem of distortion. Surv Ophthalmol. 1977 Nov-Dec; 22(3): 177-88.
[2] Moreira ATR. Astigmatismo: atualização continuada – Sociedade Brasileira de Oftalmopediatria. Arq. Bras. Oftalmol. 2001; 64(3): 2712-272.

[3] Stein HA, Freeman MJ, Stenson SM, Kara José N, Coral-Ghanem C, Oliveira PR. Guia CLAO para refração e óculos: um manual para oftalmologistas. Contact Lens Association of Ophthalmologists Inc. (CLAO). Copyright 1999.

[4] Uras R. Optica e refração ocular – coleção de manuais básicos cbo. Cultura Medica, Rio de Janeiro, 2008.

[5] Moreira SB, Moreira H, Moreira LB. Lente de contato. 3° Ed, cultura médica, Rio de Janeiro, 2004.

[6] Mannis MJ, Zadnik K, Coral-Ghanem C, Kara-Jose N. Contact Lens in Ophthalmic Practice. Springer-Verlag, New York, 2004.

[7] Kurna SA, Şengör T, Ün M, Aqui S. Success rates in the correction of astigmatism with toric and spherical soft contact lens fittings clinical ophthalmology 2010: 4 p959-966.

[8] Edmondson L, Edmondson W, Prince R. Masking astigmatism: Ciba focus night and day vs focus monthly. Optom Vis Sci 2003; 80(12): 184.

[9] Berntsen DA, Merchea MM, Richdale K, Mack CJ, Barr JT. FAAO Higher-Order Aberrations when wearing Sphere and Toric Soft Contact Lenses. Optom Vis Sci. 2009 February; 86(2): 115-122.

[10] Morgan PB, Efron SE, Efron N, Hill EA. Inefficacy of aspheric soft contact lenses for the correction of low levels of astigmatism. Optom Vis Sci. 2005; 82(9): 823-828.

[11] Richdale K, Bernsten DA, Mack CJ. Visual acuity with spherical and toric soft lenses in low- to moderate- astigmatic eyes. Optom Vis Sci 2007; 84(10): 969-75.

[12] Giovedi Filho R. Correção do astigmatismo com lentes de contato rígidas: atualização continuada – Sociedade Brasileira de Lentes de contato e córnea – SOBLEC. 2001; 64(5): 485-487.

[13] Michaud, L, Barriault, C, Dionne, A, Karwatsky, P Empirical fitting of soft or rigid gas-permeable contact lenses for the correction of moderate to severe refractive astigmatism: A comparative study Optometry (2009) 80, 375-383.

[14] Michaud L. Understanding and designing toric gas permeable contact lenses: As easy as 1-2-3. Can J Optom 2007; 69(5): 171-81.

[15] Moreira LB. Ortoceratologia nos casos com contra-indicação de cirurgia refrativa por ceratocone incipiente. Universo visual, November 2006.

[16] Hiraoka,T, Matsumoto, Y, Okamoto, F, Yamagushi, T, Hirohara, Y, Mihashi, T, Oshika, T. Corneal higher-order aberrations induced by overnight orthokeratology. Am J Ophthalmol 2005; 139: 429–436.

[17] Kang SY, Kim BK, Byun YJ. Sustainability of orthokeratology as demonstrated by corneal topography. Korean Journal of ophthalmology 2007; 21(2): 74-78.

[18] Mountford, J, Pesudovs, K. An analysis of the astigmatic changes induced by accelerated orthokeratology. Clin Exp Optom 2002; 85: 284–293.

[19] Baertschi M. Correction of high astigmatism with orthokeratology. Paper presented at the Global Orthokeratology Symposium, Chicago, July 2005.103.

[20] Swarbrick , HA. Orthokeratology review and update Clin Exp Optom 2006; 89: 3: 124-43.

[21] Durrie. D. McMinn, P. Computer-based primary visual cortex training for treatment of low myopia and early presbyopia. Trans Am Ophthalmol Soc 2007; 105: 132-140.

[22] http://www.revitalvision.com/doctors/scientificbackground/

[23] Tan, DT and Fong, A. Efficacy of neural vision therapy to enhance contrast sensitivity function and visual acuity in low myopia. J Cataract Refract Surg, 2008. Apr 34(4): 570-7.

12

Treatment Strategies and Clinical Outcomes of Aspheric Surgery for Astigmatism Using the SCHWIND Amaris Platform

Maria C. Arbelaez[1] and Samuel Arba-Mosquera[2,3]

[1]Muscat Eye Laser Centre,
[2]Grupo de Investigación de Cirugía Refractiva y Calidad de Visión,
Instituto de Oftalmobiología Aplicada, University of Valladolid, Valladolid,
[3]SCHWIND Eye-Tech-Solutions, Kleinostheim,
[1]Oman
[2]Spain
[3]Germany

1. Introduction

An optical system with astigmatism is one where rays that propagate in two perpendicular planes have different foci. If an optical system with astigmatism is used to form an image of a cross, the vertical and horizontal lines will be in sharp focus at two different distances. The term comes from the Greek α- (a-) meaning "without" and στιγμα (stigma), "a mark, spot, puncture".

There are two distinct forms of astigmatism. The first is a third-order aberration, which occurs for objects (or parts of objects) away from the optical axis. This form of aberration occurs even when the optical system is perfectly symmetrical.

The second form of astigmatism occurs when the optical system is not symmetric about the optical axis. This form of astigmatism is extremely important in vision science and eye care, since the human eye often exhibits this aberration due to imperfections in the shape of the cornea or the lens.

If an optical system is not axisymmetric, either due to an error in the shape of the optical surfaces or due to misalignment of the components, astigmatism can occur even for on-axis object points. Ophthalmic astigmatism is a refraction error of the eye in which there is a difference in degree of refraction in different meridians. It is typically characterized by an aspherical, non-figure of revolution cornea in which the corneal profile slope and refractive power in one meridian is less than that of the perpendicular axis.

Astigmatism causes difficulties in seeing fine detail. In some cases vertical lines and objects such as walls may appear to the patient to be leaning over like the Tower of Pisa. Astigmatism can be often corrected by glasses with a lens that has different radii of curvature in different planes (a cylindrical lens), contact lenses, or refractive surgery.

Astigmatism is quite common. Studies have shown that about one in three people suffers from it. The prevalence of astigmatism increases with age. Although a person may not notice mild astigmatism, higher amounts of astigmatism may cause blurry vision, squinting, asthenopia, fatigue, or headaches.

Astigmatism is an optical defect in which vision is blurred due to the inability of the optics of the eye to focus a point object into a sharp focused image on the retina. This may be due to an irregular or toric curvature of the cornea or lens. The most of the astigmatism is corneal. Astigmatism may also be caused by crystalline lens subluxation, coloboma or lenticonus. There are two types of astigmatism: regular and irregular. Irregular astigmatism is often caused by a corneal scar or scattering in the crystalline lens. Regular astigmatism arising from either the cornea or crystalline lens can be easily corrected.

The refractive error of the astigmatic eye stems from a difference in degree of curvature refraction of the two different meridians (i.e., the eye has different focal points in different planes.) For example, the image may be clearly focused on the retina in the horizontal (sagittal) plane, but not in the vertical (tangential) plane. Astigmatism causes difficulties in seeing fine detail, and in some cases vertical lines (e.g., walls) may appear to the patient to be tilted.

In With-the-rule astigmatism, the eye sees vertical lines more sharply than horizontal lines. Against-the-rule astigmatism reverses the situation. Children tend to have With-the-rule astigmatism and elderly people tend to have Against-the-rule astigmatism. The prevalence of astigmatism increases with age.

Astigmatism may be corrected with eyeglasses, contact lenses, or refractive surgery. Various considerations involving ocular health, refractive status, and lifestyle frequently determine whether one option may be better than another. In those with keratoconus, toric contact lenses often enable patients to achieve better visual acuities than eyeglasses. Once only available in a rigid gas-permeable form, toric lenses are now available also as soft lenses.

2. Aspheric ablation strategies

An aspheric lens or asphere is a lens whose surfaces have a profile that is rotationally symmetric, but is not a portion of a sphere. The asphere's more complex surface profile can reduce or eliminate spherical aberration and also reduce other optical aberrations compared to spheric lenses. Aspheric elements are used to reduce aberrations.

In prescriptions for both farsightedness and nearsightedness, the lens curve flattens toward the edge of the asphere. Aspheric ablation strategies for spherical correction are modified by means of spherical aberration compensations, whereas aspheric ablation strategies for astigmatic correction are modified by means of high-order-asitmgatism aberration compensations.

3. Ocular wavefront (OW) customized ablation strategies

The treatment plan is developed using OW customised aspheric profiles based on Hartmann-Shack sensing[1]. The high-resolution Hartmann-Shack measurements (>800 points for a 7.0-mm pupil) referred to the entire eye. Optical errors centered on the line-of-sight are described by the Zernike polynomials[2] and the coefficients of the Optical Society of America (OSA) standard[3].

Ocular Wavefront Analyzer

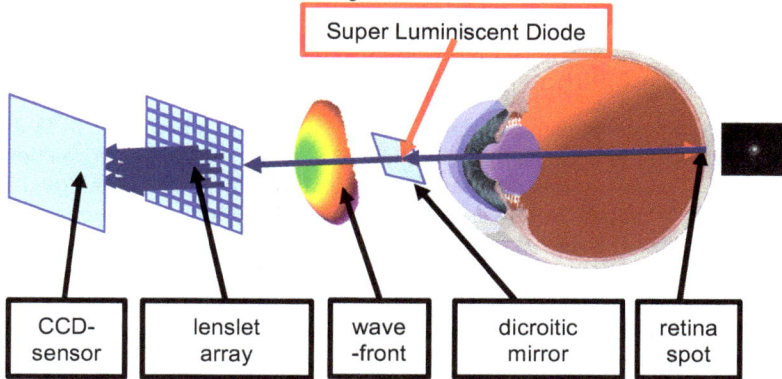

- 1452 data points in total
- >800 data points for a 7 mm pupil

Fig. 1. Principle of the OW measurement.

3.1 Treatment modality

Preoperative topography and aberrometry measurements are taken, and visual acuity, and mesopic pupil size are measured. To determine the ablation profile of the Custom Ablation Manager (CAM), manifest refraction is measured in each eye and crosschecked with objective refraction from the SCHWIND Ocular Wavefront Analyzer[4]. Each eye is planned according to the manifest refraction using the CAM Wavefront customised treatments.

The CAM aspherical profiles were developed with the aim to compensate for the induction of aberrations (especially but not only spherical aberration) observed with other types of profile definitions[5], some of these sources of aberrations are those related to the loss of efficiency of the laser ablation for non-normal incidence[6,7]. Optimization is realized by taking into account the loss of efficiency at the periphery of the cornea in relation to the center, as there is a tangential effect of the spot in relation to the corneal curvature (K (Keratometry) -reading). The software provides K-reading compensation, which considers the change in spot geometry and reflection losses of ablation efficiency.

The base-line for correcting refraction (sphere and cylinder) is aspheric, whereas the high order aberrations measured based on Hartmann-Shack sensing of the entire eye are combined with manifest refraction.

Real ablative spot shape (volume) is considered through a self-constructing algorithm. In addition, there are a randomized flying-spot ablation pattern, and controls for the local repetition rates to minimize the thermal load of the treatment[8].

A central fully corrected ablation zone is used in all eyes with a variable transition size automatically provided by the laser related to the planned refractive correction. Immediately before the ablation, the laser is calibrated per manufacturer's instructions and the calibration settings are recorded.

The CAM software is able to import, visualize, and combine diagnostic data of the eye (manifest refraction and ocular wavefront data in this case) into a customised aspherical ablation profile to optimize the corneal shape. OW based ablations attempt to reduce the wavefront aberration of the entire eye (within Optical Zone, OZ) close to a zero level, compensating, as well, for the aberration induction observed with other types of profiles.

It should be noted that opposing the preoperative wavefront aberration in laser refractive surgery constituted only a first approximation of a perfect refractive correction, as tissue removal occurs. Considerations such as treatment duration or tissue removal make even more difficult to establish a universal optimal profile. Our data suggest that Ocular wavefront customized treatments can only be successful, if the pre-existing aberrations are greater than the repeatability and the biological noise. In particular, the OW customized approach is highly efficient in eyes with greater than 0.25 microns root-mean-square (RMS) ocular HOAb, or where individual components of the OW such as coma, trefoil or spherical aberration are greater than 0.2 microns RMS.

4. Corneal wavefront (CW) customized ablation strategies

The treatment plan is developed using CW customized aspheric profiles based on corneal ray tracing (Salmon 1999[9]). Using the Keratron Scout videokeratoscope (Mattioli & Tripoli 1997[10]) (Optikon 2000 S.p.A, Rome, Italy), the topographical surface and corneal wavefront are analyzed (up to the 7th order). Considering a balanced-eye model (Q-Val –0.25) the departure of the measured corneal topography from the theoretically optimal corneal surface is calculated. Optical errors centered on the line of sight are described by the Zernike polynomials (Zernike 1934[11]) and the coefficients of the Optical Society of America (OSA) standard (Thibos et al. 2002[12]).

Ray tracing is a procedure classically performed by applying Snell's law to the corneal surface. However, it is much simpler to understand corneal wavefront in terms of optical path difference and calculate it by Huygens-Fresnel or "least time" Fermat principles (Salmon 1999[9]; Guirao & Artal 2000[13]).

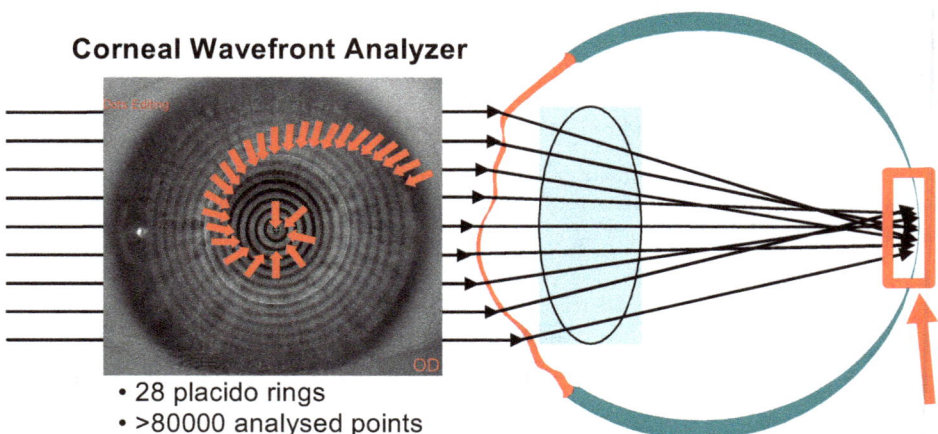

Corneal Wavefront Analyzer

• 28 placido rings
• >80000 analysed points

Fig. 2. Principle of the dderivation of the CW.

In corneal wavefront analysis, the type and size of any optical error on the anterior corneal surface are registered, thus allowing a very selective correction. The defects are corrected exactly at their origin – the anterior corneal surface. In this context, the precise localization of defects is crucial to successfully achieving optimal results in laser surgery. The corneal wavefront allows for a very precise diagnosis, thus providing an individual ablation of the cornea in order to obtain perfect results.

Applying this treatment strategy, measurement does not require pupil dilation of the eye, so that the treatment zone is not limited by the pupil and accomodation does not influence the measuring results. Mention is made that in this way forcing a fixed asphericity quotient (Q) on the eyes through the treatment is avoided. Instead, this strategy employs a dynamic postoperative expected asphericity quotient (de Ortueta & Arba-Mosquera 2008[14]), being expressed as:

$$Q_{exp} = \frac{\dfrac{1}{n^2} - \dfrac{1}{4}}{\left(1 + \dfrac{R \cdot SEq_{cp}}{n-1}\right)^3} - \frac{1}{n^2} \tag{1}$$

where Q_{exp} is the expected/predicted corneal asphericity quotient; R the apical radius of curvature of the preoperative cornea; SEq_{cp} the spherical equivalent to be corrected at the corneal plane; and n the refractive index of the cornea.

The expected quotient of asphericity does not incorporate any compensation for the effect of postop corneal biomechanics / healing response, and it is rather derived from a pure optical model of the cornea.

Preoperative topography and corneal aberrometry measurements are taken, and visual acuity, and mesopic pupil size are measured. Each eye is planned according to the manifest refraction using the CAM wavefront customized treatments. Immediately before ablation, the laser is calibrated according to the manufacturer's instructions and the calibration settings are recorded.

When evaluating the outcomes of wavefront customization strategies, wavefront aberration analysis is mandatory to be able to determine whether the customization aims could be achieved. It has been suggested, as well, that the surface ablation procedures are better suited for the wavefront guided ablation as they would avoid the induction of aberrations due to flap and interface (Chun et al. 2006[15]; Buzzonetti et al. 2004[16]). Now with the introduction of thin and ultrathin planar flaps with femtosecond laser and the newer microkeratomes such as the pendular microkeratome, this aspect of the debate will require further research.

Topography is measured under bright light conditions which might cause pupil constriction and also pupil center shift relative to normal photopic levels. Corneal wavefront customized treatments can only be successful, if the pre-existing aberrations are greater than the repeatability and the biological noise. Considerations such as treatment duration or tissue removal make it more difficult to establish a universal optimal profile.

Furthermore, coupling effects between different high order aberration terms, and between HOAs and manifest refraction is still one of the major sources of residual aberrations after refractive surgery. This topic has been discussed from a theoretical perspective by Bará et al. 2006 [17] and from a clinical perspective by MacRae 2007[18] or Buehren et al. 2007[19]. They all found mutually affecting interactions, for example, between defocus and spherical aberration, or between 3 order aberrations and low order terms, between spherical aberration and coma, or between secondary and primary astigmatisms.

The accuracy, predictability, and stability of the refractive power change, together with the minimal external impact of the CAM ablation profiles on the HOAs, leads to very good results in terms of visual quality. In summary, aspheric CW ablation profiles, designed with CAM software for the AMARIs laser platform, yield visual, optical, and refractive results comparable to those of other wavefront-guided customized techniques for correction of myopia and myopic astigmatism. The CW customized approach shows its strength in cases where abnormal optical systems are expected. Apart from the risk of minimal additional ablation of corneal tissue, systematical wavefront-customized corneal ablation can be considered as a safe and beneficial method.

5. Decision Assistant Wizard

Our definition of "Customisation" is conceptually different and can be stated as: "The planning of the optimum ablation pattern specifically for each individual eye based on its diagnosis and visual demands." It is often the case, that the best approach for planning an ablation is a sophisticated pattern, which can still be simply described in terms of sphere, cylinder, and orientation (axis). The Decision Assistant Wizard, which we present here, is based on our experience with the SCHWIND AMARIS laser. While the general principles of this Decision-Tree based planning (Fig. 3) can basically be applied to any other laser platform offering aspheric and wavefront-guided profiles, some specific aspects concerning both diagnosis and treatments may depend on other manufacturers' specifications.

We begin by acquiring four corneal topographies (Corneal Wavefront Analyzer, SCHWIND eye-tech-solutions GmbH & Co.KG, based on Keratron-Scout, OPTIKON2000, Rome, Italy) and derived CW analyses centred on the line-of-sight for each eye of the patient. We extract the mean, and discard the less representative one (the one with the poorest similarity to the mean). From those remaining three maps, we calculate the mean, and select the most representative one (the one with the highest similarity to the mean).

We continue acquiring, under non pharmacologically dilated pupils, non-cycloplegic conditions, and natural dim light conditions (to avoid pharmacologically induced pupil shifts[20],[21]), 3 aberrometries (Ocular Wavefront Analyzer, SCHWIND eye-tech-solutions GmbH & Co.KG, based on irx3, Imagine Eyes, Orsay, France) and objective refractions for each eye of the patient. To minimize the potential accommodative response of the patients, we ask them to "see-through-the-target" instead of "looking at the target." In this way, patients do not try to get a sharp image from the +1.5 D fogged target, since they were instructed to see-through-the-target. From those aberrometries, we calculate the mean, and select the most representative one (the aberrometry map with the highest similarity to the mean).

We continue assessing subjective refraction based upon non-pharmacologic and non-cycloplegic conditions, under natural photopic illumination. We use the objective refraction analyzed for a sub-pupil of 4 mm diameter, as starting refraction for this step. This is particularly useful for determining the magnitude and orientation of the astigmatism. We measure manifest refraction, uncorrected and best spectacle-corrected Snellen visual acuity[22] (UCVA and BSCVA, respectively). Further rules that we impose for accurately determining the manifest subjective refractions among equal levels of BSCVA are: taking the measurement with the least negative (the most positive) spherical equivalent (unmasking latent hyperopia), if several of them are equal in terms of spherical equivalent, we choose the measurement with the least amount of astigmatism (reducing the risk of postoperative shifts in the axis of astigmatism). This is particularly useful for determining the magnitude and orientation of the internal astigmatism as a difference between the topographic astigmatism and the astigmatism of the corneal wavefront analyses compared to the subjective astigmatism the astigmatism of the ocular wavefront analyses.

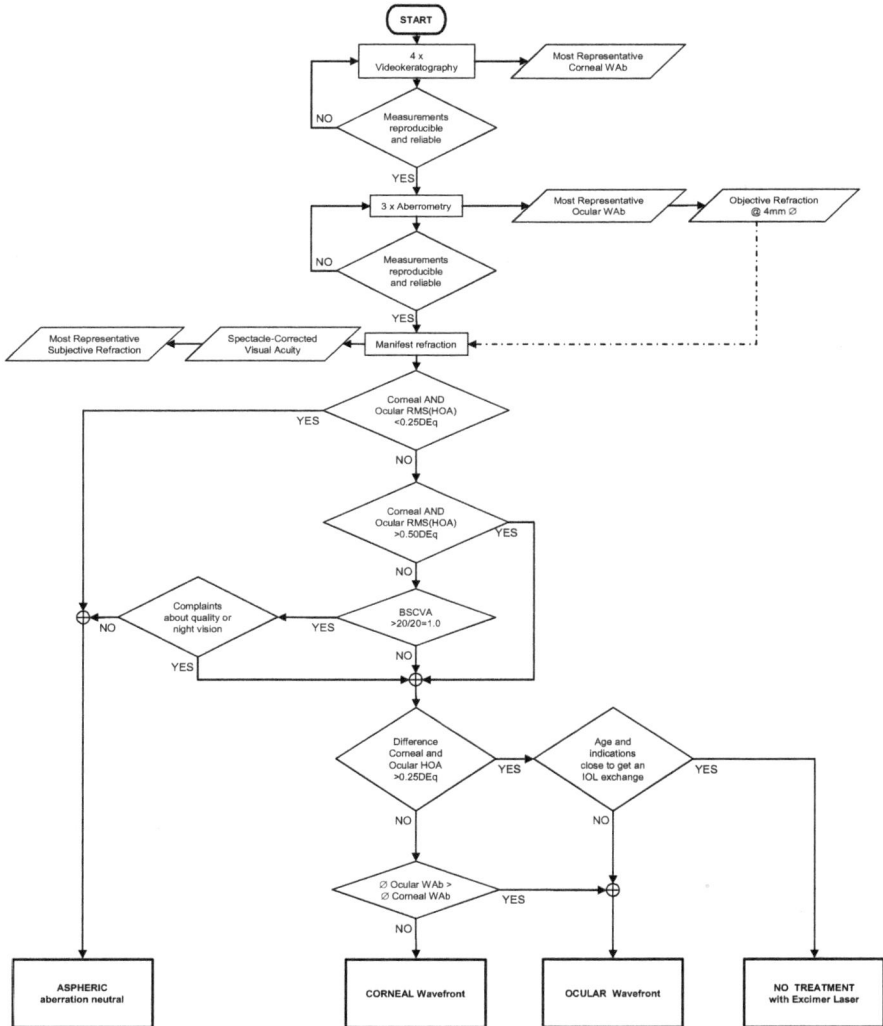

Fig. 3. Decision-Tree applied for selecting the treatment mode (Aspheric aberration neutral, Corneal-Wavefront-Guided, or Ocular-Wavefront-Guided).

The decision process starts by estimating the global optical impairment resulting from the measured wave aberrations. This is done by objectively determining the actual clinical relevance of single terms in a Zernike expansion of the wave aberration. In general, for the same magnitude of aberration, the optical blur produced by high order aberrations increases with increasing radial order and decreases with increasing angular frequencies. Based on this, the dioptric equivalent (DEq) was used.

If the global optical blur for both corneal and ocular wave-aberrations (CWAb and OWAb, respectively) are below 0.25 DEq for both eyes, then the treatment to be applied is Aspheric aberration neutral. If the global optical blur for any corneal or ocular wave-aberrations is between 0.25 DEq and 0.50 DEq for any eye, then we check the BSCVA achieved during the manifest refraction. If the BSCVA is better than 20/20 for both eyes, then we ask the patient about complaints regarding night vision or, in general, quality of vision. If the patient does not report complaints, then the treatment to be applied is Aspheric aberration neutral.

If the patient reports complaints regarding quality of vision, the BSCVA is worse than 20/20 for any eye, or the global optical blur for both corneal and ocular wave-aberrations are above 0.50 DEq for both eyes, then we compare corneal and ocular wave-aberrations. For this, we calculate the differential aberration (CWAb − OWAb, both centred at the line-of-sight) in terms of the Zernike expansion, and estimate the global optical difference. If this global optical difference between corneal and ocular wave-aberrations is below 0.25 DEq for both eyes, we consider both corneal and ocular wave-aberrations as equivalent. In this case, the treatment to be applied depends on the available diameter of the wavefront maps and the scotopic pupil size. If the diameter of the Ocular- or Corneal-WAb map (the one providing the largest diameter) is at least as large as the scotopic pupil size (in natural dark conditions) reduced in 0.25 mm, then Ocular- or Corneal-Wavefront-guided ablation is performed (the one providing the largest diameter), or Aspheric aberration neutral otherwise. Usually the size of the Ocular WAb maps is similar to the size of the scotopic pupils, whereas Corneal WAb maps are wider (up to 10 mm in diameter).

If the global optical difference between corneal and ocular wave-aberrations is above 0.25 DEq for any eye, we consider internal wave-aberration (IWAb) is relevant, then the treatment to be applied is Ocular-Wavefront-guided if the patient is neither in age nor in ophthalmic indications close to get an IOL exchange (due to e.g. lenticular opacities), otherwise no laser corneal refractive treatment is recommended (since IOL exchange is preferred).

Level of aberration	Aspheric aberration neutral	CW-guided	OW-guided
Corneal AND Ocular Wavefronts < 0.25Deq	Always	No	No
Corneal OR Ocular Wavefront between 0.25DEq and 0.50Deq	If BSCVA > 20/20 AND no complaints about quality or night vision	If (BSCVA < 20/20 OR complaints about quality or night vision) AND Internal Wavefront < 0.25DEq	If (BSCVA < 20/20 OR complaints about quality or night vision) AND no lenticular problems
Corneal AND Ocular Wavefronts > 0.50Deq	If wavefront maps smaller than scotopic pupil	If Internal Wavefront < 0.25DEq	If no lenticular problems

Table 1. Indications chart.

There are basically three types of approaches for planning a corneal refractive treatment. The first are those that have as their objective the elimination or reduction of the total aberrations of the eye. The main criticism to this approach argues that the goal "zero aberration" is inconsistent throughout the day due to accommodation, and little lasting, since aberrations change with age[23],[24],[25]. The second approach is intended to correct all corneal aberrations, since corneal aberrations do not change with age[26],[27]. However, this concept might also be wrong considering corneal aberrations interact with internal aberrations, some of them being cancelled, and producing an aberration pattern of the total eye in general different from the aberration pattern of the cornea alone. Therefore, by only removing corneal aberration we might worsen the overall aberrations, since the internal aberration might not find a corneal aberration for compensation. In case that the corneal aberration is of the same sign as the internal aberration, the correction of the corneal aberration would be useful, as it would reduce the total aberration of the eye. A third approach tries not to induce aberrations. This type of treatment is not as ambitious, but much more simple to operate. The goal of the Aberration-Free™ ablation profile is to provide a neutral high-order-aberrations (HOAb) ablation, ie to maintain the same HOAb profile both preoperatively with best spectacle correction and postoperatively without correction.

There is evidence of neural adaptation to the baseline wavefront profile. The interaction between high-order-aberrations can be beneficial to visual quality regardless of the magnitude HOAb. Based on the random nature of the HOAb induction and current research, it may be beneficial to maintain the preoperative wavefront profile for a significant number of refractive surgery candidates.

We are not postulating that customized ablation algorithms in any form (ocular-wavefront-guided, corneal-wavefront-guided, topography-guided) are not be useful. Rather, that specific populations with specific demands deserve specific treatment solutions. Aspheric treatments aimed at preservation of the preoperative HOAb show their strengths in patients with preoperative BSCVA 20/20 or better or in patients where the visual degradation cannot be attributable to the presence of clinically relevant HOAb (e.g. lens opacities).

The corneal wavefront customized approach shows its strength in cases where abnormal corneal surfaces are expected. Apart from the risk of additional ablation of corneal tissue, wavefront customized corneal ablation can be considered a safe and beneficial method. Our experience suggests that wavefront customized treatments can only be successful, if pre-existing aberrations are greater than repeatability (e.g. repeatability of diagnostic[28] and treatment devices) and biological noise (e.g. day-to-day variabilities in visual acuity, refraction, or aberration in the same subject).

Furthermore, coupling effects between different high order aberration terms, and between HOAb and manifest refraction have been found[29],[30] for example, between defocus and spherical aberration, or between 3rd order aberrations and low order terms, between spherical aberration and coma, or between secondary and primary astigmatisms. These interactions may provide some relative visual benefits[31], but may as well contribute as sources of uncertainty in the conversion of wavefront aberration maps to refractive prescriptions. Notice that for comparing OWAb and CWAb, the analysis of the IWAb as CWAb – OWAb is mandatory since RMS(IWAb) accounts for any deviation (i.e. inductions and reductions of the wave-aberration both contribute positively to increase the RMS value).

The Decision Assistant Wizard presented here may theoretically be applied to any other laser platform offering aspheric, topography-guided, and wavefront-guided profiles, if appropriate analysis functions for CWAb, OWAb, and IWAb are available. Simplified versions with limited functionalities are also possible, if, for example, neither CW-analyses (i.e. no IWAb) nor topography-guided profiles are available. The desired outcome of non-wavefront-driven refractive surgery is to balance the effects on the wave-aberration, and, to provide normal eyes with perhaps the most natural unaltered quality of vision. While Ocular Wavefront treatments have the advantage of being based on Objective Refraction of the complete human eye system, whereas Corneal Wavefront treatments have the advantage of being independent from accommodation effects or light/pupil conditions; Aspheric treatments have the advantage of saving tissue, time and due to their simplicity offer better predictability.

In highly aberrated eyes, manifest refraction may become an art, a sort of guessing around the least blurred image. In further studies, systematic deviations from the measured manifest refractions, as well as other foreseeable couplings among Zernike coefficients will be evaluated.

6. Minimization of depth and time in laser corneal refractive surgery

In laser corneal refractive surgery, one always aims to reduce the ablated tissue thickness (and, to a minor degree, to reduce the intervention time) because an ectasia of the cornea may result from excessive tissue removal. Customized laser corneal refractive surgery on aberrated eyes may yield better results than the standard procedure[18-21] but generally results in higher ablation depth, volume, and time. Therefore, optimizing the customized treatment to reduce the ablated thickness while retaining the positive aspects is pertinent.[22]

The development of new algorithms or ablation strategies for performing laser corneal refractive surgery in a customized form, minimizing the amount of ablated tissue without compromising the visual quality, and potentially maximizing visual performance without increasing risk factors would be of great value for the refractive surgery community and ultimately for the health and safety of patients. The real impact of tissue-saving algorithms in customized treatments is controversial. Minimizing the amount of tissue must be done in a way that does not compromise the refractive correction or visual performance, and it must be safe, reliable, and reproducible.

In general, for the same amount of equivalent defocus, the optical blur produced by HOAs increases with increasing radial order and decreases with increasing angular frequencies. Based on this blur effect of the single Zernike terms, we have defined a dioptric equivalent:

$$\text{DEq}_n^m = \frac{8\sqrt{2(n+1)(1+\delta_{m0})}\left|C_n^m\right|}{\text{PD}^2} \tag{2}$$

where DEq_n^m is the dioptric equivalent of the optical blur; n, the radial order of the considered Zernike term; m, the angular frequency of the considered Zernike term; δ_{m0}, the Kronecker delta function of the angular frequency and zero (1 for radially symmetric Zernike terms and 0 otherwise); C_n^m, the weight coefficient of the considered Zernike term; and PD, the analysis diameter for the optical blur.

In such a way, the dioptric equivalent produced by HOAs increases with increasing radial order and partly decreases with increasing angular frequencies. This dioptric equivalent metric is identical to the power vector notation for the low orders and allows defining a general optical blur as a general expression for the one proposed by Thibos et al[36]:

$$U_G = \sqrt{\sum \left(DEq_n^m \right)^2}$$ (3)

where U_G is the general optical blur.

We have expressed each of the Zernike terms as a dioptric equivalent in familiar units to help judge the order of magnitude of the effect. Using common clinical limits, the following classification is proposed:

$$DEq_n^m < 0.50 \text{ D} \Rightarrow \text{might be clinically relevant}$$ (4)

$$DEq_{1n}^m \geq 0.50 \text{ D} \Rightarrow \text{clinically relevant}$$ (5)

This represents the proposed objective determination of the actual clinical relevance of the single terms in a Zernike expansion of the wavefront aberration.[22]

6.1 Objective minimization of the maximum depth of a customized ablation based on the Zernike expansion of the wavefront aberration

One of the minimization approaches consists of simplifying the profile by selecting a subset of Zernike terms that minimizes the necessary ablation depth while respecting the Zernike terms considered clinically relevant. The minimize depth (MD+) function analyzes the Zernike pyramid as described in the previous section and evaluates the ablation depth of all possible free combinations of subsets of Zernike terms while fulfilling several conditions:

- Only terms of third or higher order can be disabled.
- Only terms with optical blur dioptric equivalent less than 0.5 D can be disabled.
- For each subset combination of Zernike terms, the low-order terms are recalculated using the automatic refraction balance method.

From this evaluation, the function selects the subset of Zernike terms that needs the minimum amount of maximum depth.

6.2 Objective minimization of the ablation volume of a customized ablation based on the Zernike expansion of the wavefront aberration

The other minimization approach consists of simplifying the profile by selecting a subset of Zernike terms that minimizes the necessary ablation volume while respecting the Zernike terms considered clinically relevant. The minimize volume (MV+) function analyzes the Zernike pyramid as described in the previous section and evaluates the ablation depth of all possible free combinations of subsets of Zernike terms fulfilling several conditions:

- Only terms of third or higher order can be disabled.
- Only terms with optical blur dioptric equivalent less than 0.5 D can be disabled.
- For each subset combination of Zernike terms, the low-order terms are recalculated using the automatic refraction balance method.

From this evaluation, the function selects the subset of Zernike terms that needs the minimum amount of volume for the ablation. Reduced ablation volumes lead to shorter treatment times.

One could use the equivalent defocus applied to each individual Zernike mode to compute its clinical relevance. The basis of the equivalent defocus concept is the notion that the imaging quality of an eye is determined primarily by wavefront variance, and it does not matter which Zernike mode produces that variance. This is only true when the wavefront variance is really small and the image quality is measured by the Strehl ratio. Otherwise, the relationship between wavefront variance and image quality becomes much more complex. It is important to bear in mind that 1 D of ordinary defocus does not necessarily have the same effect as 1 D of equivalent defocus because different types of aberrations affect the retinal image in different ways. Nevertheless, by expressing RMS error in terms of equivalent defocus, the data are put into familiar units that help us judge the order of magnitude of the effect.

Strictly speaking, one cannot consider the clinical relevance of every Zernike term independently without demonstrating whether a single Zernike term is alone responsible for the loss of visual quality. The visual effect of an aberration does not only depend on that specific aberration but also on other possibly present aberrations; for example, the sum of small aberrations, previously considered clinically irrelevant, could lead to a clear loss of overall optical quality. The idea of approximating a distorted wavefront by means of an equivalent dioptric error is much too controversial to be accepted without caution.

Coupling effects between different HOA terms and between HOAs and manifest refraction have been found,[44-46] for example, between defocus and spherical aberration, third-order aberrations and low-order terms, spherical aberration and coma, or secondary and primary astigmatisms. These interactions may provide some relative visual benefits[47] but may also contribute uncertainty in the conversion of wavefront aberration maps to refractive prescriptions.[48,49] One could use more sophisticated equations to model the equivalences between the optical blur produced by the different Zernike terms, but we have used a relatively simple approach driven primarily by the radial order. Different approaches for minimizing tissue ablation in refractive surgery have been proposed and extensively discussed.[22] When to use customized strategies in refractive surgery has been discussed previously as well.[18-21]

Considering that Zernike terms are either planned to be corrected or left uncorrected, visual performance is not compromised because all remaining uncorrected terms are below clinical relevance. The proposed approaches are safe, reliable, and reproducible because of the objective foundation upon which they are based. It is important to note that the selection of the Zernike terms to be included in the correction is not trivial. As mentioned, only Zernike terms considered not clinically relevant or of minor clinical relevance can be excluded from the correction, but they must not necessarily be excluded.

Actually, single Zernike terms considered not clinically relevant will only be disabled when they represent additional tissue for ablation and will be enabled when they help to save tissue. This way, particular cases are represented by the full wavefront correction by disabling all nonclinically relevant terms or by disabling all high-order terms. As per design, the MD group actually optimizes for minimum ablation depth and shows the largest savings for this aim (-8 ± 4 μm, from -20 to -1 μm), whereas the MV group actually optimizes for minimum ablation volume (time) and shows the largest savings for this aim (-8 ± 2 seconds, from -26 to -22 seconds). In this context, and as a rule of thumb, MD minimization could be used in customized myopic treatments when reducing ablation depth is directly related to decreasing the risk of keratectasia, whereas MV minimization could be used in long customized treatments when reducing ablation time is directly related to better maintenance of homogeneous corneal conditions.

7. Surgical technique selection

Excimer laser refractive surgery has evolved full circle. Surface ablations in the form of photorefractive keratectomy (PRK) swiftly evolved into intra-stromal procedure of laser in-situ keratomileusis (LASIK) due to its rapid visual recovery and minimal postoperative discomfort. However, with increasing adoption of LASIK grew the concern for post-LASIK keratectasia. The last few years have therefore, witnessed a renewed interest in alcohol assisted surface ablation procedures to avoid complications of LASIK primarily corneal ectasia and flap and interface related problems.

The decision to perform alcohol assisted LASEK or LASIK is based on preoperative central corneal thickness (measured by ultrasonic pachymetry (DGH-550 Pachette 2, DGH Technologies, USA)) and calculated depth of ablation. LASEK is performed on all patients with central pachymetry less than 500 μm. Eyes with central pachymetry above 500 μm are assigned to either LASEK or LASIK techniques, depending on the central pachymetry and the depth of ablation. The decision is based on the target of limiting the ablation to the anterior one third of the cornea (so as to achieve a residual stromal bed thickness of at least 2/3rd of pre-operative pachymetry). Patients were tested for LASIK in case they do not meet the "2/3" condition they were assigned to the LASEK group.

For corneal and conjunctival anesthesia, two drops of proparacaine HCl 0.5% (Aurocaine®, Aurolab, Madurai, India) are instilled three times before shifting the patient to the operation theatre (OT).

LASIK - Pachymetry is performed before and after flap creation (stromal bed thickness) with both the integrated online coherence pachymeter (Heidelberg, Germany) and ultrasonic pachymeter. Flap is made using LDV femtosecond laser. Contact lens is applied at the end of surgery (Biomedics 55 evolution, Ocular Sciences, Cooper Vision, Hamble, UK) in eyes with 'achieved' flap thickness less than 110 microns to avoid flap displacements, dislocations or striae.

LASEK - 17% alcohol applied for 30 seconds is used for the creation of epithelial flap. Eight or 9 mm diameter epithelial flap is made after incising the corneal epithelium with a trephine. Contact lens is applied at the end of surgery in all LASEK patients.

Postoperative Treatment – For LASIK patients, eye drop Tobradex (Alcon Inc, USA) 3 times a day is used for 1 week along with Oasis soft plugs extended duration (6404 Glendora CA) and preservative free artificial tear drops during the first three months. A bandage contact lens is used during the first night in LASIK patients with flap thickness less than 110μm. For LASEK patients, prior to epithelial healing, eye drops lomefloxacin 0.3 % (Okacin) and pranoprofen (Ofralar, Alcon Inc, USA) are used along with Oasis soft plugs extended duration. Bandage contact lens is applied in all LASEK patients for 5-7 days until complete healing of the epithelial defect. After epithelial healing, preservative free artificial tear eye drops are given along with efemoline eye drops (Fluoromethalone, Novartis Ophthalmics, Switzerland) 3 times a day for 3 months. The steroids are gradually tapered every month to once a day in the last month.

Postoperative follow-up – LASIK patients are followed on first postoperative day, at 1 month, 3 months, and 1 year. LASEK patients are examined on first postoperative day, at 1 week, 1 month, 3 months, and 1 year.

There has been a renewed interest in surface ablation modalities with epithelial repositioning like LASEK to overcome some of the flap and ectasia related complications of LASIK. Though the rate of visual recovery may be slower in surface ablation thus lacking the LASIK 'wow' effect, studies have shown that LASEK is an effective modality for surgical correction of low to moderate myopia.[8-10] However, its utility for correction of high myopia is limited.[11-13] With introduction of thin and ultrathin flaps using femtosecond laser and newer microkeratomes such as the pendular microkeratome, the indications for the 2 surgical modalities are getting indistinct. Introduction of newer ablation profiles such as customized and aspheric ablations has added another aspect to be evaluated.

It has been suggested that surface ablative procedures may be better suited for customized correction though it has not been proven clinically.[1,2,14] It has been suggested that the creation of corneal flap in LASIK patients can induce further higher order aberrations especially coma like aberrations.[15] This may be particularly relevant to thinner flaps which may have a higher incidence of flap striae. The clinical relevance of these flap induced higher order aberrations especially in relation to newer microkeratomes and femtosecond laser and the effect of flap thickness require further investigation.

The aspheric ablation profile is equally successful with both surface ablation as well as intrastromal excimer ablation minimizing the change in higher order aberrations. The latest development in excimer laser refractive is the thin and the ultrathin flap LASIK. It attempts to find the best of both worlds of standard LASIK and surface ablation. Besides pre-existing risk factors, low residual stromal bed thickness is the single most important modifiable factor that increases the risk of iatrogenic post-LASIK ectasia.[38] Thin and ultrathin flap LASIK achieves a thicker residual stromal bed and therefore is believed to decrease the risk of post-LASIK ectasia. Current study indicates that thin and ultrathin LASIK is safe, efficacious, and predictable after short term follow up of 6 months. However, future investigations with long-term follow-up are likely to prove if LASIK utilizing thin and ultrathin flaps translate into the anticipated decreased risk of post-LASIK ectasia.

8. 6D Eye-Tracker

Human eyes have six degrees of freedom to move: X/Y lateral shifts, Z levelling, horizontal/vertical rotations, and cyclotorsion (rotations around the optical axis). The analysis of these movements has been made since the middle of the 20th century. Schwiegerling and Snyder[32] measured eye motion in patients having laser in situ keratomileusis (LASIK) using a video technique and determine centration and variance of the eye position during surgery. They found a standard deviation in the eye movements in all eyes larger than 100 μm. Taylor et al.[33] determined the accuracy of an eye tracking system designed for laser refractive surgery. The system demonstrated an accuracy of 60 μm for an intact cornea and 100 μm for a cornea with a thin flap removed.

Bueeler et al.[34] investigated the lateral alignment accuracy needed in wavefront-guided refractive surgery to improve the ocular optics to a desired level in a percentage of normally aberrated eyes. To achieve the diffraction limit in 95% of the normal eyes with a 7.0 mm pupil, a lateral alignment accuracy of 70 μm or better was required. An accuracy of 200 μm was sufficient to reach the same goal with a 3.0 mm pupil. Bueeler and Mrochen[35] quantified the parallax error associated with localizing corneal positions by tracking the subjacent entrance pupil center by means of optical ray-tracing in a schematic model eye. They found tracking error can amount to 30% (or more for eye trackers mounted closer than 500 mm to the eye) of the detected lateral shift. Thus, if the eye tracker registers a lateral shift of the entrance pupil of 200 μm away from the tracking reference axis, the point of interest located on the cornea would essentially be 260 μm away from this reference axis. A laser pulse fired at that moment would be systematically displaced by 60 μm.

Measuring rotation when the patient is upright[36] to when the refractive treatments are performed with the patient supine may lead to ocular cyclotorsion,[37,38] resulting in mismatching of the applied versus the intended profiles[39,40]. Recently, some equipment can facilitate measurement of and potential compensation for static cyclotorsion occurring when the patient moves from upright to the supine position during the procedure[41], quantifying the cyclorotation occurring between wavefront measurement and laser refractive surgery[42] and compensating for it[43,44,45]. Further measuring and compensating ocular cyclotorsion during refractive treatments with the patient supine may reduce optical "noise" of the applied versus the intended profiles[46,47,48].

In recent times, many studies have discussed the methodologies and implications of ocular cyclotorsion, but not many papers pay attention to the rolling and axial movements of the eye. The more irregular a cornea is, the more important proper eye-tracking. Astigmatism is the most common aberration with a vector nature, so usually are the astigmatic problems the ones more affected or the ones which benefit the most from advanced eye tracking.

8.1 Lateral movements during ablation (1st and 2nd dimension)

AMARIS system includes a pupil-registration module for the eye-tracker subsystem, in which, the first pupil image under the AMARIS system obtained with starting the ablation is taken as reference and its location referred to the limbus is used for any further eye-tracker image in order to determine the pupil centre shift compensation (PCSC).

8.2 Eye rolling during ablation (3rd and 4th dimension)

AMARIS system includes a scleral-registration module for the eye-tracker subsystem, in which, the first few scleral-tracker images under the AMARIS system obtained with starting the ablation are taken as reference (natural rolling) and compared to any further scleral-tracker image in order to determine the eye rolling (ER).

8.3 Static cyclotorsion between upright and supine positions (5th dimension)

AMARIS system includes an eye-registration module for the eye-tracker subsystem, in which, the diagnosis image is taken as reference and compared to an eye-tracker image under the AMARIS system obtained prior to starting the ablation in order to determine the static cyclotorsion component (SCC).

8.4 Dynamic cyclotorsion during ablation (5th dimension)

AMARIS system includes an eye-registration module for the eye-tracker subsystem, in which, the first eye-tracker image under the AMARIS system obtained with starting the ablation is taken as reference and compared to any further eye-tracker image in order to determine the dynamic cyclotorsion component (DCC).

8.5 Axial displacements during ablation (6th dimension)

AMARIS system includes an scleral-registration module for the eye-tracker subsystem, in which, the first few scleral-tracker images under the AMARIS system obtained with starting the ablation are taken as reference (natural level) and compared to any further scleral-tracker image in order to determine the axial displacements (AD).

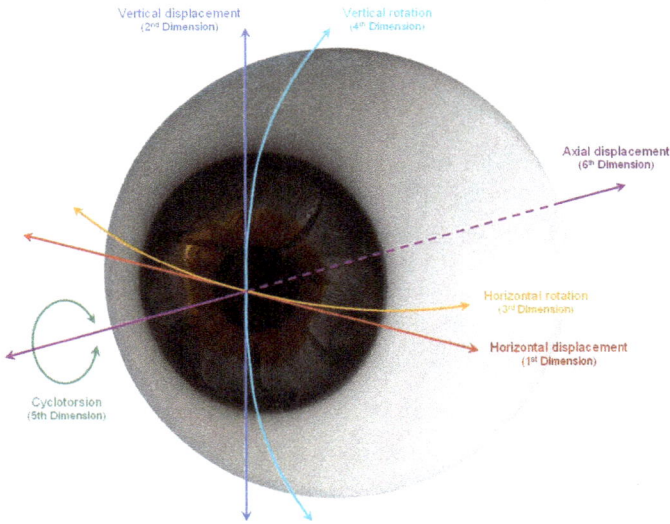

Fig. 4. Lateral movements (vertical and horizontal displacements) 1st and 2nd dimensions, Rolling movements – caused by a tilting of the head or of the eye 3rd and 4th dimensions, Rotations around the visual axis - This happens mostly when changing from upright to supine position, but also during the treatment 5th dimension, cyclotorsion, Movements along the z-axis 6th dimension. All dimensions measured and compensated for static and dynamic movements in an active/passive manner.

The AMARIS TotalTech laser includes compensation for the ocular cyclotorsions occurring from upright to supine position (static cyclotorsion from diagnosis to treatment), as well as the lateral movements, eye rollings, dynamic cyclotorsions, and displacements along the propagation axis occurring during the laser treatment. Further, the differences in pupil size and centre for and during the treatment compared to that during diagnosis[49] are also compensated for, since the theoretical impact of cyclotorted ablations is smaller than decentred ablations or edge effects[50] (coma and spherical aberration[51]). In this way, additional lateral displacements[52] due to cyclotorsions occurring around any position other than the ablation centre are avoided (induced aberrations emanating from lateral displacements always increase with decentration[53]).

A six dimensional eye-tracker is important since uncompensated pupil movements (lateral movements) induce decentrations[32] which can be visually manifested as comatic aberrations[52]. Uncompensated rolling movements induce decentrations as well[35], which can be visually manifested as comatic aberrations[52]. Uncompensated cyclotorsional movements induce aberrations[40], whereas uncompensated axial movements induce undercorrections in an asymmetrical way. Axial movements produce that the laser spots are no longer in focus when they reach the cornea, i.e. ignoring absorption processes in air, for the same energy spot diameter is larger reducing the radiant exposure and the ablation depth of the spot. Axial movements produce as well that off axis pulses hit the cornea more centrally than planned if the eye moves towards the laser system and further peripherally if the eyes moves far from the laser.

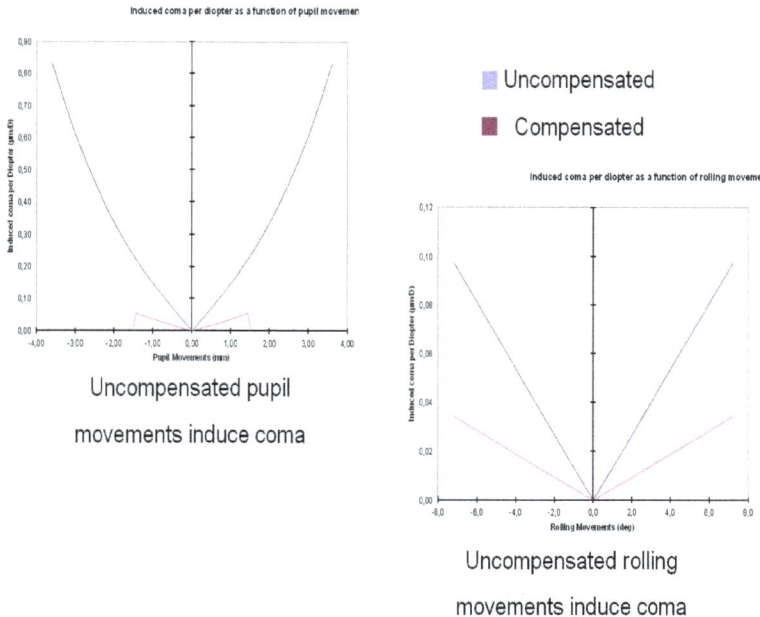

Fig. 5. A six dimensional eye-tracker is important since uncompensated pupil movements (lateral movements) induce decentrations which can be visually manifested as comatic aberrations. Uncompensated rolling movements induce decentrations as well, which can be visually manifested as comatic aberrations.

Why is 6D Eye-Tracking so important?

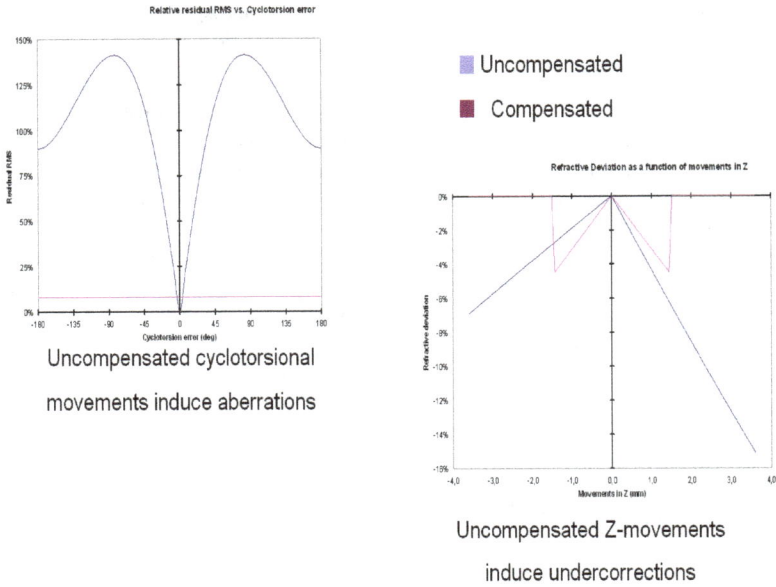

Uncompensated cyclotorsional movements induce aberrations

Uncompensated Z-movements induce undercorrections

Fig. 6. A six dimensional eye-tracker is important since uncompensated cyclotorsional movements induce aberrations, whereas uncompensated axial movements induce undercorrections in an asymmetrical way. Axial movements produce that the laser spots are no longer in focus when they reach the cornea, i.e. ignoring absorption processes in air, for the same energy spot diameter is larger reducing the radiant exposure and the ablation depth of the spot. Axial movements produce as well that off axis pulses hit the cornea more centrally than planned if the eye moves towards the laser system and further peripherally if the eyes moves far from the laser.

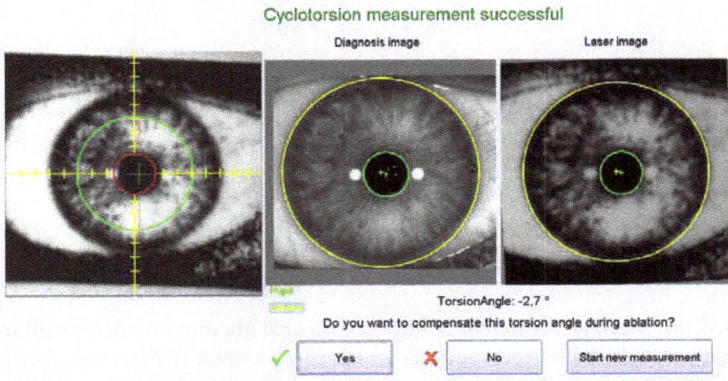

Fig. 7. Static cyclotorsion compensation.

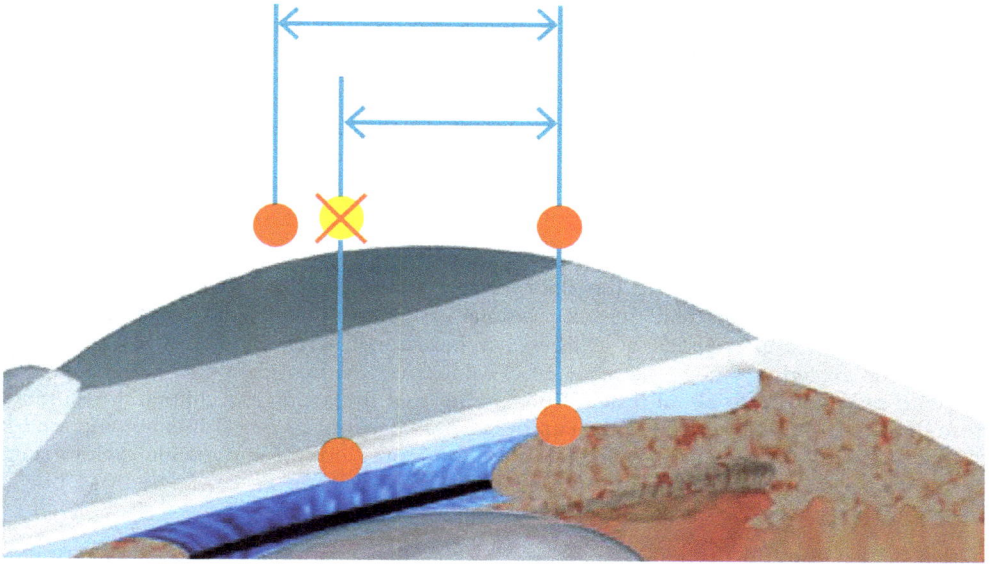

Fig. 8. Rolling compensation.

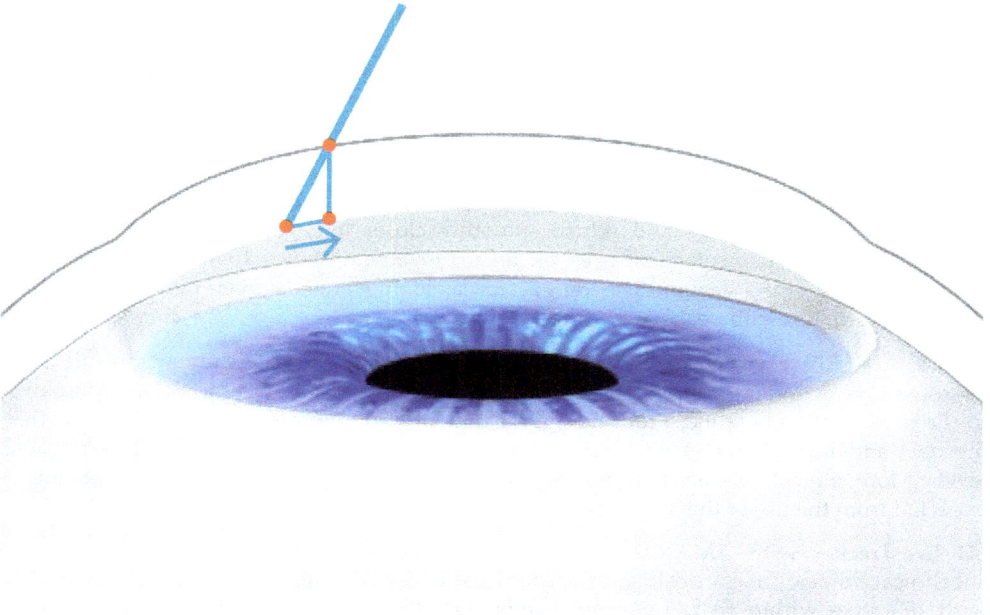

Fig. 9. Axial movements compensation.

In our experience with AMARIS system measuring the pupil displacements, we obtained an average of 150 μm. The distribution of the percentage of eyes vs. pupil displacement showed 3% of eyes had pupil displacements exceeding 1 mm. The ranges for pupil displacements over the treatment are relatively mild, but with peaks of up to about 1.5 mm.

With our system for measuring the rolling movements, we obtained an average value 5°. This value is actually the most commonly accepted value for "natural rolling" measured as angle alpha[54], lambda[55], or kappa[56]. The distribution of the percentage of eyes vs. rolling movements showes 3% of eyes had rolling exceeding 8 deg. The ranges for the rolling movements over the treatment are relatively mild, but with peaks of up to about 10 deg.

With our system for measuring the static cyclotorsional error, we obtained an average cyclotorsion of 1°, lower than the observations of Ciccio et al.,[57] who reported 4°. The distribution of the percentage of eyes vs. cyclotorsional error shows 3% of eyes had cyclotorsion exceeding 8 deg. The mean DCC values over the treatment are relatively small, but with peaks of up to about 5 deg. Considering that the average cyclotorsion resulting from the shift from the upright to the supine position is about ±4 deg,[57] it is not enough to compensate only for the static cyclotorsion without considering the dynamic cyclotorsion during the laser procedure. Finally, the effects of the DCC can be considered as optical "noise" of the applied versus the intended profiles.[58]

Without eye registration technologies,[59,60] considering that maximum cyclotorsion measured from the shift from the upright to the supine position does not exceed ±14 deg,[57] explains why "classical" spherocylindrical corrections in refractive surgery succeed without major cyclotorsional considerations. However, only limited amounts of astigmatism can effectively be corrected for this cyclotorsional error[40]. Currently available eye registration technologies, providing an accuracy of about 1 deg and measuring static and dynamic cyclotorsion components, open a new era in corneal laser refractive surgery, because patients may be treated for a wider range of refractive problems with enhanced success ratios. This requires high-resolution ablation systems as well.[61,62]

With our system for measuring the axial movements, we obtained an average of -300 μm. This negative value is fairly low, but means the patients use to push their head back at the beginning of the treatment and return smoothly closer to level during treatment. The distribution of the percentage of eyes vs. axial movement shows 10% of eyes had axial movements exceeding 1 mm. The ranges for axial movements over the treatment are relatively mild, but with peaks exceeding 1 mm.

In our AMARIS experience of over 8000 treated eyes, 91% of treatments result in a postoperative cylinder within 0.5 D, and 19% of treatments gain lines of BSCVA compared to the preoperative baseline. From the minor induction of aberrations can be inferred that mesopic and low-contrast VA have maintained, at least, the best-corrected preoperative levels. More clinical data are required before we can state how much improvement can be expected from the use of this technology.

6D Eye-Tracker with AMARIS yields excellent outcomes. Refractions are reduced to subclinical values: (mean postoperative defocus -0.12±0.17D and astigmatism 0.15±0.25D) with 70% eyes within ±0.25D of emmetropia and 19% eyes gain lines of BSCVA. Rate of registration is >90% for Cyclotorsion and >80% for Rolling and Axial movements. Mean

Rolling was within ±5° in 52% of the cases, Dynamic Rolling was within ±5° in 66% of the cases, Static Cyclotorsion was within ±4° in 69% of the cases, Dynamic Cyclotorsion was within ±2° in 72% of the cases, and Z-movement was within ±0.5mm in 69% of the cases.

6D Eye-Tracker Controls with the SCHWIND AMARIS are safe and very predictable. In summary, using SCHWIND AMARIS, six-dimensional movements of the eye can be effectively measured and compensated for both static and dynamic conditions during laser corneal ablation.

9. High speed refractive surgery

The range of repetition rates of the laser systems for refractive surgery currently available in the market runs from about 10 Hz to about 1000 Hz (median 250 Hz), with spot size diameters ranging from 6.5 mm to about 0.3 mm (median 1 mm), corresponding to treatment velocities from about 9 s/D to about 1.7 s/D (mean 5 s/D). If we compare these values to the situation at the beginning of the 21st century, a technological quantum leap is observed. In 2001, repetition rates of the laser systems for refractive surgery in the market ranged from about 10 Hz to about 300 Hz (median 50 Hz), with spot size diameters ranging from 6.5 mm to about 0.8 mm (median 2-6 mm), corresponding to treatment velocities from about 19 s/D to about 6 s/D (mean 12 s/D).

To foresee the future trends for these essential values when defining the technological capabilities of a system, four driving forces shall be considered:

- The technological progress of the last 10 years indicating an exponential improvement of the technology
- The non-linear cost-to-benefit ratio for new developments indicating a continued improvement of the technology at a slower rate
- The actual clinical needs for faster or more precise systems indicating a slow-down improvement of the technology achieving maturity and stability
- The limitations imposed by the biological tissue response to the laser interaction (e.g. thermal issues, haze development[63])

Considering these effects, we can hypothesize a scenario with repetition rates of the laser systems for refractive surgery ranging from about 300 Hz to about 1500 Hz, with spot size diameters ranging from 1.5 mm to about 0.2 mm, corresponding to treatment velocities from about 4 s/D to about 1.3 s/D.

However, due to the presence of local frequency controls, the duration of the treatments is no longer inversely proportional to the repetition rate. The duration of the treatments is inversely proportional to the repetition rate only for slow repetition rates (<180 Hz), and stabilizes asymptotically for high repetition rates (>1500 Hz).

10. Bilateral symmetry

Human vision is a binocular process. Having two eyes gives binocular summation in which the ability to detect faint objects is enhanced. It can give stereopsis in which parallax provided by the two eyes' different positions on the head give precise depth perception. Such binocular vision is usually accompanied by binocular fusion, in which a single image is seen despite each eye is having its own image of any object.

Literature suggests that marked anisometropia is uncommon, either in the magnitude of sphere or astigmatism, with few notable exceptions concluding that the axis of astigmatism does not follow any particular rule (mirror or direct symmetry) across right and left eyes.

Porter et al.[64] confirmed in a large population that although the pattern of aberrations varies from subject to subject, aberrations, including irregular ones, are correlated in left and right eyes of the same subject, indicating that they are not random defects. The Indiana Aberration Study by Thibos et al. characterized the aberration structure, and the effects of these aberrations on vision, for a reasonably large population of normal, healthy eyes in young adults, and verified the hypothesis of bilateral symmetry.

Wang et al.[65] found that anterior corneal wave aberrations varied greatly among subjects, but a moderate to high degree of mirror symmetry existed between right and left eyes. To our knowledge, very few studies in the literature have addressed the issue of symmetry of aberrations between eyes after corneal laser refractive surgery[66],[67]. Jiménez et al.[66] found that binocular function deteriorates more than monocular function after LASIK, and that this deterioration increases as the interocular differences in aberrations and corneal shape increase. They found that interocular differences above 0.4 μm RMS for 5-mm analysis diameter, lead to a decrease of more than 20% in binocular summation.

If binocular symmetry is manifested on virgin human eyes and it is important for binocular vision, it shall be interesting to assess whether existing symmetry is maintained after treating the cornea for correcting the ametropias using corneal laser refractive surgery. Further analysis of bilateral symmetry according to analysis diameter is also of interest. The analysis of bilateral symmetry should be related to binocular vision status of patients.

Cuesta et al.[68] found that even differences in corneal asphericity might affect the binocular visual function by diminishing the binocular contrast-sensitivity function. Arbelaez et al.[67] found that only four of 25 patients showed preoperatively clinically relevant differences OS vs. OD larger than 0.25 D, whereas 6-month postoperatively only 2 of 25 patients showed clinically relevant differences OS vs. OD larger than 0.25 D. 6-month postoperatively three Zernike terms lost significant correlation symmetry OS vs. OD and 4 Zernike terms gained significant correlation symmetry. However, two of them showed borderline correlations. 6-month postoperatively 6 Zernike terms significantly increased differences in symmetry OS vs. OD and 4 Zernike terms significantly decreased differences in symmetry. However, six of them showed borderline significances of the difference. 6-month postoperatively three patients lost significant correlation symmetry OS vs. OD and one patient gained significant correlation symmetry. However, two of them showed borderline significances of the difference. All these borderline situations actually shall be seen as "almost preserved" bilateral symmetry.

The presented results cannot be extrapolated to patients with symptoms of amblyopia[69], anisometropia, nystagmus, or aniseikonia[70] without further studies. Bilateral symmetry in corneal aberrations does not mean any "good or bad" point for binocular vision. We cannot evaluate exactly the role of aberrations monocularly (patients with high level of aberrations can have an excellent visual acuity and vice-versa); therefore it is more difficult binocularly.

The important question in binocular vision is "the role of interocular-differences," and if they can influence significantly binocular performance. Interocular-differences can be minor but significant for visual performance. Further studies shall help to determine the impact of this on binocular visual performance.

The more irregular a cornea is, the more important proper bilateral symmetry for adequate binocular summation. Astigmatism is the most common aberration with a vector nature, so usually are the astigmatic problems the ones more affected or the ones which benefit the most from losing or preserving bilateral symmetry.

11. Correction of high astigmatism

Because the corneal ablations for refractive surgery treatments induce aberrations (one of the most significant side-effects in myopic LASIK is the induction of spherical aberration[71], which causes halos and reduced contrast sensitivity[72]), special ablation patterns were designed to preserve the preoperative level of high order aberrations[73,74,75]. For the correction of astigmatism many different approaches have been tested, with different degrees of success, through the years[76,77,78,79,80,81].

LASIK has been successfully used for low to moderate myopic astigmatism, whether LASIK is acceptably efficacious, predictable, and safe in correcting higher myopic astigmatism is less documented, specially with regard to the effects of astigmatic corrections in HOA's[82].

The advantage of the Aberration-Free™ ablation profile is that aims being neutral for HOA, leaving the visual print of the patient as it was preoperatively with the best spectacle correction. The correction of astigmatism has been approached using several techniques and ablation profiles. There are several reports showing good results for compound myopic astigmatism using photorefractive keratectomy (PRK) and LASIK, but ablation profiles usually cause a hyperopic shift because of a coupling effect in the flattest corneal meridian. A likely mechanism of this coupling effect is probably due to epithelial remodeling and other effects such as smoothing by the LASIK flap[83]. In cases of large amounts of preoperative astigmatism, deviations from the target refractive outcome are usually attribute to "coupling factors". But, the investigation of the coupling factor remains a rather difficult task, because it seems to be dependent on various factors. Individual Excimer laser systems may have different coupling factors, cutting the flap could alter the initial prescription and also different preoperative corneal curvature (K-reading) may have an influence on the coupling factor.

The most dominant correlations of induced HOAb occurr for C[4,0], and C[6,0] versus defocus correction, for C[4,+2] versus cardinal astigmatism correction, and C[4,-2] versus oblique astigmatism correction. We evaluated the postoperative clinical outcomes and high order aberrations among eyes with astigmatism higher than 2 D that have underwent refractive surgery using the SCHWIND AMARIS laser system. SCHWIND CAM Aberration-Free Aspheric astigmatic treatments have been performed in all cases.

At six-month follow-up, 50 eyes with preoperative astigmatism higher than 2 D were retrospectively analysed. Ablations performed using the SCHWIND AMARIS flying-spot excimer laser system. LASIK flaps were created using Ziemer LDV Femtosecond laser system in all cases.

Inclusion criteria comprised:

- preoperative astigmatism higher than 2 D targeted for emmetropia
- BSCVA ≥ 20/25 (logMAR ≤ +0.1)
- <0.75 μm RMS-HO for 6-mm diameter
- successful completion of 6-month follow-up

We performed following analyses:

- UCVA
- BSCVA
- manifest subjective refraction (SR)
- corneal wavefront up to 7th order at 6-mm diameter without cycloplegia

50 eyes (100%) completed the 6M follow-up, with an average age at the time of the surgery of 28 years (from 17 to 46). 28 eyes were female, and 22 eyes male. 25 patients treated bilaterally. Mean preoperative defocus averaged -3.08 D ± 2.32 D (from -7.13 to -1.00), with mean astigmatism 3.54 D ± 0.85 D (from 2.00 to 4.75). Mean postoperative defocus averaged -0.06 D ± 0.25 D (from -0.75 to +0.75), with mean astigmatism 0.25 D ± 0.26 D (from 0.00 to 1.25). 92% of the eyes ended up in UCVA 20/20 or better. 38% of the eyes gained at least one line of BSCVA (p<.01*). >75% of the eyes within 0.50 D of astigmatism and U-vector, and >90% of the eyes within 1.00 D of astigmatism and U-vector.

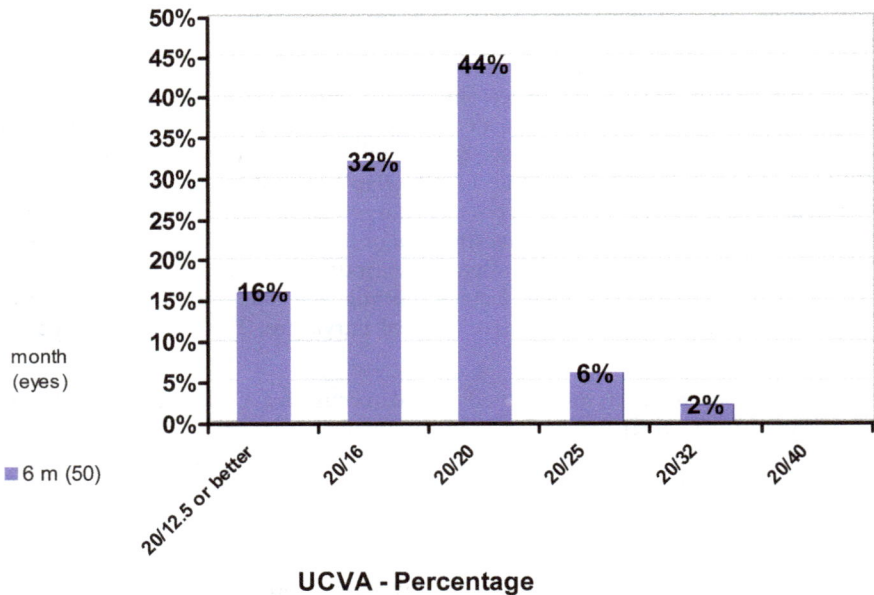

UCVA - Percentage

Fig. 10. Efficacy of the correction of moderate to high astigmatism in an aspheric astigmatic setting.

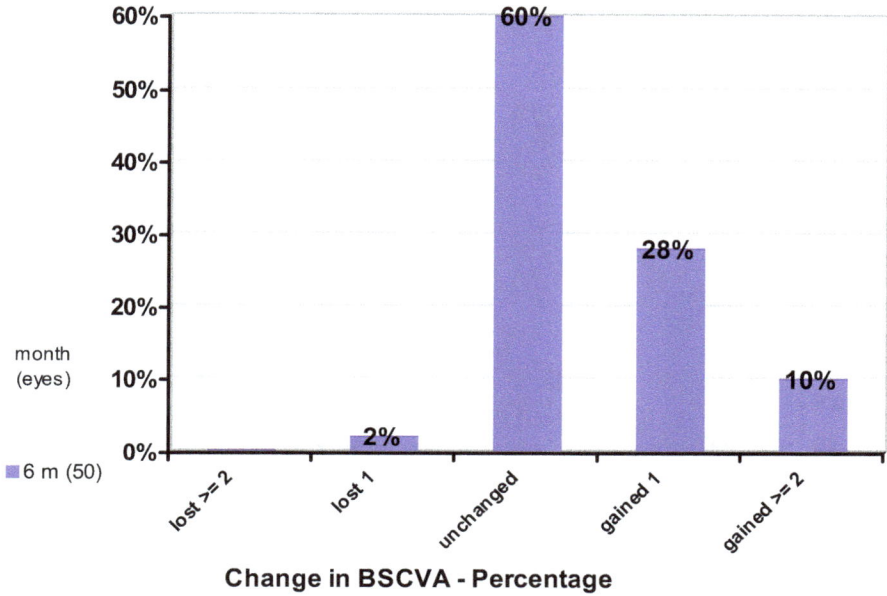

Fig. 11. Safety of the correction of moderate to high astigmatism in an aspheric astigmatic setting.

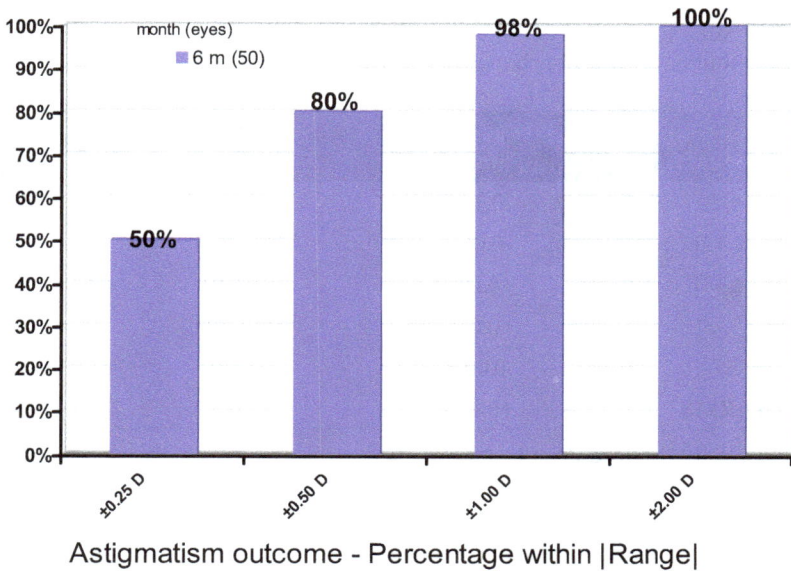

Fig. 12. Refractive astigmatic outcome of the correction of moderate to high astigmatism in an aspheric astigmatic setting.

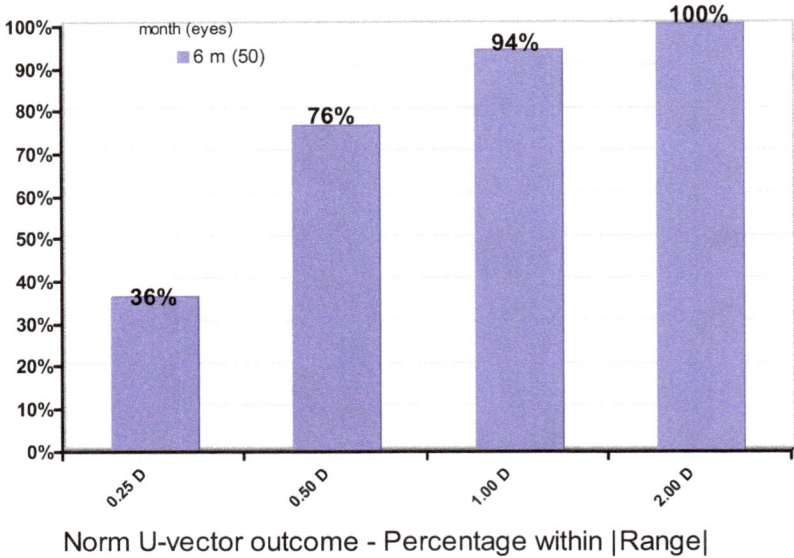

Norm U-vector outcome - Percentage within |Range|

Fig. 13. Residual blur of the correction of moderate to high astigmatism in an aspheric astigmatic setting.

A very slight undercorrection in astigmatism was observed (both cardinal and oblique).

Only 5 HO Zernike terms (out of 30) changed significantly after treatment, whereas 25 HO Zernike terms (out of 30) did not change after treatment.

Zernike term at 6-mm Ø	Preoperative (μm)	Postoperative (μm)	p-value
C[3,-3]	-0.14	-0.02	<.0001
C[4,+2]	-0.08	-0.10	<.05
C[4,+4]	+0.03	+0.01	<.05
C[5,-3]	+0.01	-0.01	<.0001
C[6,0]	0.00	+0.03	<.0001
HO-RMS	+0.47	+0.57	<.0005

Table 2. Statistically induced Zernike terms.

For all of them, the variation was well below the clinical relevance.

50 high-astigmatism treatments were analysed at 6M follow-up. Results were achieved without applying additional nomograms (residual sphere about 0 D, residual cyl about -0.25 D) (>75% within 0.50 D, >90% within 1.0 D). 6-months follow-up time shows the excellent performance of the system (48% eyes 20/16 or better UCVA, 98% eyes 20/25 or better

UCVA). Aberration-Free astigmatic treatments with SCHWIND AMARIS are safe and very
predictable (no eye lost >1 line BSCVA, 5 eyes gained >=2 lines BSCVA).

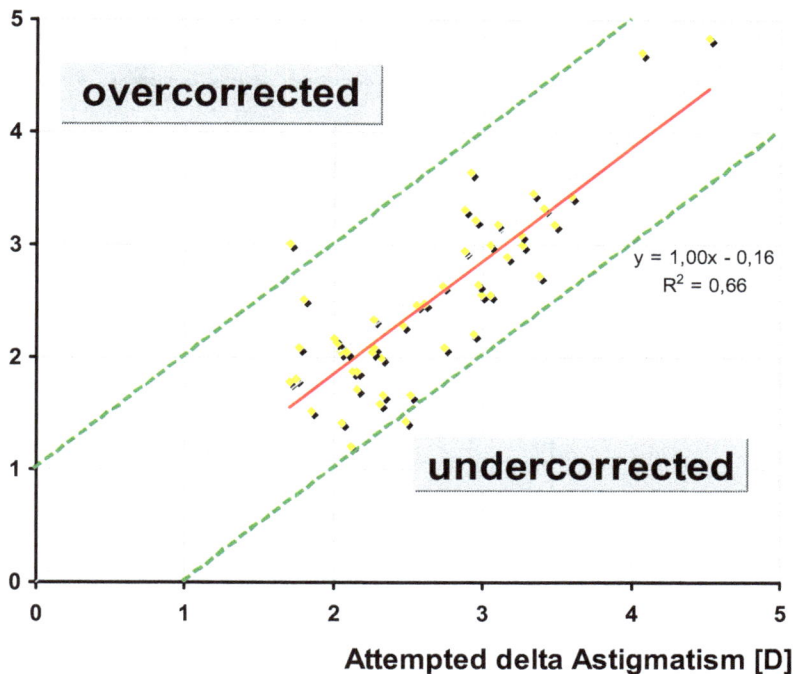

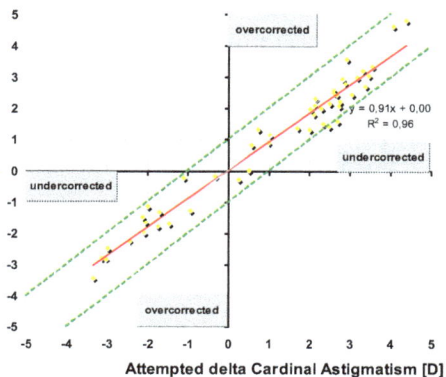

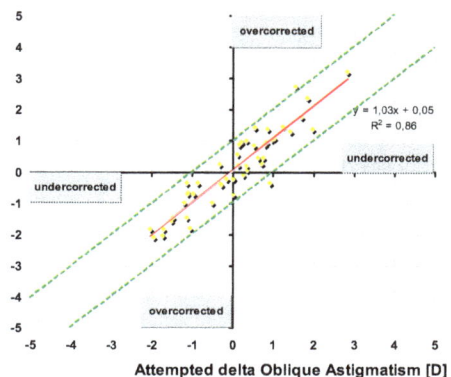

Fig. 14. Scattergram of the correction of moderate to high astigmatism in an aspheric
astigmatic setting.

From VA, 92% eyes UCVA 20/20 or better and 38% eyes improved their pre-op BSCVA, due to the minimum aberrations induction by the AMARIS-CAM profile. Despite large defocus and astigmatism magnitudes, minor significant induction of some aberration terms, well below clinically relevant magnitudes. The most dominant correlations of induced HOAb occurred for: C[4,0] vs. Defocus correction, C[4,+2] vs. Cardinal Astigmatism correction, and C[4,-2] vs. Oblique Astigmatism correction.

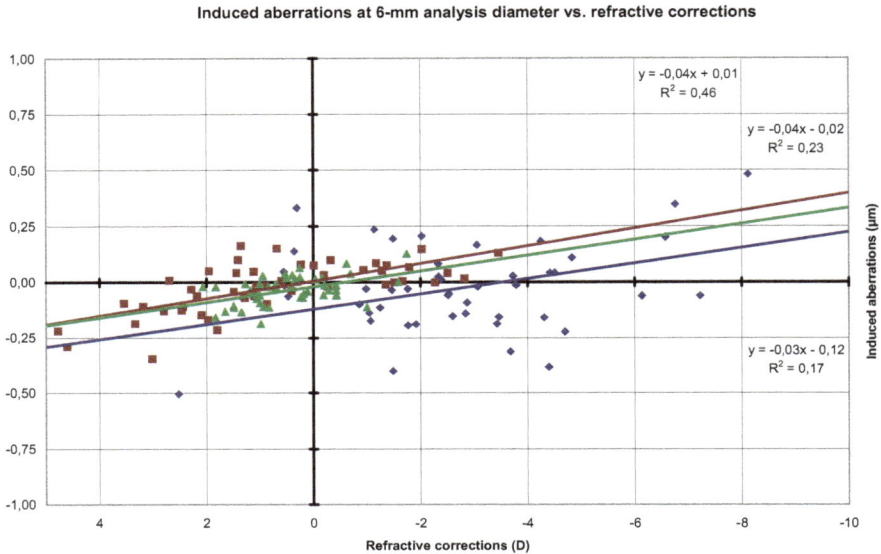

Fig. 15. Induction of aberrations after the correction of moderate to high astigmatism in an aspheric astigmatic setting.

All ablations were non-wavefront-guided treatments. Despite low aberrations, some astigmatisms were not regular. Treatments were centred at the corneal vertex. Despite myopic corrections, 40% of the treatments needed an offset >150 μm.

Laser settings were planned with the manifest astigmatism (magnitude and axis). Topographic astigmatism was not considered for the calculations. No nomogram compensations were applied. With a slight nomogram, further refinements could have been achieved.

12. References

[1] Salmon T. Measurement of Refractive Errors in Young Myopes using the COAS Shack-Hartmann Aberrometer. *Optometry and Vision Science*;2003;Vol 80
[2] Zernike F. Diffraction theory of the knife-edge test and its improved form, the phase-contrast method. *Physica I*; 1934;689-704

[3] Thibos LN, Applegate RA, Schwiegerling JT, Webb R, VSIA Standards Taskforce Members. Standards for reporting the optical aberrations of eyes. *J Refract Surg;* 2002;18:S652-S660

[4] Thibos L, Bradley A, Applegate R. Accuracy and precision of objective refraction from wavefront aberrations. *ISSN 1534-7362* , 2003 ARVO

[5] Marcos S, Cano D, Barbero S. Increase in corneal asphericity after standard laser in situ keratomileusis for myopia is not inherent to the Munnerlyn algorithm. *J Refract Surg;* 2003; 19: S592-6

[6] Dorronsoro C, Cano D, Merayo-Lloves J, Marcos S. Experiments on PMMA models to predict the impact of corneal refractive surgery on corneal shape. *Opt. Express;* 2006; 14: 6142-6156

[7] Arba Mosquera S, de Ortueta D. Geometrical analysis of the loss of ablation efficiency at non-normal incidence. *Opt. Express;* 2008; 16: 3877-3895

[8] Bende T, Seiler T, Wollensak J. Side effects in excimer corneal surgery. Corneal thermal gradients. *Graefes Arch Clin Exp Ophthalmol;* 1988; 226: 277-80

[9] Salmon TO. Corneal contribution to the Wavefront aberration of the eye. *PhD Dissertation;* 1999: 70

[10] Mattioli R, Tripoli NK. Corneal Geometry Reconstruction with the Keratron Videokeratographer. *Optometry and Vision Science* 1997; 74: 881-94

[11] Zernike F. Diffraction theory of the knife-edge test and its improved form, the phase-contrast method. *Monthly Notices of the Royal Astronomical Society;* 1934; 94: 377-384

[12] Thibos LN, Applegate RA, Schwiegerling JT, Webb R, VSIA Standards Taskforce Members. Standards for reporting the optical aberrations of eyes. *J Refract Surg;* 2002;18:S652-S660

[13] Guirao A, Artal P. Corneal wave aberration from videokeratography: accuracy and limitations of the procedure. *J Opt Soc Am A Opt Image Sci Vis.* 2000; 17: 955-65

[14] de Ortueta D, Arba Mosquera S. Mathematical properties of Asphericity: A Method to calculate with asphericities. *J Refract Surg;* 2008; 24: 119-121

[15] Chung SH, Lee IS, Lee YG, Lee HK, Kim EK, Yoon G, Seo KY. Comparison of higher-order aberrations after wavefront-guided laser in situ keratomileusis and laser-assisted subepithelial keratectomy. *J Cataract Refract Surg* 2006; 32:779-84.

[16] Buzzonetti L, Iarossi G, Valente P, Volpi M, Petrocelli G, Scullica L. Comparison of wavefront aberration changes in the anterior corneal surface after laser-assisted subepithelial keratectomy and laser in situ keratomileusis: preliminary study. *J Cataract Refract Surg* 2004; 30: 1929-33.

[17] Bará S, Arines J, Ares J, Prado P. Direct transformation of Zernike eye aberration coefficients between scaled, rotated, and/or displaced pupils. *J Opt Soc Am A.* 2006; 23: 2061-2066.

[18] MacRae S. Aberration Interaction In Aberration Interaction In Wavefront Guided Custom Wavefront Guided Custom Ablation. Wavefront Congress 2007.

[19] Bühren J, Yoon GY, Kenner S, Artrip S, MacRae S, Huxlin K. The effect of decentration on lower- and higher-order aberrations after myopic photorefractive keratectomy (PRK) in a cat model. Wavefront Congress 2007.

[20] Yang Y, Wu F. Technical note: Comparison of the wavefront aberrations between natural and pharmacological pupil dilations. *Ophthalmic Physiol Opt;* 2007; 27: 220-223

[21] Erdem U, Muftuoglu O, Gundogan FC, Sobaci G, Bayer A. Pupil center shift relative to the coaxially sighted corneal light reflex under natural and pharmacologically dilated conditions. *J Refract Surg;* 2008; 24: 530-538

[22] Snellen H. Letterproeven tot Bepaling der Gezichtsscherpte. Utrecht, Weyers, 1862

[23] Radhakrishnan H, Charman WN. Age-related changes in ocular aberrations with accommodation. *J Vis.* 2007; 7: 11.1-21

[24] López-Gil N, Fernández-Sánchez V, Legras R, Montés-Micó R, Lara F, Nguyen-Khoa JL. Accommodation-related changes in monochromatic aberrations of the human eye as a function of age. *Invest Ophthalmol Vis Sci.* 2008; 49: 1736-43

[25] Iida Y, Shimizu K, Ito M, Suzuki M. Influence of age on ocular wavefront aberration changes with accommodation. *J Refract Surg.* 2008; 24: 696-701

[26] He JC, Gwiazda J, Thorn F, Held R, Huang W. Change in corneal shape and corneal wave-front aberrations with accommodation. *J Vis.* 2003; 3:456-63

[27] Atchison DA, Markwell EL, Kasthurirangan S, Pope JM, Smith G, Swann PG. Age-related changes in optical and biometric characteristics of emmetropic eyes. *J Vis.* 2008; 8: 29.1-20

[28] Holzer MP, Sassenroth M, Auffarth GU. Reliability of corneal and total wavefront aberration measurements with the SCHWIND Corneal and Ocular Wavefront Analyzers. *J Refract Surg*; 2006; 22: 917-920.

[29] MacRae S. Aberration Interaction In Wavefront Guided Custom Wavefront Guided Custom Ablation. Wavefront Congress 2007.

[30] Bühren J, Yoon GY, Kenner S, Artrip S, MacRae S, Huxlin K. The effect of decentration on lower- and higher-order aberrations after myopic photorefractive keratectomy (PRK) in a cat model. Wavefront Congress 2007.

[31] McLellan JS, Prieto PM, Marcos S, Burns SA. Effects of interactions among wave aberrations on optical image quality. *Vision Res*; 2006; 46: 3009-3016.

[32] Schwiegerling J, Snyder RW. Eye movement during laser in situ keratomileusis. J Cataract Refract Surg. 2000 Mar;26(3):345-51.

[33] Taylor NM, Eikelboom RH, van Sarloos PP, Reid PG. Determining the accuracy of an eye tracking system for laser refractive surgery. J Refract Surg. 2000 Sep-Oct;16(5):S643-6.

[34] Bueeler M, Mrochen M, Seiler T. Maximum permissible lateral decentration in aberration-sensing and wavefront-guided corneal ablation. J Cataract Refract Surg. 2003 Feb;29(2):257-63.

[35] Bueeler M, Mrochen M. Limitations of pupil tracking in refractive surgery: systematic error in determination of corneal locations. J Refract Surg. 2004 Jul-Aug;20(4):371-8.

[36] Buehren T, Lee BJ, Collins MJ, Iskander DR. Ocular microfluctuations and videokeratoscopy. *Cornea.* 2002; 21: 346-51.

[37] Smith EM Jr, Talamo JH, Assil KK, Petashnick DE. Comparison of astigmatic axis in the seated and supine positions. *J Refract Corneal Surg.* 1994; 10: 615-20.

[38] Smith EM Jr, Talamo JH. Cyclotorsion in the seated and the supine patient. *J Cataract Refract Surg.* 1995; 21: 402-403.

[39] Bueeler M, Mrochen M, Seiler T. Maximum permissible torsional misalignment in aberration-sensing and wavefront-guided corneal ablation. J Cataract Refract Surg. 2004 Jan;30(1):17-25.

[40] Arba-Mosquera S, Merayo-Lloves J, de Ortueta D Clinical effects of pure cyclotorsional errors during refractive surgery. *Invest Ophthalmol Vis Sci.* 2008; 49: 4828-36.

[41] Chernyak DA. From wavefront device to laser: an alignment method for complete registration of the ablation to the cornea. *J Refract Surg.* 2005; 21: 463-8.

[42] Chernyak DA. Cyclotorsional eye motion occurring between wavefront measurement and refractive surgery. *J Cataract Refract Surg.* 2004; 30: 633-8.

[43] Bharti S, Bains HS. Active cyclotorsion error correction during LASIK for myopia and myopic astigmatism with the NIDEK EC-5000 CX III laser. *J Refract Surg*. 2007; 23: S1041-5.

[44] Kim H, Joo CK. Ocular cyclotorsion according to body position and flap creation before laser in situ keratomileusis. *J Cataract Refract Surg*. 2008; 34: 557-61.

[45] Park SH, Kim M, Joo CK. Measurement of pupil centroid shift and cyclotorsional displacement using iris registration. *Ophthalmologica*. 2009; 223: 166-71.

[46] Porter J, Yoon G, MacRae S, Pan G, Twietmeyer T, Cox IG, Williams DR. Surgeon offsets and dynamic eye movements in laser refractive surgery. *J Cataract Refract Surg*. 2005; 31: 2058-66.

[47] Hori-Komai Y, Sakai C, Toda I, Ito M, Yamamoto T, Tsubota K. Detection of cyclotorsional rotation during excimer laser ablation in LASIK. *J Refract Surg*. 2007; 23: 911-5.

[48] Chang J. Cyclotorsion during laser in situ keratomileusis. *J Cataract Refract Surg*. 2008; 34: 1720-6.

[49] Yang Y, Thompson K, Burns S. Pupil location under mesopic, photopic and pharmacologically dilated conditions. *Invest Ophthalmol Vis Sci*. 2002; 43: 2508-2512.

[50] Marcos S, Barbero S, Llorente L, Merayo-Lloves J. Optical response to LASIK surgery for myopia from Total and Corneal Aberration Measurements. *Invest Ophthalmol Vis Sci*. 2001; 42: 3349-3356.

[51] Marcos S. Aberrations and visual performance following standard Laser vision correction. *J Refract Surg*. 2001; 17: S596-S601.

[52] Guirao A, Williams D, Cox I. Effect of rotation and translation on the expected benefit of an ideal method to correct the eyes higher-order aberrations. *J Opt Soc Am A*. 2001; 18: 1003-1015.

[53] Uozato H, Guyton DL. Centering corneal surgical procedures. *Am J Ophthalmol*. 1987; 103: 264-275.

[54] Dunne MC, Misson GP, White EK, Barnes DA. Peripheral astigmatic asymmetry and angle alpha. Ophthalmic Physiol Opt. 1993 Jul;13(3):303-5.

[55] Salmon TO, Thibos LN. Videokeratoscope-line-of-sight misalignment and its effect on measurements of corneal and internal ocular aberrations. *J Opt Soc Am A Opt Image Sci Vis*. 2002 Apr;19(4):657-69.

[56] Hashemi H, Khabazkhoob M, Yazdani K, Mehravaran S, Jafarzadehpur E, Fotouhi A. Distribution of Angle Kappa Measurements with Orbscan II in a Population-Based Survey. *J Refract Surg*. 2010 Jan 28:1-6. doi: 10.3928/1081597X-20100114-06. [Epub ahead of print]

[57] Ciccio AE, Durrie DS, Stahl JE, Schwendeman F. Ocular cyclotorsion during customized laser ablation. *J Refract Surg*. 2005; 21: S772-S774.

[58] Bueeler M, Mrochen M. Simulation of eye-tracker latency, spot size, and ablation pulse depth on the correction of higher order wavefront aberrations with scanning spot laser systems. *J Refract Surg*. 2005; 21: 28-36.

[59] Chernyak DA. Iris-based cyclotorsional image alignment method for wavefront registration. *IEEE Transactions on Biomedical Engineering*. 2005; 52: 2032-2040.

[60] Schruender S, Fuchs H, Spasovski S, Dankert A. Intraoperative corneal topography for image registration. *J Refract Surg*. 2002; 18: S624-S629.

[61] Huang D, Arif M. Spot size and quality of scanning laser correction of higher-order wavefront aberrations. *J Cataract Refract Surg*. 2002; 28: 407-416.

[62] Guirao A,Williams D, MacRae S. Effect of beam size on the expected benefit of customized laser refractive surgery. *J Refract Surg*. 2003; 19: 15-23.

[63] Lohmann CP, Gartry DS, Muir MK, Timberlake GT, Fitzke FW, Marshall J. Corneal haze after excimer laser refractive surgery: objective measurements and functional implications. *Eur J Ophthalmol*; 1991; 1: 173-180.

[64] Porter J, Guirao A, Cox IG, Williams DR. Monochromatic aberrations of the human eye in a large population. *J. Opt. Soc. Am. A* 2001; 18: 1793-1803

[65] Wang L, Dai E, Koch DD, Nathoo A. Optical aberrations of the human anterior cornea. *J Cataract Refract Surg*. 2003; 29: 1514-21

[66] Jiménez JR, Villa C, Anera RG, Gutiérrez R, del Barco LJ. Binocular visual performance after LASIK. *J Refract Surg*. 2006; 22: 679-88

[67] Arbelaez MC, Vidal C, Arba Mosquera S. Bilateral Symmetry before and six-month after Aberration-FreeTM correction with the SCHWIND AMARIS TotalTech laser: Clinical outcomes. *J Optom;*. 2009; in press

[68] Cuesta JR, Anera RG, Jiménez R, Salas C. Impact of interocular differences in corneal asphericity on binocular summation. *Am J Ophthalmol*. 2003; 135: 279-84

[69] Mansouri B, Thompson B, Hess RF. Measurement of suprathreshold binocular interactions in amblyopia. *Vision Res*. 2008 Oct 31. [Epub ahead of print]

[70] Jiménez JR, Ponce A, Anera RG. Induced aniseikonia diminishes binocular contrast sensitivity and binocular summation. *Optom Vis Sci*. 2004; 81: 559-62

[71] Moreno-Barriuso E, Lloves JM, Marcos S. Ocular Aberrations before and after myopic corneal refractive surgery: LASIK-induced changes measured with LASER ray tracing. *Invest Ophthalmol Vis Sci* 2001; 42:1396-1403

[72] Mastropasqua L, Toto L, Zuppardi E, Nubile M, Carpineto P, Di Nicola M, Ballone E. Photorefractive keratectomy with aspheric profile of ablation versus conventional photorefractive keratectomy for myopia correction: six-month controlled clinical trial. *J Cataract Refract Surg*; 2006;32:109-16

[73] Mrochen M, Donetzky C,Wüllner C, Löffler J. Wavefront-optimized ablation profiles: Theoretical background. *J Cataract Refract Surg*; 2004;30:775-785

[74] Koller T, Iseli HP, Hafezi F, Mrochen M, Seiler T. Q-factor customized ablation profile for the correction of myopic astigmatism. *J Cataract Refract Surg*; 2006; 32:584-589

[75] Mastropasqua L, Nubile M, Ciancaglini M, Toto L, Ballone E. Prospective randomized comparison of wavefront-guided and conventional photorefractive keratectomy for myopia with the meditec MEL 70 laser. *J Refract Surg*. 2004; 20: 422-31

[76] McDonnell PJ, Moreira H, Garbus J. Photorefractive keratectomy to create toric ablations for correction of astigmatism. *Arch Ophthalmol* 1991; 109: 710-713.

[77] Argento CJ, Consentino MJ, Biondini A. Treatment of hyperopic astigmatism. *J Cataract Refract Surg* 1997; 23: 1480-1490.

[78] Barraquer C, Gutierrez AM. Results of laser in situ keratomileusis in hyperopic compound astigmatism. *J Cataract Refract Surg* 1999; 25: 1198-1204.

[79] Chayet AS, Montes M, Gómez L, Rodríguez X, Robledo N, MacRae S. Bitoric laser in situ keratomileusis for correcction of simple myopic and mixed astigmatism. *Ophthalmology* 2001; 108: 303-308.

[80] Arbelaez MC, Knorz MC. Laser in situ keramileusis for hyperopia and hyperopic astigmatism. *J Refract Surg* 1999; 15: 406–14.

[81] Vinciguerra P, Sborgi M, Epstein D, et al. Photorefractive keratectomy to correct myopic or hyperopic astigmatism with a cross-cylinder ablation. *J Refract Surg* 1999; 15: S183–5.

[82] Seiler T, Kaemmerer M, Mierdel P, Krinke H-E. Ocular optical aberrations after PRK for myopia and myopic astigmatism. *Arch Ophthalmol* 2000; 118: 17–21

[83] Huang D, Stulting RD, Carr JD, Thompson KP, Waring GO. Multiple regression and vector analysis of LASIK for myopia and astigmatism. *J Refract Surg* 1999; 15: 538-549.

13

Toric Intraocular Lenses for the Correction of Astigmatism

Milorad Milivojević,
Miroslav Vukosavljević and Mirko Resan
Eye Clinic, Military Medical Academy, Belgrade,
Serbia

1. Introduction

Astigmatism can be corrected with:

1. Glasses and contact lenses
2. Excimer laser refractive procedures (LASIK, PRK)
3. Astigmatic keratotomy
4. Limbal or corneal relaxing and clear corneal incisions
5. Toric intraocular lens

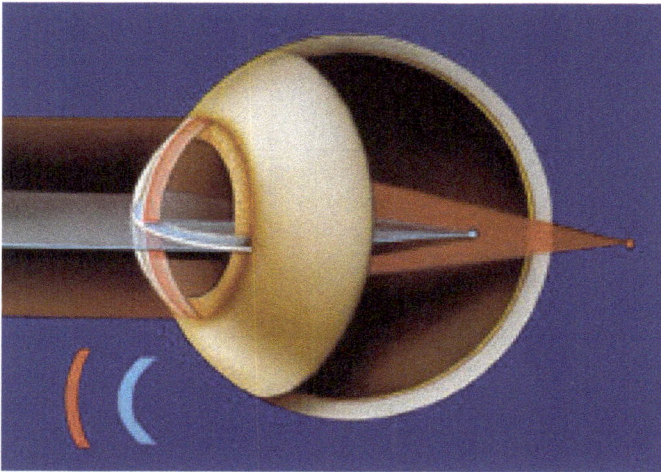

Fig. 1. Eye with astigmatism.

The ideal procedure for the correction of astigmatism should provide: precise and accurate adjustment, safety, predictable outcome, lasting effect and simplicity with an acceptable price. Conventional methods for solving problems such as glasses and/or contact lenses at the present time often do not meet the needs of patients. Whether it is the objective or subjective reasons for a large number of patients tend to avoid wearing glasses or contact lenses.

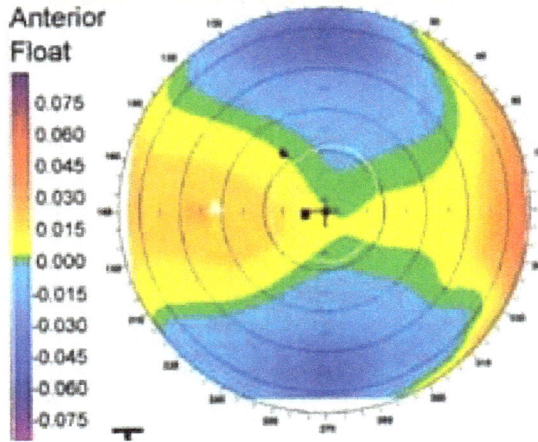

Fig. 2. The topography of corneal astigmatism.

Correcting corneal astigmatism during cataract surgery can increase spectacle independence. For the patient, this has economic benefits as well as desirable cosmetic and practical advantages. Spectacle correction of astigmatism creates meridional magnification, which when coupled with the associated back vertex distance produces retinal images that are asymmetrically magnified and distorted (1).

Company	Intraocular Lens	Range of Spherical IOL Power	Range of Cylindrical IOL Power	Range of Corneal Astigmatism Able to Correct	Percentage of Eyes Susceptible to Correction
Alcon	AcriSof Toric SN60T3/T4/T5 T6/T7T8/T9	+10.0 to +30.0(0.5)	11.5 to 6.0 (1.0)	1.0 to 4.2	34.2
STAAR	AA4203TF AA4203TL	+24.0to+28.5(0.5) +9.5 to 23.5(0.5)	2 and 3.5 2 and 3.5	1.4 and 2.4 1.4 and 2.4	17.1 17.1
Human Optics	Torica-5	-3.0 to +14.0(1.0) +15.0to+25.0(0.5) +26.0to+31.0(1.0)	2.0 to 12.0(0.5)	1.4 to 8.4	22.3
Rayner	T- flex 573T/623T	+6.0 to +26.0(0.5) -10.0 to +35.0(0.5)	1.0 to 6.0(1.0) 1.0 to11.0(0.25)	0.7 to 4.2 0.7 to 7.7	40.5 41.2
Zeiss	Acri.Comfort643TLC Acri.Comfort646TLC	0 to +40.0 -10.0 to +32.0	1.0 to 12.0(0.5) 1.0 to 12.0(0.5)	0.7 to 8.4 0.7 to 8.4	41.2 41.2

Table 1. Range of spherical and cylindrical powers and corneal astigmatism capable of correcting for the toric IOL on the market (1).

According to the literature, it is estimated that 15 to 22.2% of patients who are candidates for cataract surgery have astigmatism greater than 1.50 D. This indicates that a large number of patients still has blurred vision after cataract surgery due to residual astigmatism and require operative correction of distance vision glasses or lenses. (2,3). Since the corneal limbal relaxing incision often have an unpredictable effect on the postoperative visual acuity, and the use of Excimer laser refractive surgery is often not feasible because of it is often contraindicated in elderly people, expensive procedure, requires high technological equipment and expertise of medical personnel. Toric intraocular lenses are the correction of choice for high levels of astigmatism. They promise a predictable method of astigmatic correction with minimal impact to the cornea. However, the effectiveness of a toric IOL is dependent on its orientation. (1,4)

2. Surgical aspects of implantation of toric intraocular lenses

Cataract surgery with implantation of toric intraocular lenses is identical to the normal procedure and requires no special training (4). The difference is reflected in the preoperative treatment, and in celebration of the cylinder axis, which is adjusted to the patient's eye. Toric IOLs need precise positioning to achieve optimal visual results. In accordance with the corneal measurements, reference markers on opposite sides of the pupil need to be established to demarcate the correct axis for IOL orientation. Eye rotation occurs in a supine position and so these markers need to be established pre-operatively. The slit lamp beam axis graticule can be dialed to the correct axis or a bespoke eyepiece graticule can be used to determine where to place the markers, which can be applied to the cornea or conjunctiva using ink or with scratches. Ink should be applied at the last possible minute as it can diffuse by 10° or disappear before implantation is complete. As an alternative, a Neodymium:Yttrium-Aluminum-Garnet (Nd:YAG) laser can be used to mark the cornea. It has been suggested that this improves the accuracy and definition of the markers. Specific toric axis marking instruments exist. One step methods, such as the Devgan Axis Marker (Accutome, Pennsylvania, USA) and the Gerten Pendulum Marker (Geuder, Heidelberg, Germany) are used pre-operatively to determine the required axis. They are dependent on a vertical head position when applied to the cornea. Two-step methods require marking the cornea at the zero and 180 degree positions pre-operatively and then aligning a degree gauge with these markings intra-operatively to establish the correct position (1). The iris architecture is intricate and full marking is done manually or by using the instrument in a sitting position (1,5). Another difference lies in the fact that the shaft of toric IOL to coincide with the axis of the cylinder, marked preoperatively. This is achieved by the end of the operation during the removal of viscoelastic. There are two main surgical factors that can influence IOL rotation. In the early post-operative period careful wound construction is essential. Following surgery, the IOP can fluctuate and in 6.3 per cent of patients, it drops to below 5 mmHg. It is important to emphasize that it is necessary to remove viscoelastic a rotation for maximum stability. Viscoelastic lag could lead to undesirable postoperative implant rotation, and therefore should be brought into question and the desired outcome (1).

Consideration of IOL haptic design is very important when trying to prevent postoperative lens rotation. Over time, the capsular bag contracts to enclose and secure the IOL, however, before this contraction occurs there is potentfor rotation (6). To prevent rotation immediately after implantation, it is important to maximize the contact between the IOL haptic and the capsular bag. A polymethyl methacrylate (PMMA) IOL creates the most friction with the bag, followed by acrylic, with silicon causing the least (7). It is believed that if the implant rotates by more than 30 degrees postoperatively, the effect of cylindrical lenses is lost. The third difference relates to the calculation of the refractive lens, the strength and axis cylinder. As a rule, keratometry very carefully set manually, not automatic keratometer. Must also be taken into account and astigmatism, which will occur as a consequence of the main corneal incision. IOL manufacturers have developed calculators to determine the refractive power lens (as spherical and cylindrical components), and determine the shaft in which the implant should be placed. The data are entered to the calculator are manually specified value keratometry, spherical components required strength, where you are planning a major incision. These calculators are easily and freely available for use on the Internet (8).

3. The outcome of intraocular implantation of toric IOL

When it comes to the outcome of implantation of toric intraocular lenses, it is essential to assess the following parameters:

3.1 Rotational stability in capsular bag

3.1.1 Plate haptic IOLs

Plate haptic IOLs demonstrate excellent long-term stability. In comparison with open-loop haptics, plate haptic IOLs are not as susceptible to the effects of compression from the capsular bag.

The first commercially available toric IOL was the STAAR 4203TF (STAAR Surgical, Company, California, USA), which achieved FDA approval in 1998. It is a biconvex, silicone, plate haptic toric IOL, 10.8 mm in length, with two 1.15-mm positioning holes. The lens is available with a torus of either 2.00 or 3.50 D, which corrects levels of corneal astigmatism between 1.50 and 3.50 D. The lens demonstrates excellent long-term stability once fixation within the capsular bag has been established, 30 however, in the early postoperative period, the lens demonstrates a relatively high incidence of rotation. In its FDA trial, 24 per cent of the lenses rotated more than 10°, 12 per cent more than 20° and 8 per cent more than 30° (9).

The AT-TORBI (Carl Zeiss Meditec, Berlin, Germany) (previously the ACri comfort toric IOL) is an acrylic, bi-toric, plate haptic IOL, 11 mm in length, possessing two positioning holes on the haptic. It is a microincisional lens, and it can be inserted through a 1.5-mm incision. The AT-TORBI has a 6.0-mm optic, and can correct high levels of astigmatism, as it is available with a torus of 1.00 to 12.00 D in 0.50-D steps. Large-scale studies are required to demonstrate the effectiveness of this lens but early results are very promising. In a pilot study involving 21 eyes with 2.00 to 9.00 D of corneal astigmatism, only one lens rotated more than 5° between day one and six months post-operatively, with 76.1 per cent of these subjects achieving a postoperative uncorrected vision of 20/40 or better (10).

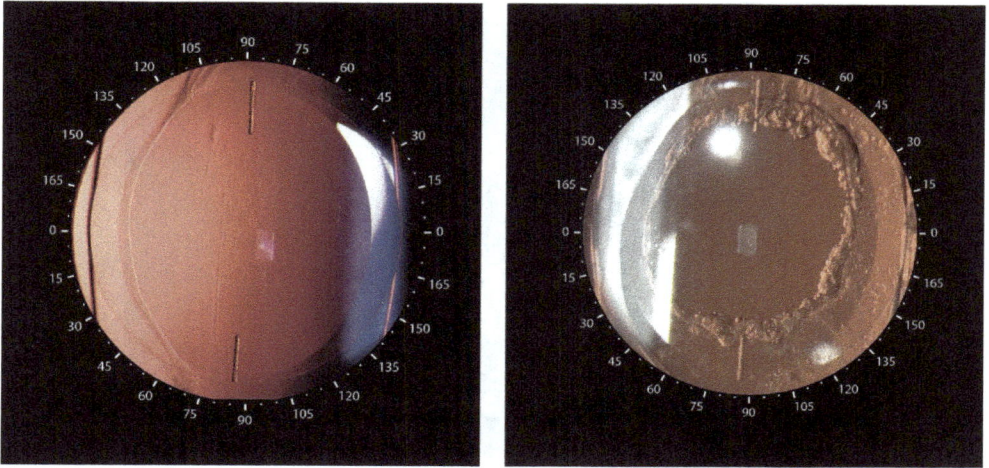

Fig. 3. Slit-lamp retroillumination photographs of a Staar toric intraocular lens with a superimposed digital protractor before (left) and after (right) a circular neodymium–yttrium-aluminum-garnet posterior capsulotomy (9).

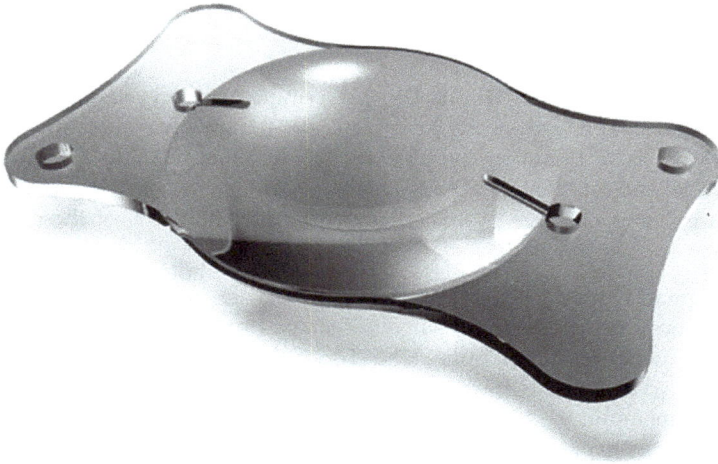

Fig. 4. The ACri comfort toric IOL (10).

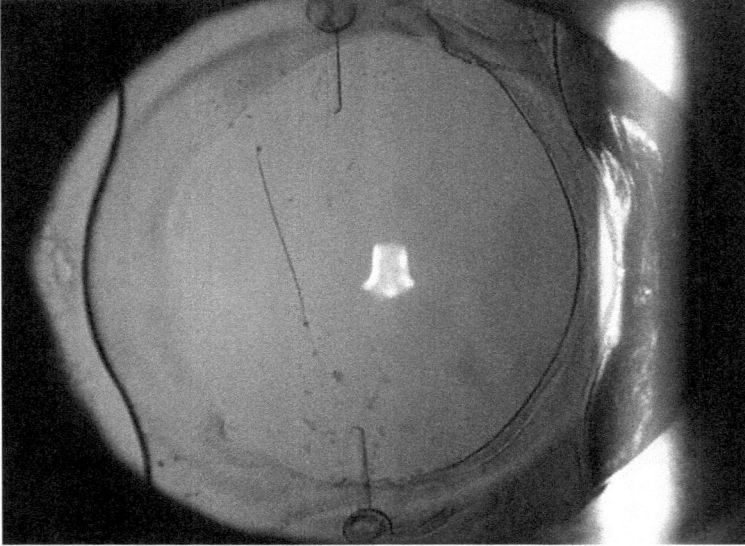

Fig. 5. The ACri comfort toric IOL in situ 3 months postoperatively (10).

3.1.2 Open loop haptic lenses

Open loop haptic lenses compared with previous models (plate haptic IOLs) demonstrate excellent early rotational stability in comparison to plate haptics. The longer loop haptics ensure immediate contact between haptic and capsular bag, maximizing friction in the early postoperative period, however, they are susceptible to late rotation caused by the compression of the capsular bag (11).

The AcrySof toric IOL (Alcon, Fort Worth, USA) is a single-piece acrylic toric IOL with open loop L-shaped haptics. It has a posterior toric surface with three available toric powers 1.50, 2.25 and 3.00 D. It is a 13mm in length with a 6.0mm optic. The AcrySof toric has demonstrated excellent rotational stability results. During its FDA trial, 81.9% of lenses rotated less than 5° and only 2.9% rotated over 10° and only 0.8% of these lenses were repositioned (2,8).

The Torica S (Human Optics, Erlangen, Germany) otherwise known as the Microcyl Toric 6116 (Human Optics), is a three-piece, silicon, Z-shaped open loop haptic toric IOL. It is 11.6mm in length with a 6.0mm optic. The Torica S has a novel haptic design with undulations designed to increase the friction between lens and bag. It has been reported that these undulations maintain the IOLs position but make it difficult to rotate the lens within the bag. To prevent the haptic undulations from causing trauma when rotating the lens, it is recommended that they are compressed against the optic and held away from the capsular bag until the lens is in the required position. In a study of 21 eyes (14 subjects) no lens rotated more than 5°(12).

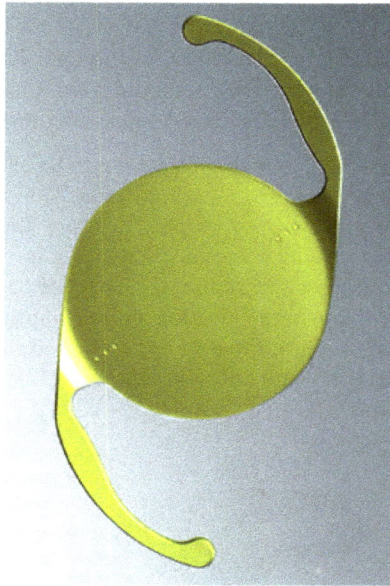

Fig. 6. AcrySof toric IOL.

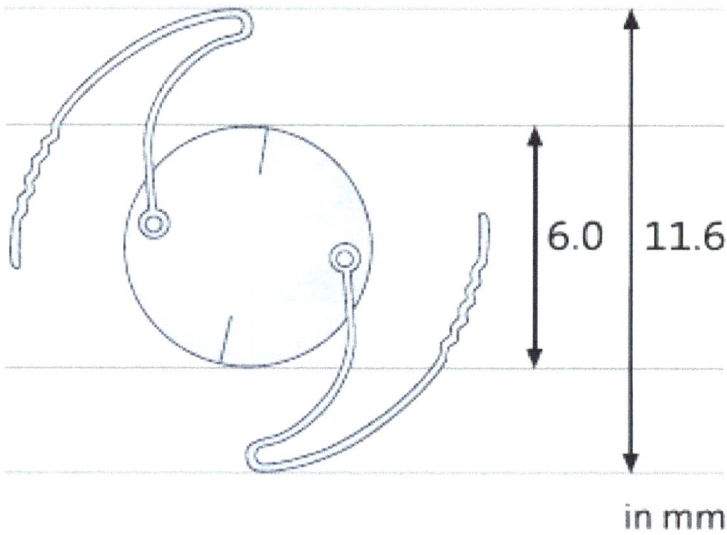

Fig. 7. The Torica-S IOL.

3.1.3 Closed loop haptics IOLs

Closed-loop haptics are a relatively new addition to the toric IOL market. These lenses are typically longer than the plate haptics, which should give good initial contact. The loops have a second insertion on the IOL that may resist capsular compression.

The T-flex toric (Rayner, Hove, UK) is a single-piece, acrylic, closed-loop haptic with anti-vaulting haptic technology. It is available in two sizes; the 573T has a 5.75-mm optic and 12 mm haptics, and the 623T has a 6.25-mm optic and 12.5 mm haptic. The anterior surface of the optic houses the toric surface, which is available with a torus of one to 11 D. The anti-vaulting haptic technology is designed to reduce the effect of compression using a lock and key system. Compression will push the outside of the haptic against the inner haptic, locking it into place. It has been reported that in a group of 10 subjects no lens rotated more than 5° between one week and two years after implantation (13).

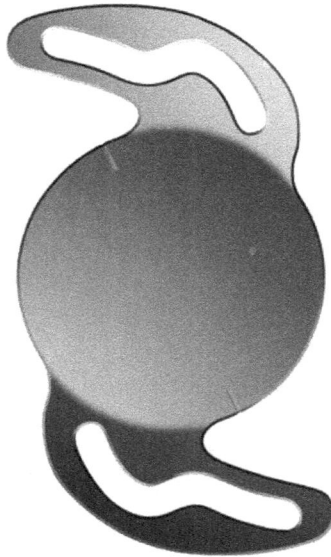

Fig. 8. Rayner T-*flex*® Aspheric Toric IOL.

The Akreos (Bausch & Lomb, Rochester, USA) aspheric platform is a single piece acrylic, closed loop haptic IOL. It has a 6.0-mm optic and is 11 mm in length with a 360° square edge. The IOL is currently being assessed for its viability as a platform for housing a toric surface. A multicenter study has examined the rotational stability of the Akreos haptic housing from one day to six months post-operatively in 97 eyes. This lens was shown to be stable, as 96 per cent of the IOLs rotated no more than 5° and 99% no more than 10° (14).

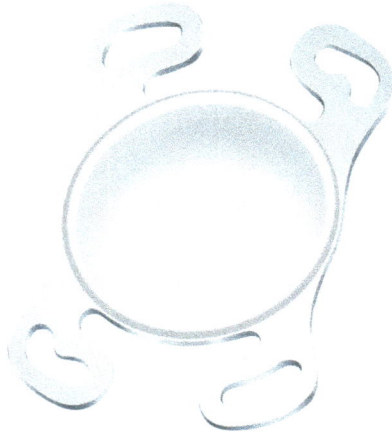

Fig. 9. Akreos™ aspheric IOL.

Tsinopoulos and colleagues (15) reported a new procedure for intra-operative toric intraocular lens (IOL) axis assessment in order to achieve optimal implantation. IOL implantation procedure was directly recorded. An assessor estimated the angle formed by the marked 0–180 axis and the toric IOL axis after implantation with the use of the appropriate software. If IOL implantation was assessed to be inaccurate, the surgeon was advised to correct IOL positioning by rotating the IOL clockwise. The assessment procedure was repeated until accurate IOL positioning was achieved.

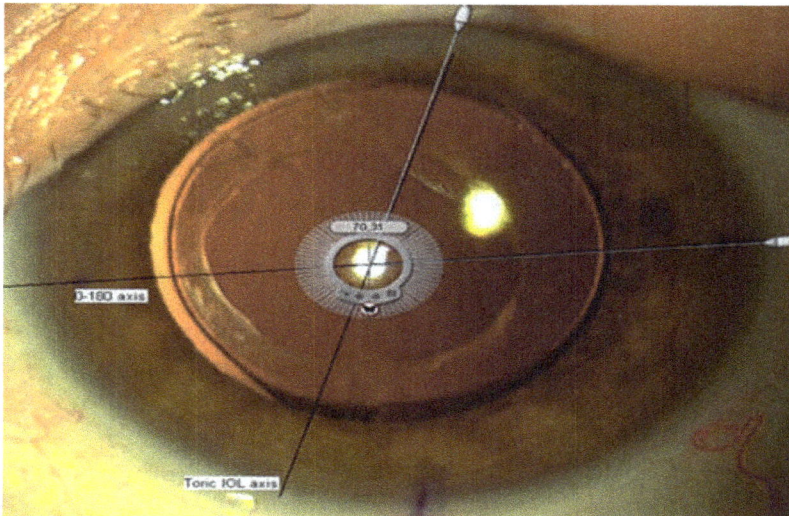

Fig. 10. Intra-operative toric implantation assessment with the use of the appropriate software (15).

3.2 The reduction of absolute residual astigmatism

The average absolute residual astigmatism after implantation of toric intraocular lenses is less than 0.55D. In patients who have significant astigmatism, and implanted them classic spherical lenses residual astigmatism is an average of 1.22D (1).

3.3 Uncorrected visual acuity at distance

Ninety-four percent of patients achieve visual acuity ≥ 0.5 with no correction, which is a remarkable result. Also, these patients have a greater vision improvement at all levels compared with patients who have conventional spherical lens. In 97% of patients whose toric lenses implanted in both eyes maximize distance vision without correction (1,2).

3.3.1 Stability and predictability of outcome

Patients who have significant astigmatism after cataract surgery have the option for correcting glasses or contact lenses. However, for many patients who expect excellent postoperative vision this is unacceptable solution.

Relaxing incisions that had previously been strongly represented in the correction of astigmatism now use fewer surgeons (40%) for the following reasons:

- Unpredictable results in a significant number of cases
- The problem of regression, astigmatism, especially in patients with severe preoperative astigmatism
- Inability to correct high astigmatism
- Paracentral incisions can correct high astigmatism, but more complications
- Healing of incisions can be problematic, since it is predominantly an elderly patient
- Patients with steep corneas and asymmetriastigmatism are not good candidates (1,16).

When speaking of the Excimer laser for the correction of astigmatism, the method is effective and safe, but laser is expensive and this way the correction is often unavailable for most patients (17).

3.3.2 Economic evaluation of toric intraocular lens

Pineda and colleagues (18) assessed the economic value of improved uncorrected visual acuity among patients with cataract and preexisting astigmatism treated with toric intraocular lenses (IOLs) compared with conventional monofocal IOLs. They concluded that toric IOLs reduce lifetime economic costs by reducing the need for glasses or contact lenses following cataract removal. These results can inform physicians and patients regarding the value of toric IOLs in the treatment of cataract and preexisting astigmatism.

Laurendeau and collegues (19) in their study concluded that bilateral toric IOL implants in astigmatic patients decreased spectacle dependence for distance vision and the need for complex spectacles. The economic consequences for patients depended on the national spectacle costs usually incurred after cataract surgery.

4. Conclusion

Toric intraocular lenses are accurate, reliable, predictable, permanently correcting astigmatism in cataract patients who are operated, while the flow of the operation is not extended, or require special training for surgeons already trained. Rotational stability of an IOL is the primary determinant of the refractive outcome. The surgeon should also keep in mind that the final outcome is very important and proper selection of patients, including patients with irregular astigmatism due to the scar tissue forming of the cornea, keratoconus, pellucid marginal degeneration, etc,. New available aspheric toric lens offer a better quality of vision postoperatively (reduction of spherical aberration, further improving contrast sensitivity, and uncorrected visual acuity at a distance). Toric IOLs reduce lifetime economic costs by reducing the need for glasses or contact lenses following cataract removal.

5. References

[1] Buckhurst PJ. Wolffsohn JS. Davies LN, Naroo SA. Surgical correction of astigmatism during cataract surgery. Clin Exp Optom 2010; 93: 409–418.

[2] Bauer NJC, De Vries NE, Webers CAB, Hendrikse F, Nuijts RMMA. Astigmatism management in cataract surgery with the AcrySof toric intraocular lens. J Cataract Refract Surg 2008; 34:1483–1488.

[3] Masket S, Wang L, Belani S. Induced astigmatism with 2.2- and 3.0-mm coaxial phacoemulsification incisions. J Refract Surg 2009; 25: 21–24.

[4] Amesbury EC, Miller KM. Correction of astigmatism at the time of cataract surgery. Curr Opin Ophthalmol 2009; 20: 19–24.

[5] Graether JM. Simplified system of marking the cornea for a toric intraocular lens. J Cataract Refract Surg 2009; 35: 1498–1500.

[6] Patel CK, Ormonde S, Rosen PH, Bron AJ. Postoperative intraocular lens rotation: a randomized comparison of plate and loop haptic implants. Ophthalmology 1999; 106: 2190–2195.

[7] Oshika T, Nagata T, Ishii Y. Adhesion of lens capsule to intraocular lenses of polymethylmethacrylate, silicone and acrylic foldable materials: an experimental study. Br J Ophthalmol 1998; 82: 549–553.

[8] AcrySof Toric Single-Piece Natural IOL Product Information. Fort Worth, TX: Alcon Laboratories, Inc.; 2005.

[9] Jampaulo M, Olson MD, Miller KM. Long-term Staar toric intraocular lens rotational stability. Am J Ophthalmol 2008; 146: 550–553.

[10] Alio JL, Agdeppa MCC, Pongo VC, Kady BE. Microincision cataract surgery with toric intraocular lens implantation for correcting moderate and high astigmatism: pilot study. J Cataract Refract Surg 2010; 36: 44–52.

[11] Chang DF. Comparative rotational stability of single-piece open-loop acrylic and plate-haptic silicone toric intraocular lenses. J Cataract Refract Surg 2008; 34: 1842– 1847.

[12] De Silva DJ, Ramkissoon YD, Bloom PA. Evaluation of a toric intraocular lens with a Z-haptic. J Cataract Refract Surg 2006; 32: 1492–1498.

[13] Narendran R, Vyas A, Bacon P. Centration, rotational stability and outcomes of Rayner T-flexTM toric lens implantation: 2 year results. Proceedings of the XXVII congress of the ESCRS, Barcelona, 2009.

[14] Buckhurst PJ, Wolffsohn JS, Naroo SA, Davies LN. Rotational and centration stability of an aspheric intraocular lens with a simulated toric design. J Cataract Refract Surg 2010; 36: 1523-1528.

[15] Tsinopoulos IT, Symeonidis C, Tsaousis KT, Tsakpinis D, Ziakas NG, Dimitrakos SA. Intra-operative assessment of toric intra-ocular lens implantation. Indian J Ophthalmol 2011; 59: 60-62.

[16] Kaufmann C, Peter J, Ooi K, Phipps S, Cooper P, Goggin M. Limbal relaxing incisions versus on-axis incisions to reduce corneal astigmatism at the time of cataract surgery. J Cataract Refract Surg 2005; 31: 2261-2265.

[17] Sanders DR, Sanders ML. Comparison of the toric implantable collamer lens and custom ablation LASIK for myopic astigmatism. J Refract Surg 2008; 24: 773-778.

[18] Pineda R, Denevich S, Lee WC, Waycaster C, Pashos CL. Economic evaluation of toric intraocular lens. Arch Ophthalmol. 2010; 128: 834-840.

[19] Laurendeau C, Lafuma A, Berdeaux G. Modelling lifetime cost consequences of toric compared with standard IOLs in cataract surgery of astigmatic patients in four Europian countries. Journal of Medical Economics 2009; 12: 230-237.

14

Comparing Nomograms of Two Symmetric and Two Asymmetric Intacs® Segments Implantation for Treatment of Pellucid Marginal Degeneration

Luis A. Rodriguez and Anny E. Villegas*

Corneal Clinic, Centro Medico Docente La Trinidad (CMDLT), Caracas
Venezuela

1. Introduction

Non-inflammatory progressive corneal ectasia and thinning disease are among the most common abnormalities that refractive surgeons diagnose. Pellucid Marginal Degeneration (PMD) is another ectatic pathology that is rarely detected. PMD is a bilateral, non-inflammatory, progressive peripheral inferior corneal thinning disorder (1,2). Diagnosis is based on the presence of corneal thinning with ectasia characterized by a peripheral band of thinning of the inferior cornea with 1 to 2 mm of normal cornea between this area and the limbus (2,3). The area of thinning typically is epithelialized, clear, avascular, and without lipid deposit. Like keratoconus, PMD is a bilateral progressive disorder although eyes may be asymmetrically affected. Topographic examination is very useful to differentiate this ectatic disorder. The topographic appearance shows a classical "butterfly" pattern that demonstrates large amounts of against-the-rule astigmatism as measured by simulated keratometry and inferior thinning. PMD can also be diagnosed by performing a pachymetric map of the entire cornea, as well as by elevation corneal maps using placido-ring-based videokeratoscopy technology (1).

The etiology of PMD is not clear, and it is not known whether PMD, keratoconus and keratoglobus are distinct diseases or phenotypic variations of the same disorder (4). PMD is usually asymptomatic except for progressive deterioration in uncorrected visual acuity caused by irregular astigmatism (5). Slit-lamp examination shows a peripheral band of thinning with a protrusion ("beer-belly" contour) of the inferior cornea (6,7,8). Topographically, this protrusion in the peripheral inferior cornea has high keratometry powers, radiating toward the center from the inferior oblique meridians, typically in the inferior peripheral cornea. There is an area of flattening in the center of the cornea (5). In transmission electron microscopy of the cornea, abnormal fibrous long-spacing (FSL) collagen with a periodicity of 100 to 110 nm in PMD is revealed, which contrasts with 60 to 64 nm found in normal corneas (9). A study reported in 2002 describes associations with

---

* None of the authors has a financial or proprietary interest in any material or method mentioned in this article.

vernal keratoconjunctivitis, Marfan's syndrome, ocular hypertension, keratoconus, keratoglobus and hydrops (23).

In the early stages, spectacles and contact lenses are the usual treatment approaches; however, in patients who cannot be rehabilitated with these options, a surgical procedure is necessary (10). Different surgical options include crescentic wedge resection, crescentic lamellar keratoplasty, penetrating keratoplasty, epikeratophakia and thermokeratoplasty. However, all these techniques have disadvantages: unpredictability, irreversibility, long period of rehabilitation and significant complication rates (11-16). Authors suggest the use of intracorneal rings (ICR) in glasses/contact lens-intolerant patients affected by early and moderate PMD with against-the-rule astigmatism and inferior peripheral corneal thickness of >450 μm (10). Since ICR mechanically lifts the inferior ectasia of PMD, flattens the soft ectatic corneal tissue, and decreases asymmetrical astigmatism, visual acuity is expected to improve following this procedure (17). Intacs® works on the principle of tissue addition. Peripheral distention is directly proportional to the degree of central corneal flattening, and by an arc-shortening effect it manages to change the shape and power of the central cornea in ectatic eyes without weakening the central or the paracentral cornea (17,18). The aspheric shape of the natural cornea reduces aberrations and minimizes refractive error fluctuations as the pupil changes its size, and therefore reduces visual disturbances such as glare and halos. It is important to observe that Intacs® maintains an aspheric cornea. After placement of ring segments, central cornea has been shown to maintain a prolate shape because Intacs® flattens the peripheral cornea more than the central cornea (19). The major objective of corneal ring segment inserts is to reshape the abnormality by neither removing corneal tissue nor touching the central cornea (20). Various reports have been published illustrating either the symmetrical (inserting two same-size segments) or the asymmetrical (inserting two different size segments) Intacs® implantation techniques for the management of PMD. Both these techniques have been independently shown to improve UCVA, BSCVA and topographic findings (9,10).

Intacs® are polymethylmethacrylate crescent-shaped segments with arc length of 150° and inner and outer diameters of 6.8 mm and 8.1 mm respectively. The ring segments are available in sizes ranging in thickness from 0.25 to 0.45 mm (Table 3).

2. Patients and methods

Symmetric ring segments were implanted in ten (10) eyes and asymmetric ring segments were implanted in nine (9) eyes. Swanson nomogram was used to calculate segment thickness in each eye.

De-Centered Cones (Posterior Float 50% outside the 3 mm optical zone)**		
Spherical Equiv	Inferior Intacs®	Superior Intacs®
+1.00 to -2.00	.250 mm	.300 mm
-2.00 to -3.00	.250 mm	.350 mm
-3.00 to -4.00	.300 mm	.400 mm*
-4.00 and -5.00	.300 mm	.450 mm*
-5.00 and higher	.350 mm	.450 mm*

**Keratoconus, Pellucid Marginal Degeneration or "Pellucid Like" Nomogram (24)

Comparing Nomograms of Two Symmetric and Two Asymmetric Intacs® Segments Implantation for
Treatment of Pellucid Marginal Degeneration

235

The election of using asymmetric and symmetric ring segments was based on spherical equivalent and was randomly chosen.

Besides the demographic details, key parameters evaluated during the preoperative and postoperative examination included: slitlamp microscopy, manifest refraction, spherical equivalent (SE), uncorrected visual acuity (UCVA), corneal pachymetry, tonometry, flat and steep keratometry readings and topography (Orbscan II). Postoperatively patients were evaluated at one month, three months, six months and one year.

3. Surgical procedure

Intacs® implantation was performed under topical anesthesia. After the patients were prepared through corneal hydration with balanced saline solution and sterile fields, the geometric center of the cornea was measured and marked. A radial 2 mm incision was performed in the steep corneal meridian with a diamond knife that was calibrated to 85% corneal depth. A vacuum centering guide - sloped shelf ring connected to a KV2000 vacuum system (Addition Technology® 155 Moffett Park Drive, Suite B-1 Sunnyvale, CA 94089-1330 U.S.A.) was positioned to stabilize the globe. Clockwise and counterclockwise stromal dissectors were introduced into the base of the incision to create stromal tunnels. Intacs® of selected thicknesses were placed in the stromal tunnels from each side of the incision. The incision site was closed with one interrupted 10-0 nylon suture. Post-operative medication included an antibiotic/steroid combination taken every six (6) hours for two (2) weeks. All procedures were uneventful and performed by the same surgeon, (LAR).

4. Statistical analysis

The two groups were analyzed for any bias with respect to age, size of segments, initial values of visual acuity, astigmatism, spherical equivalent, flat and steep keratometry readings. Both groups were found to be comparable.

Our study was descriptive and results were represented as averages and percentages (±standard deviations). Confidence intervals were set at 95%.

Paired t test was used to compare the two groups with respect to changes in the following parameters: visual acuity, astigmatism, spherical equivalent, keratometries (flat and steep readings). Visual acuity was expressed in log mar (Snellen equivalent). One-way Anova test was applied to compare the changes in values throughout time in both the symmetric and asymmetric groups. Bonferroni post test was applied in cases where the values were statistically significant. Any value of P less than or equal to 0.05 (P >0.05) was considered statistically significant.

5. Results

Preoperative values in asymmetric group: UCVA 1.00 (log mar); astigmatism: -4.00D; SE: -2.90D, K (flat) 43.09 D; K (steep) 47.02D. (Table 1) UCVA 0.85 (log mar); astigmatism: -4,50D; SE: -2.74D; K (flat) 43.03 D; K (steep) 47.05D. (Table 2)

Tables 1 and 2 show an improvement in visual acuity, reduction in astigmatism, spherical equivalent and decrease in steep and flat keratometry post-op.

Parameter	Initial			Final		
	Mean	SE	CI 95%	Mean	SE	95% CI
Visual Acuity (LogMAR)	1.00	0.14	0.67 – 1.33	0.22	0.04	0.13 – 0.30
Astigmatism	-4.00	0.49	-5.13 - -2.88	-2.11	0.39	-5.25 - -0.55
Spherical Equivalent	-2.90	1.02	-3.08 - -0.06	-1.57	0.62	-3.08 - -0.06
Keratometry Flat	43.09	0.49	41.95 – 44.23	40.79	0.63	39.33 – 42.25
Keratometry Steep	47.02	0.6	45.63 – 48.40	44.51	1.06	42.07 – 46.96

SE: Standard Error; 95% CI: Confidence Interval of mean 95% (Lower – Upper)

Table 1. Initial and Final Values for Visual Acuity (LogMAR), Astigmatism, Spherical Equivalent and Keratometry (Flat and Steep) in Patients with Diagnosis of Pellucid Marginal Degeneration with Insertion Asymmetrical Intacs ® Segments

Parameter	Initial			Final		
	Mean	SE	CI 95%	Mean	SE	95% CI
Visual Acuity (LogMAR)	0.85	0.19	0.42 – 1.28	0.28	0.09	0.09 – 0.48
Astigmatism	-4.50	0.44	-5.5 - -3.5	-3.30	0.54	-4.53 - -2.07
Spherical Equivalent	-2.74	1.08	-5.17 - -0.3	-0.58	0.40	-1.49 – 0.33
Keratometry Flat	43.03	0.27	42.41 – 43.65	42.12	0.50	40.98 – 43.25
Keratometry Steep	47.05	0.79	45.27 – 48.84	45.07	0.48	43.98 – 46.15

SE: Standard Error; 95% CI: Confidence Interval of mean 95% (Lower – Upper)

Table 2. Initial and Final Values for Visual Acuity (LogMAR), Astigmatism, Spherical Equivalent and Keratometry (Flat and Steep) in Patients with Diagnosis of Pellucid Marginal Degeneration with Insertion Symmetrical Intacs ® Segments

The characteristics of the implanted segments were the following:

Asymmetric segments implanted: 300/250 (3), 450/300 (2), 350/250 (2), 450/250 (2).

Symmetric segments implanted: 450 (1), 400 (1), 350 (1), 300 (4), 250 (3).

The asymmetric group had an average age of 29.67 ± 3.42 years, and the symmetric group had an average age of 34.5 ± 3.42 years. The study showed a non-significant statistical difference between the groups (p=0.357).

Visual Acuity in the symmetric group was better than the asymmetric group. In order to compare the two groups and showed a non-significant statistical difference between the two groups (p=0.550). Figure 1

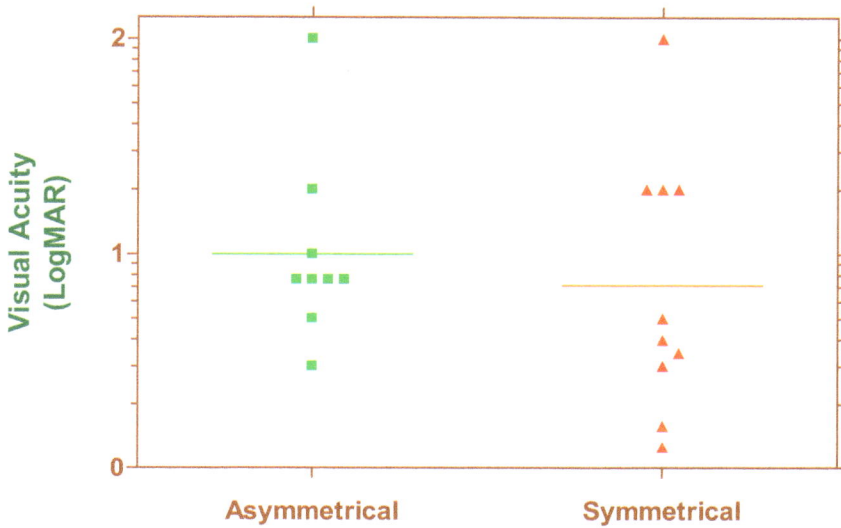

Fig. 1. Initial Values of Visual Acuity in Patients with Diagnosis of Pellucid Marginal
Degeneration with Insertion of Symmetrical or Asymmetrical Intacs ® Segments

Spherical equivalent and steep keratometry showed no significant statistical difference in
astigmatism between the two groups (p=0.456; p=0.914; p=0.647 respectively). Figure 2, 3
and 4

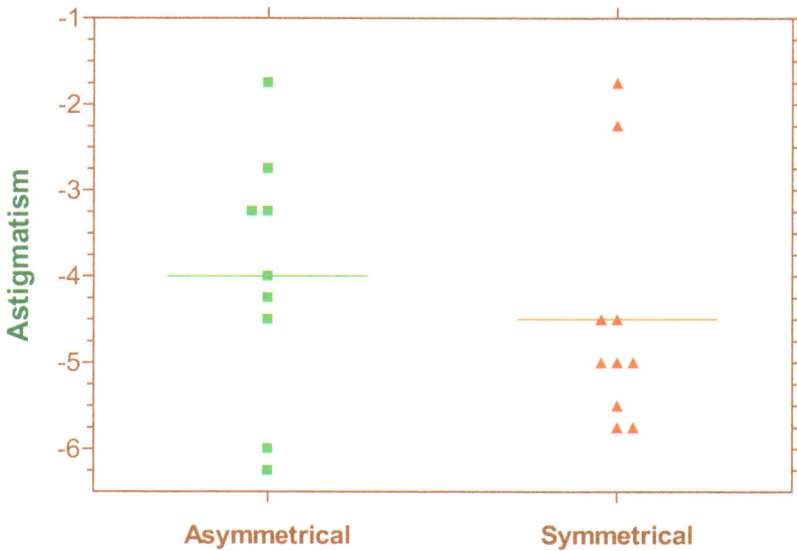

Fig. 2. Initial Values of Astigmatism in Patients with Diagnosis of Pellucid Marginal
Degeneration with Insertion of Symmetrical or Asymmetrical Intacs ® Segments

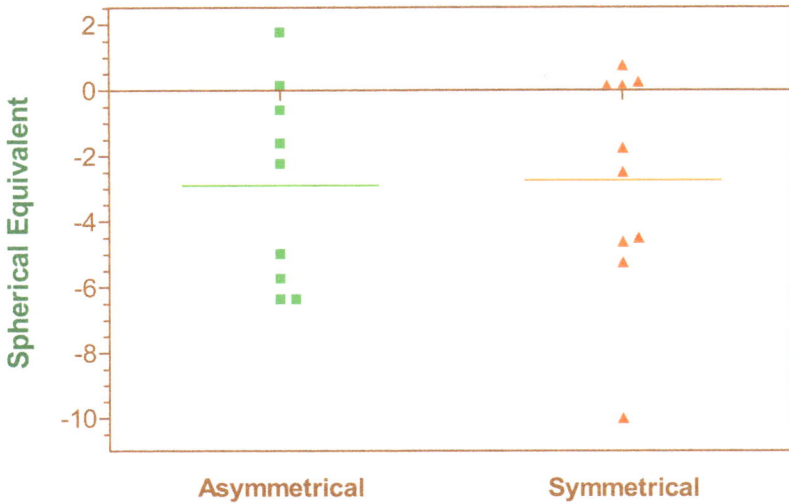

Fig. 3. Initial Values of Spherical Equivalent in Patients with Diagnosis of Pellucid Marginal Degeneration with Insertion of Symmetrical or Asymmetrical Intacs ® Segments

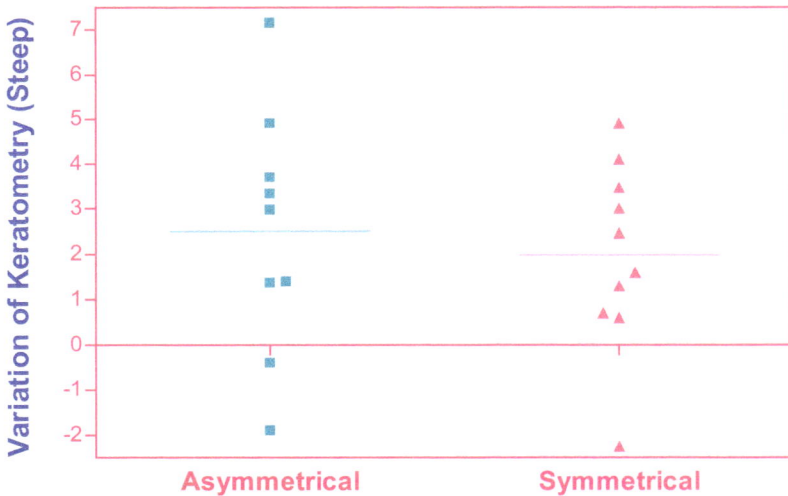

Fig. 4. Variation of Keratometry (Steep) in Patients with Diagnosis of Pellucid Marginal Degeneration with Insertion of Symmetrical or Asymmetrical Intacs ® Segments

After comparing the groups with flat keratometry, a significant statistical difference was found (p=0.025). This variation was greater in the asymmetric group. Figure 5

In Figure 6 and 7 the evolution of visual acuity for the asymmetric and symmetric group can be seen. After applying one-way Anova, a significant statistical difference was evidenced (p<0.0001 and p=0.0003). We subsequently applied the Bonferroni multiple comparison test

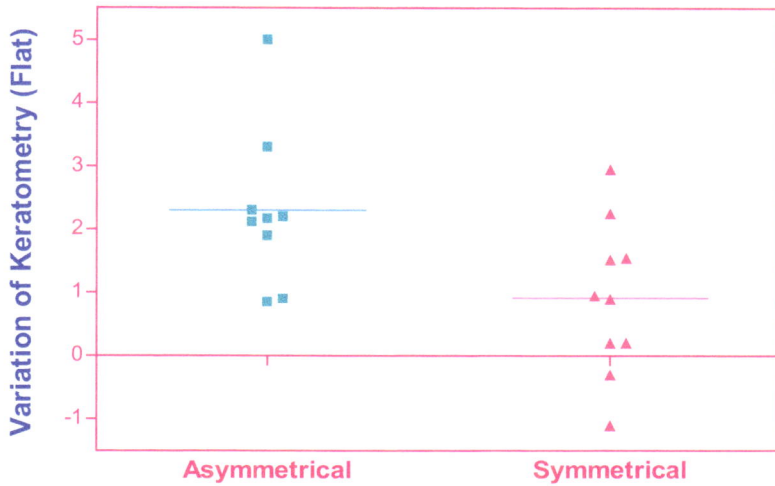

Fig. 5. Variation of Keratometry (Flat) in Patients with Diagnosis of Pellucid Marginal
Degeneration with Insertion of Symmetrical or Asymmetrical Intacs ® Segments

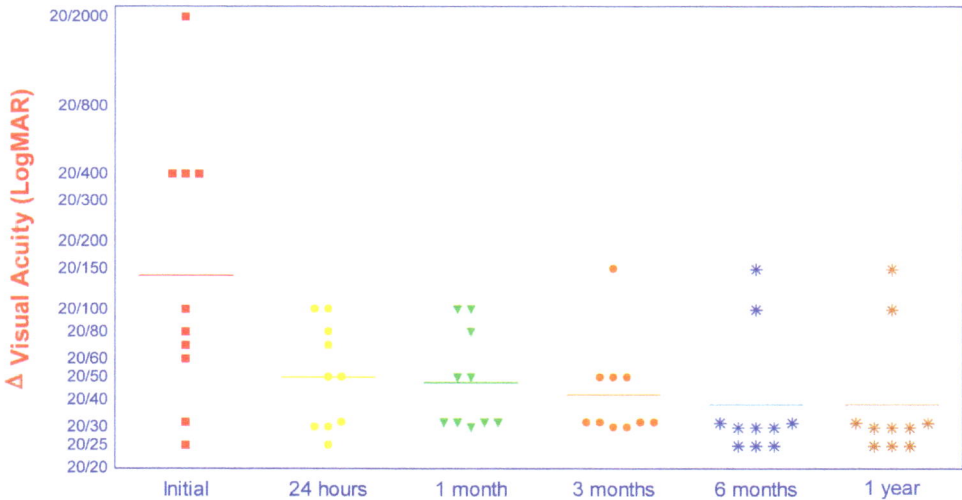

Fig. 6. Time Course of Visual Acuity (LogMAR) in Patients with Diagnosis of Pellucid
Marginal Degeneration with Insertion of Asymmetrical Intacs ®

in order to compare each post-operatory time period. No significant statistical differences
were seen.

In Figure 8 and 9 the evolution of astigmatism for the asymmetric and symmetric group was
shown. With the application of one-way Anova, a significant statistical difference was
observed in asymmetric group (p=0.031) while no significant statistical difference was found
postoperatively (p =0.074) in symmetric group. The Bonferroni multiple comparison test

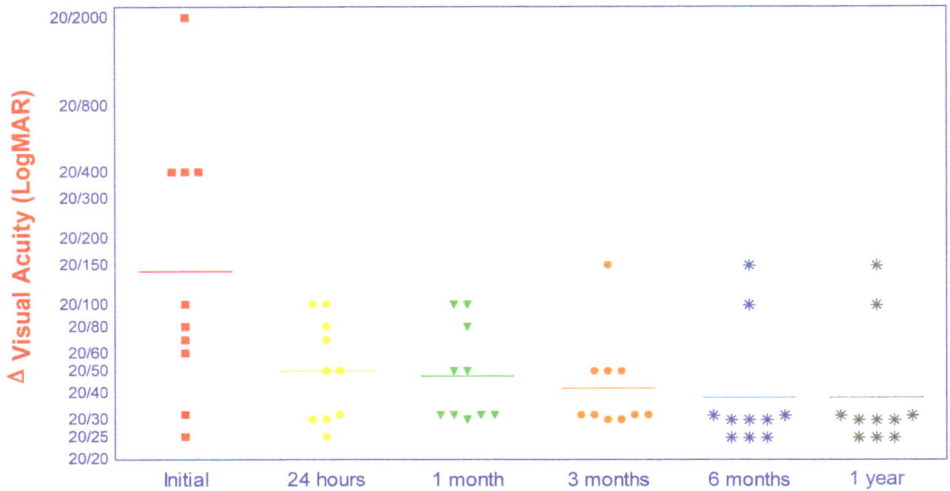

Fig. 7. Time Course of Visual Acuity (LogMAR) in Patients with Diagnosis of Pellucid Marginal Degeneration with Insertion of Symmetrical Intacs ®

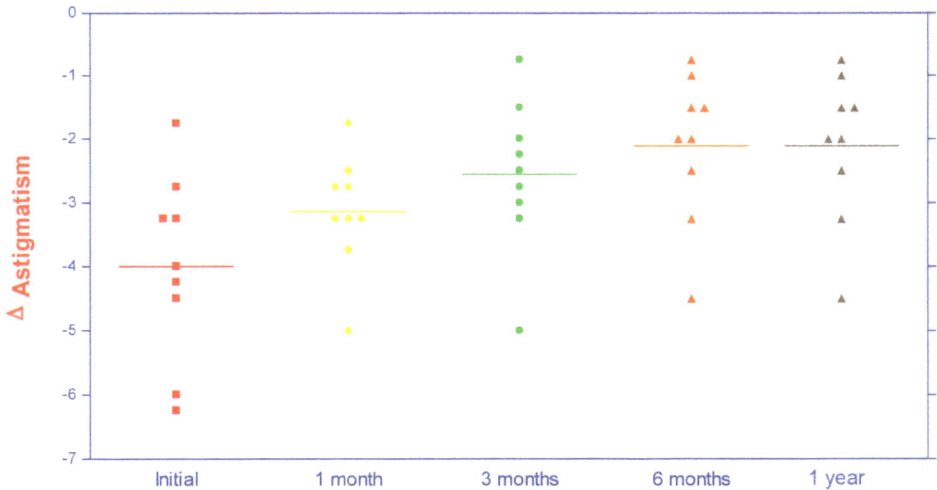

Fig. 8. Time Course of Astigmatism in Patients with Diagnosis of Pellucid Marginal Degeneration with Insertion of Asymmetrical Intacs ®

showed no significant statistical difference between initial and one month, and significant statistical differences between initial and three months and between initial, six months and one year respectively.

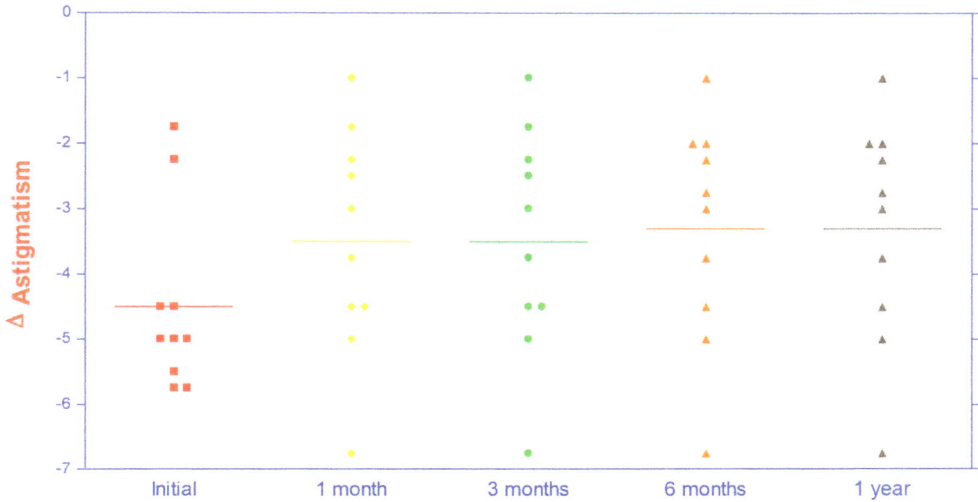

Fig. 9. Time Course of Astigmatism in Patients with Diagnosis of Pellucid Marginal
Degeneration with Insertion of Symmetrical Intacs ®

Figures 10 and 11 analyzed the variation of spherical equivalent for the asymmetric and
symmetric group. After applying one-way Anova, a significant statistical difference was
observed in both groups (p=0.030; p=0.020). In addition we used the Bonferroni multiple
comparison test in order to compare each time period and thereby established that the only
difference was between initial and first month postoperatively in asymmetric group and
initial with six month and first year in symmetric group.

In Figure 12 the evolution of flat keratometry in the asymmetric group is graphed. After the
application of one–way Anova, a significant statistical difference was evidenced (p=0.005).
We then applied the Bonferroni multiple comparison test in order to compare all the
postoperative time periods. The difference found was observed in the comparison between
the initial with three months and the initial with six months. No difference was found upon
comparing initial with one month, nor when comparing the various time periods after initial
(one month, three months, and six months) respectively. No significant statistical difference
was observed in symmetric group (p=0.543) figure 13.

In Figure 14 the variation in steep keratometry in the asymmetric group was observed. After
applying one-way Anova, a significant statistical difference was observed (p=0.003). In
addition we applied the Bonferroni multiple comparison test in order to compare each time
period, and the only difference found was when comparing initial with one month.

In Figure 15 we observed the evolution of steep keratometry in the symmetric group. No
significant statistical difference was found when one–way Anova was applied (p=0.080).

With respect to the variation in visual acuity (log mar), astigmastism and spherical
equivcalent, when both groups were compared with the student's t test, no significant
statistical difference was found between them (p=0.366; p=0.412; p=0.344 respectively).
Figure 16, 17 and 18.

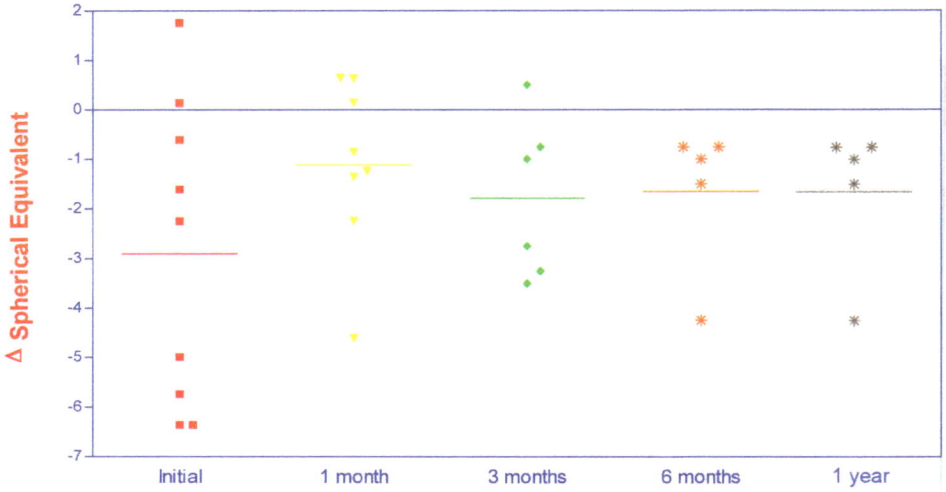

Fig. 10. Time Course of Spherical Equivalent in Patients with Diagnosis of Pellucid Marginal Degeneration with Insertion of Asymmetrical Intacs ®

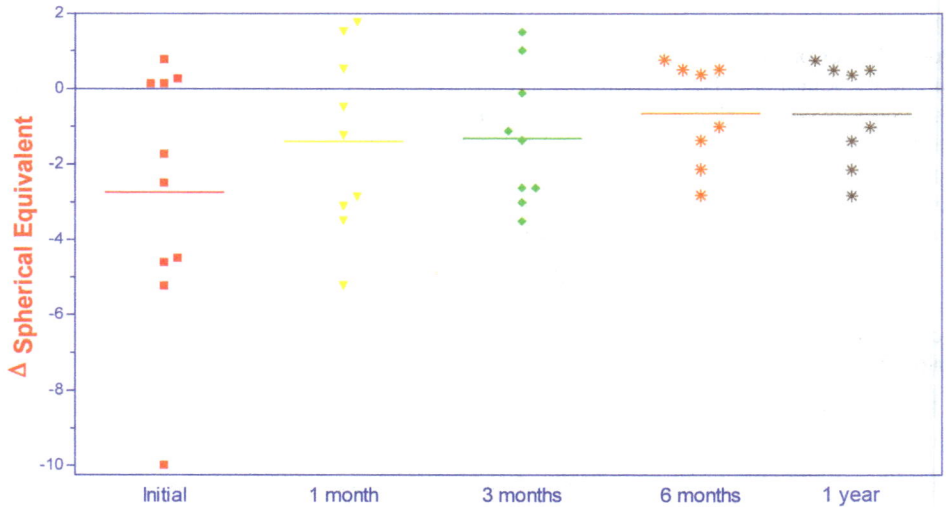

Fig. 11. Time Course of Spherical Equivalent in Patients with Diagnosis of Pellucid Marginal Degeneration with Insertion of Symmetrical Intacs ®

Comparing Nomograms of Two Symmetric and Two Asymmetric Intacs® Segments Implantation for
Treatment of Pellucid Marginal Degeneration

243

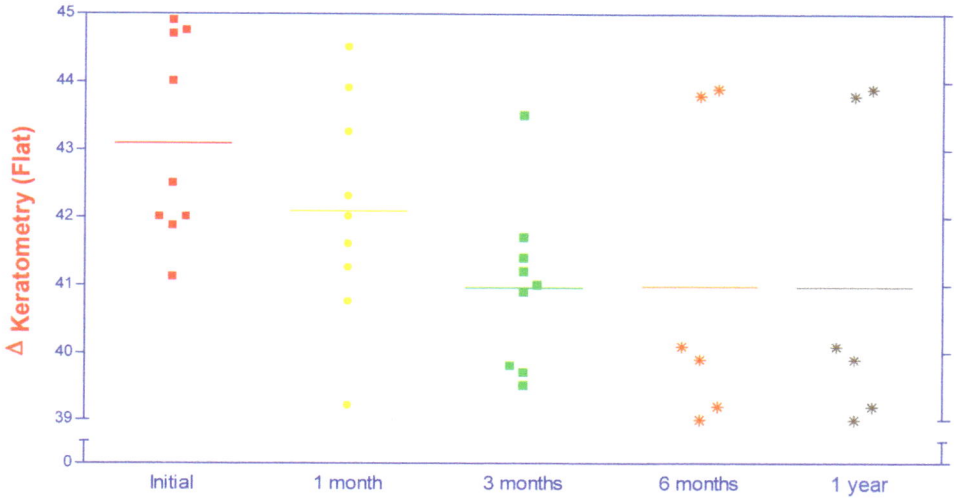

Fig. 12. Time Course of Keratometry (Flat) in Patients with Diagnosis of Pellucid Marginal
Degeneration with Insertion of Asymmetrical Intacs ®

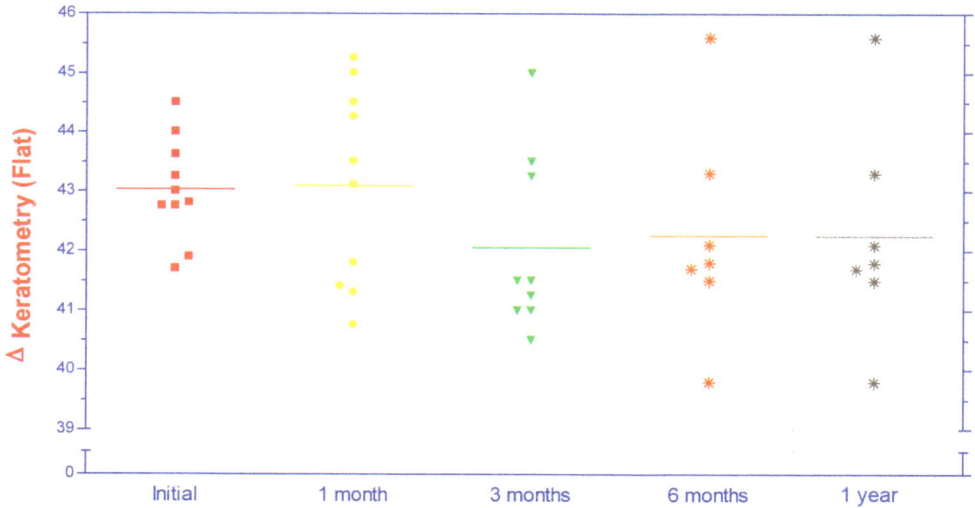

Fig. 13. Time Course of Keratometry (Flat) in Patients with Diagnosis of Pellucid Marginal
Degeneration with Insertion of Symmetrical Intacs ®

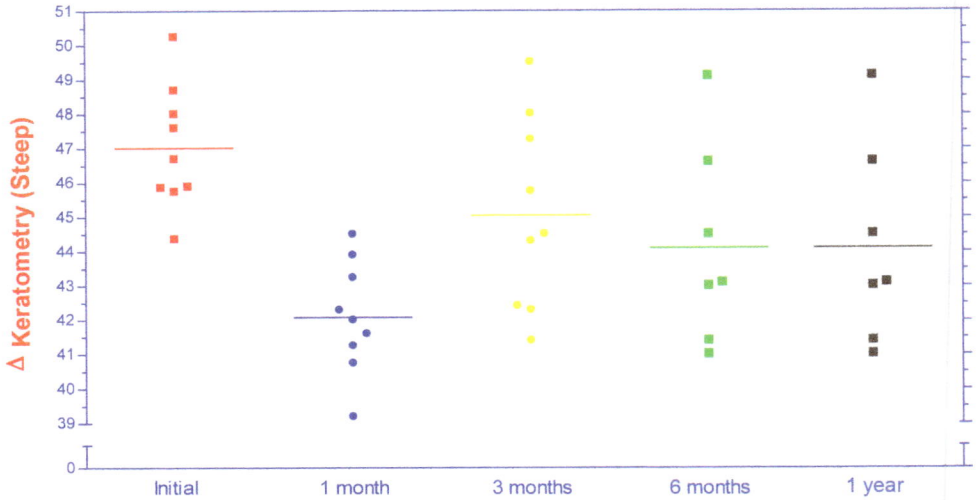

Fig. 14. Time Course of Keratometry (Steep) in Patients with Diagnosis of Pellucid Marginal Degeneration with Insertion of Asymmetrical Intacs ®

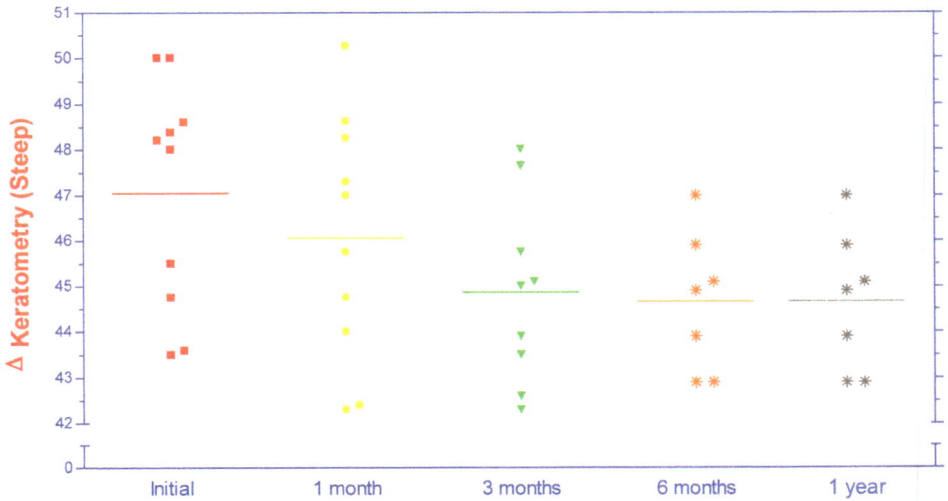

Fig. 15. Time Course of Keratometry (Steep) in Patients with Diagnosis of Pellucid Marginal Degeneration with Insertion of Symmetrical Intacs ®

Comparing Nomograms of Two Symmetric and Two Asymmetric Intacs® Segments Implantation for
Treatment of Pellucid Marginal Degeneration

245

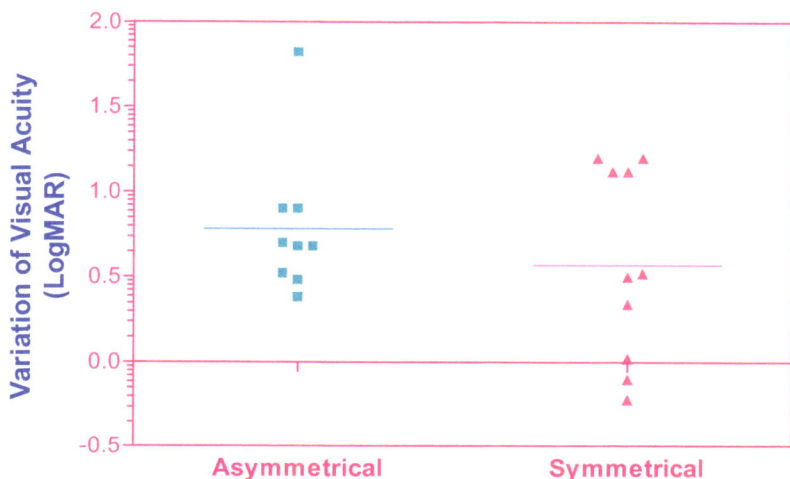

Fig. 16. Variation of Visual Acuity (LogMAR) in Patients with Diagnosis of Pellucid
Marginal Degeneration with Insertion of Symmetrical or Asymmetrical Intacs ® Segments

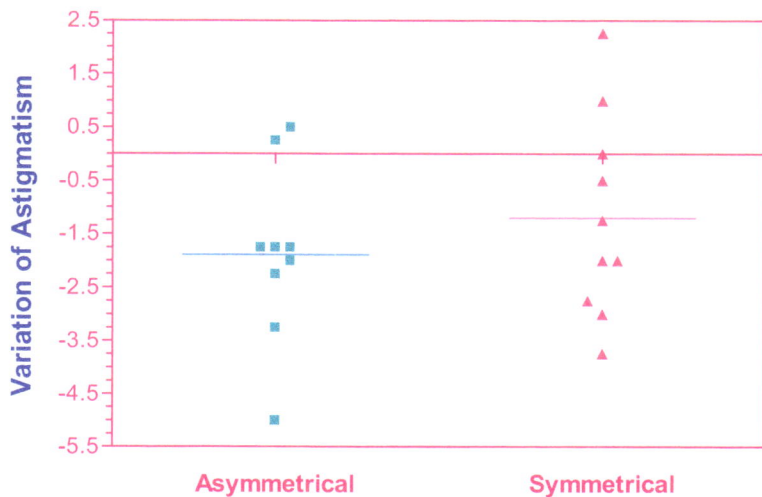

Fig. 17. Variation of Astigmatism in Patients with Diagnosis of Pellucid Marginal
Degeneration with Insertion of Symmetrical or Asymmetrical Intacs ® Segments

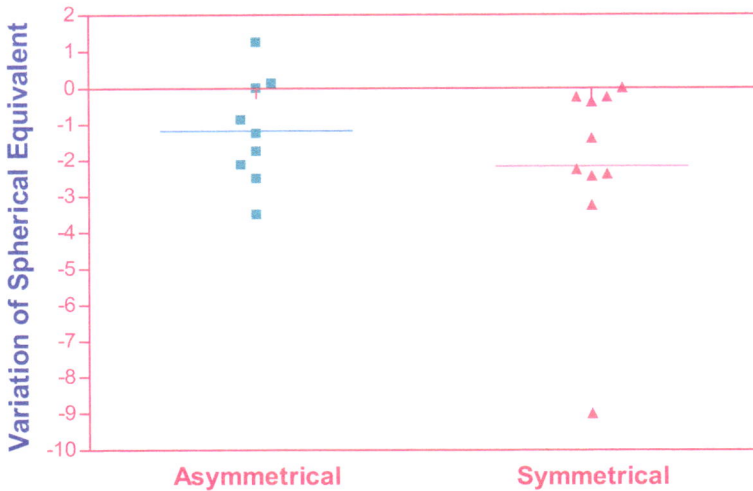

Fig. 18. Variation of Spherical Equivalent in Patients with Diagnosis of Pellucid Marginal Degeneration with Insertion of Symmetrical or Asymmetrical Intacs ® Segments

5.1 Results in asymmetric group

At the end of follow-up period (one year), mean UCVA was 0.22 log mar, ±0,04 (20/30) (95% IC=0.13-0.30). Statistically significant differences were noted throughout the follow-up period (p < 0.0001)

Astigmatism value at final follow-up was -2.11D ±0.39 (95% IC= -5.25 – 0.55). P values at all of the postoperative follow-up periods were statistically significant (p=0.001). The maximum improvement in astigmatism was at three months postoperative.

Spherical equivalent mean value was -1.57D ± 0.62 (95% IC=-3.08- 0.06). The changes in mean spherical equivalent during the follow-up period were statistically significant (p=0.030) with maximum improvement at one month postoperative.

Keratometry flat meridian was 40.79D±0.63 (95% IC= 39.33- 42.25). All the changes in mean readings in flat keratometry were statistically significant (p=0.005). Maximum improvement was between three and six months postoperative.

Keratometry steep meridian was 44.51D±1.06 (95% IC= 42.07 – 46.96). The changes in mean readings in steep keratometry were statistically significant (p=0.003) with maximum improvement at first month.

5.2 Results in symmetric group

Mean UCVA was 0.28 log mar, ±0.09 (20/40) (95% IC=0.09-0.48). Statistically significant differences were noted throughout the follow-up period (p < 0.0003)

Astigmatism value at final follow-up was -3.30D ±0.54 (95% IC= -4.53 – 2.07). At first year, the difference was not statistically significant (p=0.074).

Spherical equivalent mean values were -0.58D ± 0.40 (95% IC=-1.49 – 0.33). The difference was statistically significant (p=0.020) with maximum improvement at six months postoperative.

Keratometry flat meridian value was 42.12D±0.50 (95% IC= 40.98- 43.25). At first year, the difference was not statistically significant (p=0.543).

Keratometry steep meridian was 45.07D±0.48 (95% IC= 43.98 – 46.15). At first year postoperative the difference was not statistically significant (p= 0.080).

5.3 Comparing results of both groups

Initial visual acuity values were not statistically different between both groups (p=0.550).

Astigmatism initial values were not statistically significant between both groups. (p=0.456). Spherical equivalent values were not statistically significant between both groups (p=0.914). Keratometries (flat and steep) meridian initial values were not statistically significant between both groups (p=0.905 symmetric group), (p=0.972 asymmetric group).

UCVA was not statistically significant between the groups (p=0.366). The difference of final post-op values in astigmatism for the groups was not statistically significant. (p=0.412). The difference of spherical equivalent values at six months post-op between the groups was not statistically significant (p=0.344). The difference of keratometry flat values at six months post-op between the groups was significant (p=0.025) with a better result in the asymmetric group. Keratometry steep values at one year postoperatively in both groups were not statistically significant. (p=0.647).

6. Discussion

Pellucid marginal degeneration (PMD) is a disease with a complicated prognosis in patients who are intolerant to contact lenses (10). Different procedures have been used to treat PMD with unpredictable results. Symmetric and asymmetric Intacs® segments are relatively new devices that reinforce the cornea through the arc-shortening effect of the corneal lamellae that produces flattening of the central cornea. The goal of using Intacs® for PMD is to reshape the cornea without removing tissue by lifting the inferior ectasia, flattening the soft ectatic corneal tissue and decreasing astigmatism. With this treatment, tissue and endothelium is maintained with the benefit that an additive surgical approach is used that adds rigidity and reinforces the ectatic cornea, flattening the central area, and positioning the optical zone in the center of the pupil. This procedure is also reversible. Mularoni et al. proposed a treatment with two asymmetric intracorneal segments in patients with intolerance to contact lenses and early and moderate PMD. Results were great improvement in UCVA, BSCVA and topographical findings (10). Colin J. and Malet F. implanted two symmetric Intacs® segments and followed the progress for two years post operatively obtaining favorable results. The findings in this study indicated that Intacs® segments are an effective long-term treatment for keratoconus and associated ectasia (21). Kymionis et al. reported a case of PMD treated with Intacs® symmetric segments which reported an improvement in corneal topographic pattern. ICR insertion can reduce the corneal steepening and astigmatism associated with PMD (9). Rodriguez Prats et al. reported a reduction of steepening and astigmatism associated with PMD by implanting one inferior segment (17). Sharma M. and Boxer Wachler noted that placement of inferior segment Intacs® alone was more suitable than double segments Intacs® insertion for peripherally located cones (22). Alió et al found that by implanting either one or two segments produced a similar effect in the reduction of the refractive cylinder and the keratometric readings (19). Both methods have similar results especially when concerning the visual acuity.

In our study, we compared implanting two segments in an asymmetric group to implanting two segments in a symmetric group, with a slightly better result in UCVA in the asymmetric group. When we evaluated BCVA, UCVA, spherical equivalent, astigmatism and keratometric readings, the differences between preop and postop values in all parameters were significantly reduced in both groups with statistically significant differences.

We noted that when analyzing nomograms of the symmetric and asymmetric groups, there were no statistically significant differences when comparing the results of both procedures. This is mainly due to similar spherical equivalent and showed that both nomograms were effective. Both groups tolerated spectacles and contact lenses well after the procedures.

In the asymmetric group we implanted intracorneal segments that were thicker in the protrusion area and thinner in the flatter area, taking spherical equivalent into account. This could possibly have led to an overcorrection with the implantation of the thicker segment. When implanting thicker segments in the thinner protrusion area, great skill was used so as not to perforate the cornea or extrude the segment. In the symmetric group we implanted two same thickness segments, also dependent on spherical equivalent. In symmetric implantations there are more articles available that reported success in keratoconus and other ectasias. By implanting thinner segments in the protrusion area, undercorrection was a possibility. The advantage of implanting two segments was that corneal prolate is maintained.

7. References

[1] Sridhar MS, Mahesh S, Bansal AK, Nutheti R, Rao GN Pellucid marginal corneal degeneration. Ophthalmology 2004; 1102-7

[2] Rabinowitz YS, Keratoconus. Surv Ophthalmology 1998; 297-319

[3] Karim Rasheed, Yaron Rabinowitz, MD, Pellucid Marginal Degeneration. Emecine

[4] Santos RM, Bechara SJ, Kara-Jose N. Corneal topography in asymptomatic family members of a patient with pellucid marginal degeneration. Am J Ophthalmology 1999; 205-207.

[5] Kymionis GD, Aslanides IM, Siganos CS, Pallikaris IG. Intacs® for early pellucid marginal degeneration. J Cataract Refract Surg 2004; 230-233

[6] Schlaeppi V., La dystrophie marginale inferieure pellucid de la cornee. Mod Probl Ophthalmology 1957; 672-677

Comparing Nomograms of Two Symmetric and Two Asymmetric Intacs® Segments Implantation for
Treatment of Pellucid Marginal Degeneration

249

[7] Maguire LJ, Klyce SD, McDonald ME, Kauffmann HE, Corneal topography of pellucid marginal degeneration. Ophthalmology 1987; 519-24

[8] Maeda N, Klyce SD, Tano Y. Detection and classification of mild irregular astigmatism in patients with good visual acuity. Surv Ophthalmology 1998; 53-8

[9] Rodriguez MM, Newsome DA, Krachmer JH.Pellucid marginal cornea degeneration: a clinical pathologic study of two cases. Exp Eye Res 1981; 277-288

[10] Mularoni A, Torreggiani A, Di Biase A, Laffi GL, Tassinari G, Conservative Treatment of Early and Moderate Pellucid Marginal Degeneration. Ophthalmology 2005; 660-666

[11] Rodriguez-Gonzales-Herrero ME, Gutierrez Ortega AR, De Imperial Mora-Figueroa Jm, Surgical treatment of pellucid marginal degeneration associated with cataract [letter]. J Cataract Refract Surg 2000; 309-11

[12] Cameron JA, results of lamellar crescentic resection for pellucid marginal degeneration. IS J Ophthalmology 1992; 296-302

[13] Kremer I, Sperber LT, Laibson PR. Pellucid marginal degeneration treated by lamellar and penetrating keratoplasty [letter]. Arch Ophthalmology 1993; 169-70

[14] Colin J, Cochener B, Savary G, Malet f. Correcting keratoconus with intracorneal rings. J Cataract Refract Surg 2000; 1117-22

[15] Holmes-Higgins DK, Burris TE, INTACS® Study Group. Corneal surface topography and associated visual performance with INTACS® for myopia. Phase III clinical trial results. Ophthalmology 2000; 2061-71

[16] Kymionis GD, Siganos CS, Kounis G, et al. Management of post-LASIK corneal ectasia with Intacs® insert: one year results. Arch Ophthalmology 2003; 332-6.

[17] Rodriguez-Prats J, Galal Ahmed, Garcia-Lledo Magdalena, et al. Intracorneal rings for the correction of pellucid marginal degeneration Cataract Refract Surg 2003; 1421-1424

[18] Burris TE, Baker PC, Ayer CT, et al. Flattening of central corneal curvature with intrastromal corneal rings of increasing thickness: an eye-bank eye study. J Cataract Refract Surg 1993; 182-7.

[19] J.L. Alió, A Artola, A. Hassanein, H Haroun, A Galal, One or two Intacs® segments for the correction of keratoconus. J Cataract Refract Surg 2005; 943-953

[20] Colin J, Velou S, Implantation of Intacs® and a refractive intraocular lens to correct keratoconus. J Cataract Refract Surg 2003; 832-834

[21] Colin J, Cochener B, Savary G, et al. Intacs® inserts for treating keratoconus: one-year results. Ophthalmology 2001; 1409-1414

[22] Sharma M, Boxer Wachler BS. Comparison of single-segment and Double-segment Intacs® for keratoconus and post-LASIK ectasia. Am J Ophthalmology 2006; 891–895

[23] M.S Sridhar, S Mahesh, A.K Bansal, Rishita Nutheti, G.N. Pellucid marginal corneal degeneration. International Center for Advancement of Rural Eye Care, L.V. Prasad Eye Institute, Hyderabad, India. Presented as a poster at: American Academy of Ophthalmology and Pan-American Association of Ophthalmology Joint Meeting, October 20–23, 2002; Orlando.

[24] Swanson M. Developing Solutions for the Ectatic Cornea. Uploaded 2010. Available on web site: http://www.swannkeratoconus.com/main/mnoms.html

15

Etiology and Clinical Presentation of Astigmatism

Sanja Masnec Olujić
Ghethaldus Ophthalmology Policlinics, Zagreb
Croatia

1. Introduction

A perfect point image of an object point is called a stigmatic image. The term „stigmatic"is derived from the Greek word stigma, which refers to a sharply pointed stylus (Liesegang et al., 2002). Thus, a stigmatic optical system is one able to focus all the light rays from a point source onto a single point. However, in most cases, images are not stigmatic.

In paraxial optics, the focus is stigmatic, and all paraxial rays (those extremely close to the optical axis) focus onto a point. With nonparaxial rays, the focus is generally not stigmatic. Deviations from stigmatic imaging are called aberrations, and, one of a number of ways to classify such aberrations is clinically: into spherical aberrations, regular astigmatism and irregular astigmatism.

Astigmatism is the unequal refraction of the same eye in two different meridians. Unlike the basic types of refraction- emetropia, myopia and hyperopia- where all the light rays enter one focus (on the retina, behind it, or in front of it), in astigmatism there is no a single focus. In basic types of refraction, the cornea is spherical and it refracts equally in all the meridians.

In astigmatism variations in the curvature of the cornea or lens along different meridians prevent the light rays from focusing onto a single point. Corneal refraction depends on the corneal curvature. If the cornea is more curved, the power of refraction is higher and vice versa. Corneal and lenticular astigmatism can complement or cancel each other. Their summation represents the so called "total astigmatism".

Due to the lack of a single focus, an astigmatic eye is not able to see clearly without correction. Astigmatic patients complain of visual disturbances in both far (in myopia) and near vision (in hyperopia), which causes astenopic problems (headache, dizziness, fatigue etc). Additionally, regular, symmetric objects might seem to them irregular, and /or elongated.

2. Astigmatism types

Astigmatism can be regular or irregular. It can also be divided into myopic, hyperopic and mixed/compound astigmatism (where one of the main meridians is hyperopic and the other one myopic).

2.1 Regular astigmatism

In regular astigmatism each meridian refracts regularly and equally, but differently from the other meridians. One of the meridians refracts the most and another one the least. Those two meridians are called the main meridians, and they are perpendicular to each other.

In most cases, one of the main meridians is located vertically and the other one horizontally, but there can also be oblique, still maintaining the 90° angle to each other.

In the remaining meridians, located between the both two main meridians, refraction changes gradually –increases or decreases (Fig 1).

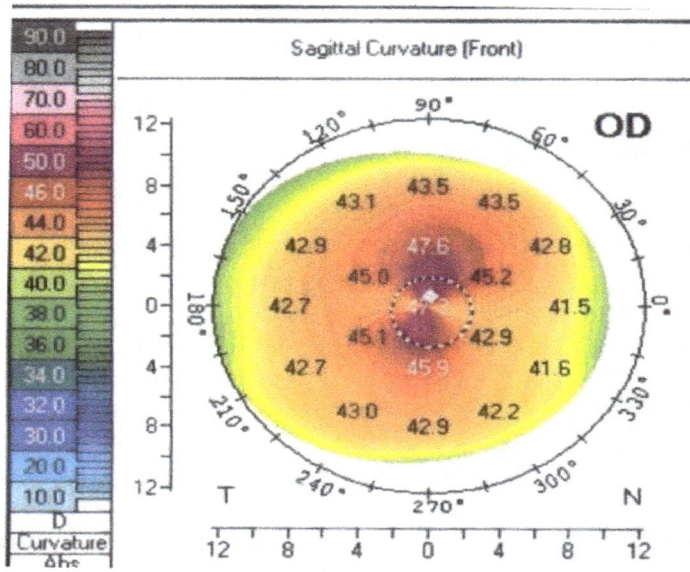

Fig. 1. With-the-rule astigmatism of 5.4 D shown on the topographical map of the anterior corneal surface , with quantitative information on the corneal curvature, astigmatism and its meridians.

Vertical meridian, in most of cases, refracts more then the horizontal, most likely due to the pressure of eyelids onto the cornea. This type of astigmatism is called *with- the- rule* astigmatism and is more common in children (Mohindra et al., 1978).

If the horizontal meridian refracts more, this is called *against- the- rule* astigmatism and is more common in older adults.

The difference in refraction of the two main meridians represents the amount of astigmatism and is represented in diopters (D).

When that difference is no more than 1/2 -3/4 diopters it is a so-called physiological astigmatism and a correction is usually not needed, as it does not lead to visual deterioration or subjective symptoms. Mostly, it is neutralized by the lenticular astigmatism (Parunovic et al., 1995).

Astigmatism over ¾ D can lead to visual disturbances and other subjective symptoms, because the lenticular astigmatism, which rarely exceeds 1-1.5 D, is not able to compensate for the corneal astigmatism.

Regular type astigmatism is rarely greater than 6-7 D.

For a better understanding of astigmatism and its correction, the most important optical concept is the **conoid of Sturm.**

The refractive power, as mentioned above, changes from one meridian to the next, and an astigmatic surface cannot bring a pencil of light rays to a point focus. Two focal lines instead of a single focus are formed. This complex geometrical envelope of a pencil of light rays refracted by a circular spherocylindrical lens is called the **conoid of Sturm.**

The conoid of Sturm has two focal lines, each parallel to one of the main meridians of the spherocylindrical lens. All the light rays in the pencil pass through each of the focal lines. The cross sections of the conoid of Sturm at various points along its length are mostly elliptical, including the portion of the conoid external to the two focal lines. At the dioptric mean of the two focal lines there is a circular cross section of the conoid of Sturm. This circular patch of light rays is called the *circle of least confusion*, and represents the best overall focus for the spherocylindrical lens. The circle of least confusion is the position where all the rays would be brought to focus if the lens had a spherical power equal to the average spherical power of all the meridians of the spherocylindrical lens (Michaels, 1980).

This average spherical power of a spherocylindrical lens represents the spherical equivalent of the lens, and can be calculated by the following equation:

Spherical equivalent = sphere + cylinder/2.

About 50% of infants in their first years of life show astigmatism of over 1D (Bennet et al., 1939; Mohindra et al., 1978).

Some authors have suggested that this high astigmatism helps the infant to bracket the position of best focus while it learns to accommodate (Howland et al., 1978).

In adults, this high incidence of astigmatism is much smaller. Different studies show that about 15 % of adults have astigmatism greater than 1D, and only 2 % of more then 3D (Yanoff & Duker, 2004).

In the leater group, it is most likely that much of the high astigmatism is due to some form of intraocular surgery, such as cataract surgery (particularly when extracapsular cataract extraction is performed), corneal transplants, corneal lacerations repair, ...etc.

Regular astigmatism can be congenital and acquired. Congenital astigmatism is usually inherited. Acquired astigmatism is mostly against-the rule and as mentioned above, can result from various intraocular surgeries.

Most oftenly, astigmatism is static, but it can also change during the life time. With –the – rule astigmatism tends to lessen over the years, and the position of the main meridians can also slightly change during the lifetime.

Regular astigmatism is correctable by cylindrical spectacle lenses and contact lenses.

In with-the rule astigmatism, a correcting plus cylinder lens should be used at or near the 90° axis. In against-the rule astigmatism, a correcting plus cylinder lens should be used at or near the 180° axis.

2.2 Irregular astigmatism

Irregular astigmatism appears when the refraction of light is unequal and irregular in the same meridian of the eye.

That is usually a consequence of pathological changes especially to the cornea (maculae centrales corneae, ulcus, pannus, keratoconus etc) or lens (cataract, posterior capsular opacification, lens subluxation etc).

The visual acuity of such an eye is deteriorated and sometimes monocular diplopia or poliopia occurs. All eyes have at least a small amount of irregular astigmatism, but the term is used clinically only for the stronger irregularities, such as those mentioned above, or occurring with keratoconus.

In the past, irregular astigmatism was not a field of strong interest by clinicians, as it was not very common, and was not treatable. It could not be corrected with spectacles, and rigid contact lenses could alleviate the problem to some extent only if the irregular astigmatism was corneal in origin.

With the development of keratorefractive surgical procedures, it became increasingly of interest, as keratorefractive surgeries may produce visually significant irregular astigmatism, or be used to treat it.

2.2.1 Keratoconus

Keratoconus (conical cornea) is a condition characterized by a progressive corneal steepening, usually inferior to the center of the cornea (Fig. 2.). As a result of a noninflammatory thinning of the corneal stroma eventually myopia is induced, together with irregular astigmatism, leading to an impairment in the quality of vision.

Keratoconus is a bilateral, usually asymmetric, noninflammatory corneal ectasia, which belongs to a group of corneal shape disorders, together with pellucid marginal corneal degeneration and keratoglobus.

By keratometry keratoconus is classified as:

1. mild (< 48 D)
2. moderate (48-54 D)
3. severe (> 54 D).

Epidemiology and pathogenesis

Keratoconus occurs in all ethnic groups with no male or female preponderance.

Rarely, it can be congenital (Smolin, 1987).

In majority of the cases, its onset is at puberty and then progresses until the third to fourth decade of life, with an incidence of approximately 1 per 2000 in the general population, and a prevalence of 54.5 per 100,000 (Hofstetter, 1959; Kennedy et al., 1986).

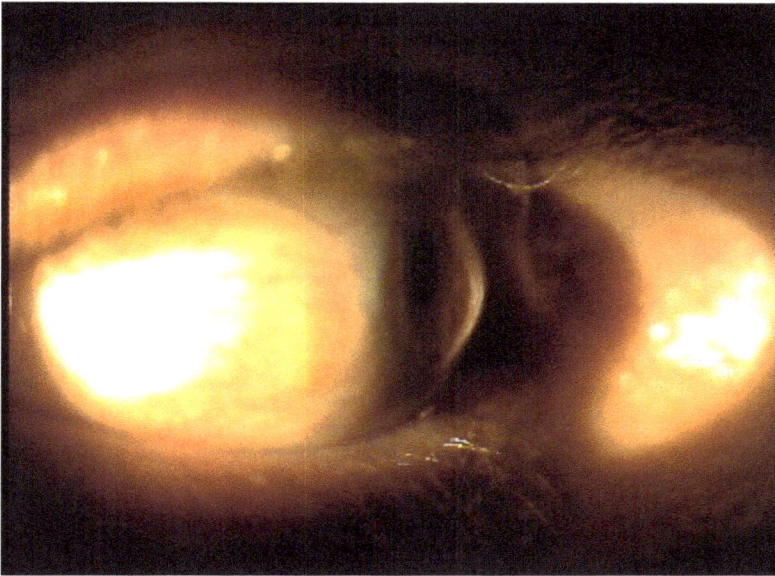

Fig. 2. Keratoconus (conical cornea)

In some cases it may also start later in life and progress at any age.

The etiology of the disease can be divided into three groups:

1. inherited
2. sporadic
3. acquired (secondary or in association to / with other diseases).

The inheritance of keratoconus is still not defined completely. Before the presence of videokeratography it was believed that more than 90 % of cases were sporadic, but recent studies revealed evidence that suggests an autosomal dominant pattern of inheritance (Gonzales & McDonnell, 1992).

Corneal thinning appears to result from a loss of structural components in the cornea, but why this happens is still not clear.

Recent biochemical studies of cornea with keratoconus suggest that enzyme abnormalities in the corneal epithelium, such as increased expression of proteases and other catabolic enzymes (Sawagamuchi et al., 1989) and decreased levels of inhibitors of proteolytic enzymes, may play a role in corneal stromal digestion and degradation (Fukuchi et al., 1994).

Investigations of corneal α1 proteinase inhibitor and α2 macroglobulin (also proteinase inhibitor) support the hypothesis that the degradation process may be aberrant in keratoconus (Sawagamuchi et al., 1994)

Evidence has been provided regarding abnormalities in gene promoters involved in these enzyme activities (Maruyama et al., 2001).

Other studies have reported abnormalities in corneal collagen and its cross-linking, as a potential cause of keratoconus (Bron, 1988).

Some authors have proposed a role for an IL-1 system in the cornea in the pathogenesis of keratoconus. It is suggested that the increased expression of the IL-1 receptor sensitizes the keratocytes to IL-1 released from the epithelium or endothelium, causing a loss of keratocytes through apoptosis and a decrease in stromal mass over time (Wilson et al., 1996).

It is most commonly a single disorder, although much evidence exists that it could be a phenotypic expression of many causes, or part of other multisystem or systemic disorders, as well as ocular non-corneal disorders (Rabinowitz, 1998, table 1).

Multisystem Disorders	Ocular Disorders
Alagille' s syndrome	Aniridia
Albers-Schonberg disease	Anetoderma and bilateral subcapsular cataracts
Angelman syndrome	Ankyloblepharon
Apert' s syndrome	Bilateral macular coloboma
Autographism	Blue sclerae
Anetoderma	Congenital cataracts
Bardet-Biedl syndrome	Ectodermal and mesodermal anomalities
Crouzon' s syndrome	Floppy eyelid syndrome
Down syndrome	Gyrate atrophy
Ehlers-Danlos syndrome	Iridoschisis
Goltz-Gorlin syndrome	Lebers congenital amaurosis
Hyperornithemia	Persistent pupilarry membrane
Icthyosis	Posterior lenticonus
Kurz syndrome	Retinitis pigmentosa
Laurence-Moon-Bardet-Biedl syndrome	Retinal disinsection syndrome
Marphan' s syndrome	Retrolental fibroplasia
Mulvihil-Smith syndrome	Vernal conjunctivitis
Nail patella syndrome	Atopic keratoconjunctivitis
Neurocutaneous angiomatosis	Axenfeld' s anomaly
Neurofibromatosis	Avellino' s dystrophy
Noonan' s syndrome	Chandler' s syndrome
Osteogenesis imperfecta	Corneal amyloidosis
Oculodentodigital syndrome	Deep filiform corneal dystrophy
Pseudoxanthoma elasticum	Essential iris atrophy
Rieger' s syndrome	Fleck corneal dystrophy
Rothmund s syndrome	Fuchs corneal dystrophy
Tourette' s disease	Iridocorneal dystrophy
Turner' s syndrome	Lattice dystrophy
Xeroderma pigmentosum	Microcornea
Congenital hip dysplasia	Pellucid marginal degeneration
False chordae tendineae of left ventricle	Posterior polymorphous dystrophy
Joint hypermobility	Terriens marginal degeneration
Mitral valve prolapse	
Measles retinopathy	
Ocular hypertension	
Thalesselis syndrome	

Table 1. Diseases associated with keratoconus, as reported by different authors

The most common association is with Down syndrome, connective tissue disorders, and Leber's congenital amaurosis (Cullen & Butler, 1963; Iwaszkiewicz, 1989).

Acquired etiologies can be divided into those which are attributed to inflammatory conditions, such as vernal conjunctivitis and those secondary to eye rubbing which can also release inflammatory mediators, such as Leber's congenital amaurosis and Down syndrome.

Many authors report a high incidence of mitral valve prolapse (58%) in patients with advanced keratoconus, while others report of eye rubbing in systemic atopy and cytokine interleukin-1, as a mediator of stromal degradation. Other factors, such as contact lens wear, may play a role in the development of the cone (Krachmer et al.,1984; Sharif et al., 1992).

Also, some studies report 6-8% of cases with positive family history or evidence of familiar transmission (Hallerman & Wilson, 1977; Krachmer et al., 1984).

Ocular manifestations

Early stages of the disorder may not present any symptoms. Cornea may appear normal on slit-lamp examination and there may be no symptoms of the disease. It maya be suspected by an ophthalmologist because the patient cannot be refracted to a 20/20 corrected vision. There might only be a mild steepening of keratometry mires, inferiorly or centrally. In such cases, anterior topography of the central and paracentral cornea will confirm the suspected diagnosis (Krachmer et al, 1984). In advanced cases, there can be a significant visual disturbance followed by a significant visual loss, but, fortunately, patients with keratoconus never become totally blind. Symptoms, as well as clinical signs, are variable and depend on the stage of the progression and on the severity of the disease.

The corneal manifestations include steepening (centrally or paracentrally, most commonly inferiorly or inferotemporally), thinning of the corneal apex, conical protrusion, a ring of iron deposits partially or completely accumulating in the epithelium surrounding the cone (Fleischer's ring), anterior scars at the level of Bowman's membrane, enlarged corneal nerves, increased intensity of the corneal endothelial reflex, and deep vertical lines in stroma and Descemet' s membrane, that disappear momentally under digital pressure during slit-lamp examination (Vogt' s striae).

The steeping of the cornea leads to clinical signs, which include the V-shaped protrusion of the lower eyelid on downgaze due to the ectatic cornea (Munson's sign, Fig. 3.), sharply focused light beam at the nasal limbus, produced by lateral illumination (Rizzuti's sign), and a dark reflex using the retroillumination techniques in the area of the cone, when observing the cornea with the pupil dilatation (Charleaux' s sign), and an irregular "scissor" reflex on retinoscopy.

Some patients with advanced keratoconus may occasionally experience sudden visual loss and pain due to the acute rupture of Descemet's membrane (acute hydrops). In such cases the conjunctive may be injected, and diffuse stromal edema appears. These breaks in Descemet's membrane result in acute overhydration and a stromal imbibing of aqueous. The overlying corneal epithelium may become edematous. The edema may last for months and, after the resolution of redness and relief of pain over time, can be replaced by scarring (and the corneal steepness may be reduced).

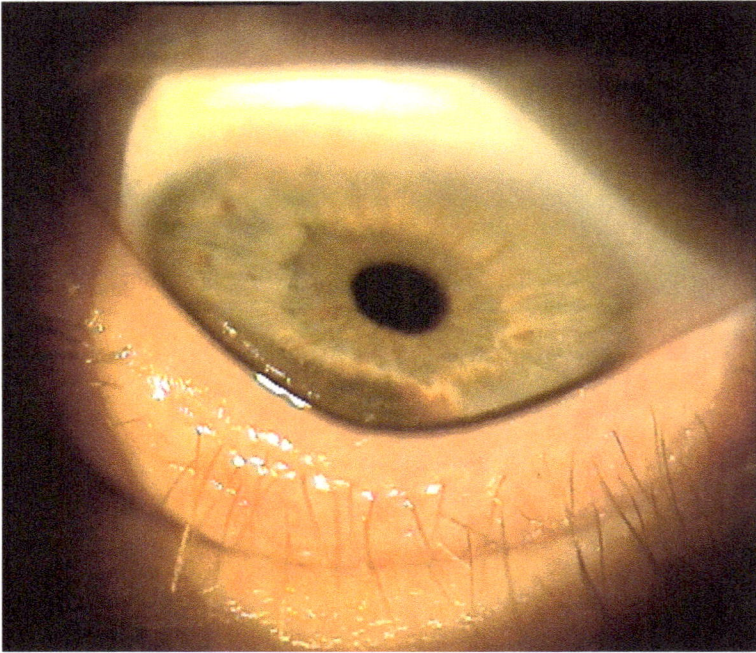

Fig. 3. V-shaped protrusion of the lower eyelid on downgaze due to the ectatic cornea (Munson' s sign)

Histopathology

The classic histopathological triad in keratoconus includes the thinning of the corneal stroma, breaks in Bowman' s layer and iron deposits in the basal layers of the corneal epithelium. Also, every other layer of the cornea can be pathologically affected, depending on the stage of the keratoconus. The endothelium is usually not affected, and the Descemet's membrane is rarely affected, other than in cases of acute hydrops.

Two types of cone morphology may be present. The first one is a „nipple" type cone, located centrally, characterized by small size (5 mm) and steep curvature; the second one is an „oval" type cone, located inferiorly or inferotemporally, characterized by larger size (5-6 mm), and an ellipsoid shape (Perry et al., 1980).

These can be distinguished in most cases on slit-lamp examination, or in the anterior corneal topography.

Diagnosis

To confirm the diagnosis several devices are available from handheld keratoscopes (placido disks), computer-assisted videokeratoscopes to (more recently) computerized videokeratography (Fig.4).

Computer-assisted topographic modeling systems allow the clinicians to detect subtle and minor variations in power distribution of the anterior and posterior corneal surface. The *forme fruste*, or subclinical keratoconus, recognized by Placido disk-based topography, requires caution and is considered a contraindication to refractive surgery. With regard to the identification of forme fruste keratoconus, classification programs on corneal topographers may assist in differentiating between keratoconus suspects, corneal distortion, and even patients having undergone refractive surgery, and normal variations of corneal topography.

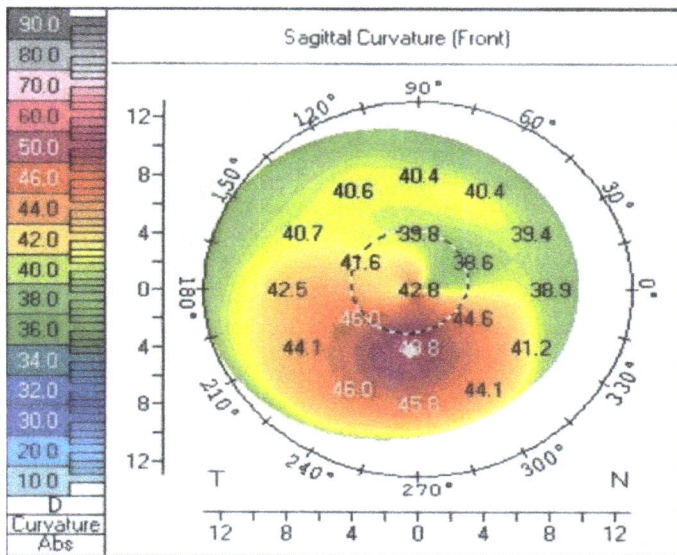

Fig. 4. Color-coded map of peripheral keratoconus. Note the inferior steepening

Rabinowitz has suggested that the diagnosis of keratoconus can be made when keratometry is greater than 47.20 D, the steepening of the inferior cornea compared with the superior cornea is more than 1.2 D, and the skewing of the radial axis of astigmatism is greater then 21° (Rabinowitz YS, 1995).

Differential diagnosis

The differential diagnosis of keratoconus includes other corneal ectasia disorders, such as pellucid marginal corneal degeneration and keratoglobus, and the posttraumatic or post-surgical (after refractive or cataract surgery) corneal ectasia or protrusion of the cornea after corneal ulceration thinning.

Treatment

Treatment of keratoconus starts with spectacles in very early stages, for astigmatism and myopia, and rigid gas permeable contact lenses in cases of inadequate visual acuity correction with spectacles. Contact lenses represent the treatment of choice in 90% of patients (Buxton et al., 1984).

In case of contact lens failure due to a lack of adequate visual acuity, or induced corneal abrasion, apical scarring, neovascularization due to hypoxia, poor lens tolerability and discomfort and lens displacement, surgical procedure is indicated. The most frequent surgical procedure is penetrating keratoplasty, which refers to the full-thickness replacement of diseased corneal tissue with a healthy donor. The main difficulty during surgery is suturing to the thin corneal bed.

Lamellar keratoplasty is also effective, but is not as frequently used as the penetrating keratoplasty, due to technical challenges and it being more time consuming. It is a procedure in which a partial-thickness graft of donor tissue (donor stroma or sclera) is used to provide tectonic stability and /or optical improvement.

There are generally two types of lamellar keratoplasty: anterior and posterior. In the anterior lamellar keratoplasty, the transplanted tissue does not include corneal endothelium and this procedure avoids endothelial rejection. The aim in deep lamellar and posterior lamellar keratoplasty is to replace diseased corneal endothelium while keeping the anterior corneal surface intact, as well as reducing refractive error and irregular astigmatism. In a short amount of time, deep lamellar endothelial keratoplasty (DLEK), Descemet-stripping endothelial keratoplasty (DSEK), Descemet-stripping automated endothelial keratoplasty (DSAEK) and Descemet' s membrane endothelial keratoplasty (DMEK) have become the techniques of choice for partial corneal transplant surgeries.

Descemet's membrane endothelial keratoplasty (DMEK) and Descemet-stripping automated endothelial keratoplasty (DSAEK) are new types of partial-thickness corneal graft operations, in which only the innermost corneal layers are replaced. Visual recovery is quicker, there is less physical restriction on activities and no related suture problems.

The results of lamellar techniques are far better than epikeratoplasty which has been abandoned due to the suboptimal visual outcomes. A keratoconic patient has a 10-20% chance, over her/his lifetime, of needing a corneal transplant (Smiddy et al., 1988; Tuft et al.,1994).

Intracorneal ring segments Intacts can be also used in cases without corneal scarring to reduce myopia and astigmatism. The purpose of Intacts segment implantation is to defer the need for corneal transplantation and restore contact lens tolerance. The placement of Intacts generates the response that interrupts the biomechanical disease progression, and a biomechanical response that allows visual improvement over six months. The improvement in visual acuity and refraction is accomplished by shortening the path length of the portion of the collagen lamellae that are central to the segments. The redistribution of corneal curvature leads to a redistribution of corneal stress, interrupting the biomechanical cycle of the keratoconus progression.

A relatively new method of treating progressive corneal ectasia is **corneal collagen crosslinking (CXL).** Its clinical use has been rapidly increasing since it was originally introduced in 1997 as the first treatment that could improve the biomechanical stability of the weakened cornea. This method is based on combined action of the photo-sensitizer riboflavin (vitamin B2) and ultraviolet A light, which induce the formation of new covalent bonds between the collagen fibers.

This method has been widely accepted since the first introduction by Spoerl and his co-workers at Dresden University in Germany, in 1997 (Spörl et al., 1997).

The recent advances in diagnostic devices resulted in the detection of more subtle corneal changes, suggesting that the sublinical forms are more common than fully developed keratoconus. The iatrogenic post-LASIK ectasia is the second most common corneal ectasia. It usually appears as a result of refractive surgery performed in predisposed individuals or in patients with an undetected early form of keratoconus. Before the introduction of corneal collagen crosslinking, the only treatment that could halt the progression of keratoconus in most cases was the penetrating keratoplasty.

Studies which have been conducted so far demonstrated the beneficial effect in halting the progression of the diseases, with a very low complication rate (Koller et al., 2009; Tomkins & Garzozi, 2008).

The term „crosslinking"refers to the formation of bonds between natural polymer molecules.

The original crosslinking technique described by Wollensak and co-workers is still being used today, with the minor modifications. (Wollensak et al., 2003).

The photopolymerizing effect is induced by the combined action of riboflavin as a photo-sensitizer, and long wavelength ultraviolet (UVA) light of 370 nm. This particular wavelength was chosen so that riboflavin can achieve a maximal absorption while still remaining bellow harmful radiation levels. During the exposure, riboflavin is excited into a triplet state, generating the so-called reactive oxygen species which, in turn, induce the formation of new covalent bonds (disulphide /s-s) between the amino acids of neighboring collagen fibers.

After the application of a local anesthetic, a lid speculum is inserted and central corneal abrasion up to 9.0 mm in diameter is made. According to the protocol of the Institute for Refractive and Ophthalmic Surgery in Zürich, Switzerland, 0.1% riboflavin solution containing 10 mg of riboflavin-5-phosphate diluted in 10 ml of a 20% dextran solution is instilled every 3 minutes, for 30 minutes. After that, central corneal thickness (CCT) is measured. For safety reasons, additional riboflavin 0.1% hypoosmotic drops without dextran should be applied in corneas whose thickness is less than 400 µm. Otherwise, UVA light should not be applied. The cornea is then irradiated for 30 minutes with an UVA illumination device. The device must provide a homogenous UV radiation with irradiance of 3 mW/ cm^2 at the working distance of 5 cm. During irradiation, the cornea is moistened every 3 minutes with the riboflavin 0.1% drops. The total dosage delivered to the cornea in that way is 5.4 J/cm^2. At the end, antibiotic ointment is applied and bandage lens inserted to facilitate the epithelial healing.

Beside the standard CXL, as described above (with removal of the epithelium), the treatment can also be the transepithelial CXL (without removal of the epithelium). The later has less complications, such as death of keratocytes. Not being invasive, it is very well tolerated.

Indications for cross-linking today are clinical and instrumental progression (refractive, topographic, pachimetric, aberrometric) of corneal ectasia disorders such as keratoconus and pellucid marginal degeneration in the last 6-12 months, iatrogenic keratectasia after refractive lamellar surgery and corneal melting not responding to conventional therapy.

Contraindications include corneal thickness of less than 400 μm, central corneal opacity, epithelial healing disorders, such as map dot dystrophy and rheumatic disorders, refractive keratotomy, previous herpes simplex virus keratitis (UV-A may induce herpes reactivation), corneal melting disorders, concurrent infection, severe ocular surface disease, and pregnancy.

In recent years, corneal collagen crosslinking has become a standard treatment for the progressive corneal ectasia in numerous centers throughout the world. Additional basic and clinical research is necessary in order to establish more precise indications and to demonstrate the permanence of the treatment. Despite the evidence in support of the safety of new procedure, future studies are necessary to define its limitations and its long-term efficacy. It has the potential to reduce corneal curvature by approximately 1.0-1.5 D.

Despite the fact that no sight-threatening complications were recorded in the large prospective studies, there are some sporadic reports of stromal haze resistant to topical steroid treatment (Mazzota et al., 2007), diffuse lamellar keratitis in post-LASIK ectasia, herpetic keratitis and iritis (Kymionis et al., 2007), Acanthamoeba keratitis with corneal perforation (Rama et al., 2009), and microbial keratitis (Pollhammer & Cursiefen, 2009; Zamora & Males, 2009). Other potential complications include delay in reepithelization, sterile infiltrates, potential for induction of herpes simples virus and dendritic ulcer, and ocular surface disorders and tear dysfunction (Corkin, 2009).

The reliable data on the turnover rate of the collagen fibers are still insufficient due to the almost complete absence of corneal remodeling (Wollensak & Iomdina., 2009).

However, data such as the increased resistance to the enzymatic degradation in the crosslinked corneas support the theory of the long –lasting effect of the treatment (Spoerl et al., 2004).

2.3 Other corneal ectasias

Pellucid marginal corneal degeneration

Pellucid marginal corneal degeneration is a variant of keratoconus, characterized by a peripheral band of thinning of the inferior cornea and protrusion from the 4 to 8 o'clock position but a 2 mm uninvolved surface of the cornea between the thinning and the limbus.

It has also been described in scleroderma (Sii et al., 2004) and in Sjögren syndrome (Fernández-Barboza et al., 2009).

The thickness of the central cornea is usually normal but with marked against-the-rule astigmatism. It can nicely be recognized by videokeratography due to the typical „butterfly"appearance that represents a large degree of against-the-rule astigmatism (Maguire et al., 1987).

Treatment includes spectacles or contact lenses. Due to the extensive against-the-rule astigmatism, the success rate for fitting those patients with the hard contact lens is lesser than in patients with keratoconus. In case of inadequately vision corrected patients or in case of lens intolerability, large, eccentric penetrating keratoplasty may be considered.

Keratoglobus

In keratoglobus, in contrast to the localized thinning centrally or paracentrally in keratoconus, the entire cornea is thinned out, especially near the limbus, and has a globular protrusion (Krachmer et al., 1984).

It comes in two forms: a congenital or juvenile form and an acquired, adult form. The congenital form can be part of Ehlers-Danlos syndrome type VI, or part of the corneal syndrome associated with blue sclera and red hair (Royce et al., 1990).

The adult form can be associated with blepharitis, vernal keratoconjunctivitis, and orbital diseases than cause proptosis (Cameron, 1993).

It has a recessive pattern of inheritance and is often associated with blue sclerae and other systemic features, such as Ehlers-Danlos syndrome and other systemic connective tissue abnormalities. These kinds of corneas can be so thinned that they are prone to corneal rupture from a minimal trauma.

It was also described in thyroid orbitopathy (Jacobs et al., 1974), and was acquired in pellucid marginal degeneration after extracapsular cataract extraction (Rumelt & Rehany, 1998).

Treatment includes protection from trauma, and protective spectacles are strongly recommended. Hard contact lenses are contraindicated. Lamellar epikeratoplasty should be considered to reinforce thin corneas, and in case of acquired keratoglobus, central penetrating keratoplasty may be successful.

Terrien's marginal corneal degeneration

Terrien's marginal degeneration is a bilateral, slowly- progressive condition with marginal corneal ectasia associated with corneal neovascularisation, lipid deposition along the central edge, thinning and opacification. The cause is unknown, but it is likely to be different from the causes of most degenerations that occurs with age. It can occur at any age, but most frequently in men, 20-40 years old. Two types have been described. First one is slowly-progressive and mostly asymptomatic, and occurs in older population. The second one occurs in younger patients, it is more inflammatory in type and may be associated with episcleritis and scleritis (Iwamoto et al., 1972).

Terrien's marginal degeneration initially starts superiorly with peripheral corneal haze, gradually vascularizes, and is followed by corneal thinning that starts between the limbus and line of lipid deposition. Characteristically, a steeper sloping of the cornea occurs at the advancing edge, without the overlying edge like as in Mooren's ulcer (see below).

The thinning progresses circumferentially, but the overlying epithelium is intact.

Unlike the Mooren's ulcer, usually there is no pain or inflammation, but occasionally, it may present with recurrent painful episodes of inflammation. Perforation may occur, but is rare.

A pseudopterygium may occur in an oblique axis in some patients.

Irregular astigmatism is characteristic in the progressive flattening of vertical meridian, and the high degree of against-the rule astigmatism.

Treatment includes the use of rigid gas-permeable contact lenses. More severe thinning may require crescentic, full-thickness or lamellar keratoplasty (Hahn & Kim, 1993).

Mooren's ulcer

Mooren's ulcer is a progressive, crescentic, peripheral corneal ulceration. Two clinical types have been documented. One type occurs primarily in the older population, it is typically unilateral and more responsive to local therapy. The other is bilateral, painful, progressive corneal destruction, mostly in younger individuals, more resistant to systemic immunosuppression. The pathogenesis of Mooren's ulcer is unknown but appears to involve an autoimmune reaction against a specific target molecule in the stroma, which may occur in genetically susceptible individuals (Gottsch et al., 1999).

It has a characteristic extensive, "overhanging" edge which is absent in Terrien's disease, and progresses with a stromal, yellowish infiltrate at the advancing margin. Over time, overlying epithelial defect develops, followed by stromal melting. In the second type, the inflammation may affect all the layers of cornea and perilimbal tissue, and perforation can occur.

Patients complain of severe pain, photophobia and tearing.

In chronic cases, topographical maps show severe irregular astigmatism and peripheral steepening as a result of peripheral corneal thinning and scarring. Unlike the other forms of peripheral ulcerative keratitis, no clear zone between the ulcer and limbus can be seen.

Treatment includes local, systemic, and surgical therapy. Local therapy includes topical corticosteroids, followed by conjunctival resection if inflammation is not controlled, as well as topical cyclosporine drops. Systemic immunosuppressive treatment of the more aggressive bilateral disease has included corticosteroids, cyclosporine and methotrexate (Brown & Mondino, 1984; Foster, 1985).

Other surgical procedures include epikeratoplasty, lamellar keratoplasty, delimiting keratotomy, conjunctival flap and patch grafts of periostium.

2.4 Residual astigmatism (non-corneal astigmatism)

Corneal astigmatism of more than 2D is present in 5% of general population, while at least 93% of the population has at least 0.5D of corneal astigmatism. The percentage of residual astigmatism is between 10% and 80% (Parunovic et al., 1995).

Spherical rigid contact lens can correct total astigmatism if the correction of cylinder with the spectacles is the same value as the value of corneal astigmatism. In some cases there is a difference in value between astigmatism corrected with the spectacles and corneal astigmatism. Astigmatism that rises from this difference is called residual astigmatism, and does not correlate with the anterior surface of the cornea. Residual astigmatism is in most cases lenticular, but can also be derived from a badly fitted contact lens (a decentrated or deformed contact lens).

Lenticular astigmatism may also be caused by lens subluxation, like in Marfan's syndrome (Konradsen et al., 2010; Yeung & Weissman, 1997), changes in lens contour, like in anterior and posterior lenticonus in Alport' s syndrome (Al-Mahmood et al., 2010; Blaise et al., 2003; Hentati et al., 2008; Kim et al., 2010), lenticular trauma etc.

Residual, lenticular astigmatism is most always against-the-rule astigmatism, rarely more than 1D, and usually is masked by correction of total refractive astigmatism. Residual astigmatism (RA) is calculated by subtracting the value of corneal astigmatism (CA) from the value of astigmatism corrected by the spectacles (SC), according the formula: RA = SC - CA.

Example:
Keratometry: 43.00 / 43.50 x 90
Spectacle correction: -2.00 /-1.50 x 180
Residual astigmatism = (- 1.00 x 180) - (- 0.50 x 180) = - 0.50 x 180

2.5 Surgically induced astigmatism

One of the possible complications of cataract surgery (especially extracapsular and intracapsular cataract extraction), as well as penetrating keratoplasty, is induced astigmatism, which is a major cause of functional disturbance and insufficient uncorrected visual acuity.

The aim of cataract surgery today is rapid visual rehabilitation, the best possible uncorrected visual acuity, and minimal postoperative astigmatism.

The phacoemulsification procedure results in less surgically induced astigmatism than extracapsular cataract extraction, in which the incision is much larger.

Clear corneal incision (CCI) is the most used type of incision in phacoemulsification surgery, because it is less time-consuming and doesn't require cauterization or wound suturing. The location of the CCI affects the degree of postoperative astigmatism.

CCI is made deliberately in the steepest meridian if astigmatism is addressed. It can be made at superior, oblique or temporal locations.

Temporal CCI induces regular astigmatism 90 degrees away from the incision (with-the-rule astigmatism) thus minimizing the postoperative astigmatism (Cilino et al., 1997; Cravy, 1991; Hayashi et al., 1994). It is known to induce the least postoperative astigmatism. Also, the smaller the CCI, the lesser the induced astigmatism.

Oblique scleral tunnel incision predictably reduces astigmatism by simultaneously producing corneal flattening and steepening (Simsek et al., 1998).

Some studies have shown that a small superior CCI induces greater postoperative astigmatism than a small supero-oblique CCI, and a small supero-oblique CCI induces higher postoperative astigmatism than a small temporal CCI (Mendivil, 1996; Reiner et al., 1999; Wirbelauer et al.,1997).

Some authors reported that, although temporal CCI is reported to result in the least induced astigmatism, locating the incision superotemporally or superonasally may ease surgical manipulations during the phacoemulsification cataract surgery for a right-handed surgeon who works from the 12 o' clock position relative to the patient (Ermis et al., 2004).

Performing the procedure from the patient's temporal side may not be possible with the most operating tables, and locating the CCI temporally in left eye may be difficult for a right-handed surgeon who sits at the 12 o' clock position.

Several groups of authors analyzed refractive astigmatism in patients who have had phacoemulsification cataract surgery performed by the oblique clear corneal incision. They provided evidence that the supero-oblique clear corneal incision does not induce the clinically significant amount of oblique astigmatism (Jacobs et al., 1999; Brian et al., 2001; Masnec et al., 2007).

Also, evidence is provided that the superotemporal or superonasal CCI has minimal effect on corneal astigmatism (Masnec et al., 2007).

Further studies on more patients should provide definitive conclusions about the influence of the superotemporal or superonasal clear corneal incision on postoperative astigmatism.

Many studies investigated the influence of different factors, such as the type of a surgery, length of incision and its type (curved, straight, frown), location and width of incision (central vs. peripheral-limbal or scleral), presence or absence of a suture and the suturing method, on postoperative astigmatism (Azar et al., 1997; Roman et al., 1998; Simsek et al.,1998; Wirbelauer et al.,1997)..

Any incisions that are made in the cornea have the potential to change the curvature and therefore the dioptric power of the cornea in that meridian.

The location as well as the width of the incision affects the degree of postoperative astigmatism.

Typically, corneal incisions cause flattening at the axis where they are made. The basic concepts are:

• The larger the incisions, the greater the flattening

The larger the arc length of the corneal incisions, the more effect it has in flattening the cornea at that meridian. Due to the coupling effect, arc lengths of more than 90° are ineffective.

• The more central the incisions, the greater the flattening

Most surgeons prefer performing limbal relaxing incisions (LRIs) at the periphery of the clear cornea. Due to this location, they tend to be more forgiving, heal better, and are less likely to cause irregular astigmatism. But, due to the distance from the central cornea and increased thickness of the cornea at the periphery, these incisions have less effect than astigmatic keratotomy (AK) incisions, which are more centrally placed.

• For penetrating incisions, the shorter the tunnel length, the greater the flattening

Creating an "astigmatically neutral" clear corneal incision during cataract surgery requires the incision to have a sufficient tunnel length. This reduces the compromise of the corneal structure at the incision site and induces little change in the corneal astigmatism. For increasing the astigmatic effect of the corneal incisions, the surgeon can make the tunnel length shorter; however, this results in an incision that may be more prone to leaking during the postoperative period. Surgeon can also vary the position of the corneal incision so that it is placed on the steep axis and, therefore, any induced flattening will help the patient by reducing astigmatism.

• For nonpenetrating incisions, the deeper the incision, the greater the flattening

Most nomograms for LRIs call for nonpenetrating incisions that are placed perpendicularly to corneal tissue. With incisions that are made at 80% or 90% of the corneal thickness, as measured by pachymetry, there is a significant flattening of the corneal astigmatism. As the incisions become more shallow, their effect is lesser, and incisions at less than half corneal depth have little effect on the corneal curvature and power (Budak et al., 1998; Gills et al., 2003; Nichamin, 2006; Thornton, 1994; Wang et al., 2003).

3. Conclusion

Beside the congenital astigmatism which is usually inherited, acquired form of astigmatism can be a result of various intraocular surgeries.

Regular astigmatism is correctable by cylindrical spectacle lenses and contact lenses. In case of irregular astigmatism, cylindrical lenses usually do not help and rigid contact lenses may be useful.

That is usually a consequence of pathological changes of cornea, such as keratoconus, or the lens.

In the past, irregular astigmatism was not very interesting for clinicians because it was not very common and not treatable. However, with the development of keratorefractive surgical procedures, it became increasingly of interest as, in many cases, keratorefractive surgeries produce visually significant irregular astigmatism and, at the same time, may also be able to treat it.

Special focus still remains on keratoconus, a disorder characterized by progressive corneal steepening due to the loss of structural components in the cornea, but its cause is still unclear. It is difficult to treat, and a keratoconic patient has a 10-20% chance, over their lifetime, of needing a corneal transplant. Still, in 90 % of patients contact lenses represent the treatment of choice.

In recent years, corneal collagen crosslinking has become a standard treatment for the progressive corneal ectasia in numerous centers throughout the world, because much evidence has been provided that it can improve biomechanical stability of the weakened cornea.

Additional basic and clinical research is necessary in order to establish more precise indications and to demonstrate the permanence of the treatment. Despite the evidence in support of the safety of this new procedure, future studies are necessary to define its limitations and its long-term efficacy.

4. References

Al-Mahmood, AM., Al-Swailem, SA., Al-Khalaf A., Al-Binali GY. (2010). Progressive Posterior Lenticonus In a Patient with Alport Syndrome. *Middle East Afr J Ophthalmol*, Vol. 17, No. 4 (2010), pp. 379-381

Azar, DT., Stark, WJ., Dodick, J., Khoury, JM., Vitale, S., Enger, C., & Reed, C. (1997). Prospective, randomized vector analysis of astigmatism after three-, one-, and no-suture phacoemulsification. *J Cataract Refract Surg*, Vol. 23, (1997), pp. 1164-73

Bennet, AG., & Rabbits, RB. (1989) *Clinical Visual Optics*, (2nd ed.) , Butterworths, London

Blaise, P., Delanaye, P., Martalo, O., Pierard, GE., Rorive, G., Galand, A. (2003). Anterior lenticonus: diagnostic aid in Alport syndrome. J Fr Ophthalmol, Vol. 26, No.10. (Dec 2003), pp. 1075-82

Brian, J., Jacobs, BS., Bruce, I., Gaynes, OD., Phar, MD., Thomas, A., & Deutch, MD. *J Cataract Refractive Surg*, Vol. 27, (2001), pp. 1176-9

Bron, AJ. (1988). Keratoconus. *Cornea*, Vol. 7, (1988), pp. 163-9

Brown, SI., Mondino BJ. (1984). Therapy of Mooren s ulcer. *Am J Ophthalmol*. Vol. 98. (1984), pp. 1-6

Budak, K., Friedman, NK., Koch, DD. (1998). Limbal relaxing incisions with cataract surgery. . *J Cataract Refract Surg*, Vol. 24, (1998), pp. 503-508

Buxton, JN. (1978) .Contact lenses in keratoconus. *Contact Intraocular Lans Med J*, Vol. 4. (1978), pp. 74

Buxton, JN., Keates, RH., & Hoefle FB. (1984). The contact lens correction of keratoconus. *The CLAO Guide to Basic Science and Clinical Practice : Contact lenses,* (ed), Grune and Stratton, Orlando

Cameron, JA., Cotter, JB., Risco, JM., & Alvarez, H. (1991). Epikeratoplasty for keratoglobus associated with blue sclera. *Ophthalmology*, Vol. 98, (1991), pp. 446-52

Cameron, JA. (1993). Keratoglobus. *Cornea*, Vol. 12, (1993), pp. 124-30

Cameron, JA. (1993). Corneal abnormalities in Ehlers-Danlos syndrome type VI. *Cornea*, Vol. 12, (1993), pp. 54-9

Caporossi, A., Mazzotta, C., Baiocchi, S., & Caporossi, T. (2010). Long-term results of riboflavin ultraviolet a corneal collagen cross-linking for keratoconus in Italy: The Siena eye cross study. *Am J Ophthalmol*, (Feb 2010)

Chan, CC., Sharma, M & Wachler, BS. (2007). Effect of inferior-segment Intacts with and without C3-R on keratoconus. *J Cataract Refract Surg*, Vol. 33, No. 1. (Januar 2007), pp. 75-80

Chang, DF.(2008). Mastering refractive IOLs-the art and science, Slack, ISBN 978-1-55642-859-3

Cillino, S., Morreale, D., Mauceri, A., Ajovalasit, C., & Ponte, F. (1997). Temporal versus superior approach phacoemulsification: short-term postoperative astigmatism. *J Cataract Refract Surg*, Vol. 23, (1997), pp. 267-71

Collin, J., Cochenee, B., & Savary, G. (2001). Intacts inserts for treating keratoconus: one - year results. *Ophthalmology*, Vol. 108, (2001), pp. 1409-14

Corkin, R. (2009). CXL Indications and Patient Selection. *Cataract & Refract Surg Today*, (April 2009), pp.33-35

Cravy, TV. (1991). Routine use of a lateral approach to cataract extraction to achive rapid and sustained stabilisation of postoperative astigmatism. *J Cataract Refract Surg*, Vol. 17, (1991), pp. 415-23

Cullen, JF., & Butler, HG. (1963). Mongolism (Down s syndrome) and keratoconus. *Br J Ophthalmol*, Vol .47, (1963), pp. 321-30

Cupak, K. (2004). *Oftalmologija* (2nd ed), Naknadni zavod globus, ISBN 953-167-163-x, Zagreb

Dana , MR., Putz, JS., & Viana, MAG. (1992). Contact lens failure in keratoconus menagement. *Ophthalmology*, Vol. 99, (1992), pp. 1187-92

Ermis, SS., Inan, UU., & Ozturk, F. (2004). *J Cataract Refract Surg*, Vol. 30, (2004), pp. 1316-19

Ernest, PH., Lavery, KT., & Kiessling, LA. (1994). Relative strenght of scleral corneal and clear corneal incisions constructed in cadaver eyes. *J Cataract Refract Surg*, Vol. 20, (1994), pp. 626-9

Ernest, PH., Fenzl, R., Lavery, KT., & Sensoli, A. (1995) Relative stability of clear corneal incisions in a cadaver eye model. *J Cataract Refract Surg*, Vol. 21, (1995), pp. 39-42

Fernández-Barboza, F., Verdiguel-Sotelo K., Hernández-Löpez, A. (2009). Pellucid marginal degeneration and corneal ulceration, associated with Sjögren syndrome. *Rev Med Inst Mex Seguro Soc*, Vol. 47.(2009), pp. 77-82

Filip, O., Golu, T., & Filip I. (1994). Keratoconus in Albers-Schonberd diases. *Ophthalmologia*, Vol 38. (1994), pp. 247-251

Foote, CS. (1968). Mechanisms of photosensitized oxidation. There are several different types of photosensitized oxidation which may be important in biological systems. *Science*, Vol. 162, No. 857 (November, 1968), pp. 963-70

Foster, CS. (1985). Systemic immunosuppressive therapy for progressive bilateral Mooren' s ulcer. *Ophthalmology*, Vol. 92, (1985), pp. 1436-9

Fukuchi , T., Yue, B., Sugar, J.,S.(1994). Lysosomal enzyme activities in conjunctival tissues of patients with keratoconus. *Arch Ophthalmol*, Vol. 112, (1994), pp: 1368-1374

Gills, JP., Rowsey, JJ. (2003). Managing coupling in secondary astigmatism keratotomy. In: Fine, IH., Packer, M., Hoffman, RS. Eds. *A Complete Surgical Guide for Correcting Astigmatism.* (2003). Thorofare, Slack Incorporated, Nj pp. 131-140

Gills, JP., Wallace, RB., Miller, K. (2003). Reducing pre-existing astigmatism with limbal relaxing incisions. In: Gills, J, ed. *A Complete Surgical Guide for Correcting Astigmatism.* (2003). Thorofare, Slack Incorporated, Nj pp. 99-119

Gonzales, V., & McDonell PJ. (1992). Computer-assisted corneal topography in parents of patients with keratoconus. *Arch Ophthalmol*, Vol. 110, (1992), pp. 1412-4

Gottsch, JD., Li, Q., Ashraf, F. (1999) Cytokine-induced calgranulin C expression in keratocytes. *Clin immunol*, Vol. 91 (1999), pp: 34-40

Grewal, DS., Brar, GS., Jain, R., Sood, V., Singla, M., & Grewal, SP. (2009). Corneal collagen crosslinking using riboflavin and ultraviolet-A light for keratoconus: one year analysis using Scheimpflug imaging. *J Cataract Refract Surg*, Vol. 35, No. 3 (March 2009), pp. 425-32

Hafezi, F., Kanellopoulos, J., Wiltfang, R., & Seiler, T. (2007). Corneal collagen crosslinking with riboflavin and ultraviolet A to treat induced keratectasia after laser in situ keratomileusis. *J Cataract Refract Surg*, Vol. 33, No. 12 (December 2007), pp. 2035-40

Hahn, TW., Kim, JH. (1993). Two step annular tectonic lamellar keratoplasty in severe Terrien s marginal degeneration. *Ophthalmic Surg*. Vol. 24, (1993), pp. 831-4

Hallerman , W . & Wilson, EJ. (1977). Genetische Betractungen uber den Keratoconus. *Klin Monatsb Augenheilk, Vol.* 170, (1977), pp. 906-908

Hayashi, K., Nakao, F., & Hayashi, F. (1994). Corneal topographic analysis of superolateral incision cataract surgery. *Cataract Refract Surg,* Vol. 20, (1994), pp. 392-9

Hentati, N., Sellami, D., Makni, K., Kharrat, M., Hachicha, J., Hammadi, A., Feki, J. (2008). Ocular findings in Alport syndrome: 32 case studies. *J Fr Ophthalmol,* Vol. 31, No. 6. (Jun 2008), pp. 597-604

Hofstetter, H. (1959). A keratoscopic survey of 13,395 eyes. *Am J Optom Acad Optom,* Vol. 36. (1959), pp. 3-11

Howland, HC., Atkinson, J., Braddick, O., & French, J. (1978). Astigmatism measured by Photorefraction. *Science,* Vol. 202, (1978), pp. 331-3

Iwamoto, T., DeVoe AG., Farris RL. (1972). Electron microscopy in cases of marginal degenerations of cornea. *Invest Ophthalmol Vis Sci.,* Vol 11, (1972), pp. 241-57

Iwaszkiewicz, E. (1989). Keratoconus II. Coexisting diseases and theories on its etiology and pathogenesis. *Klin Oczna,* Vol. 91, (1989), pp. 210-211

Jacobs, BJ., Gaynes, BI., & Deutch, TA. (1999). Refractive astigmatism after oblique clear corneal phacoemulsification cataract incision. *J Cataract Refract Surg,* Vol. 25. (1999), pp. 949-52

Jacobs, DS., Green WR., Maumenee, AE. (1974). Acquired keratoglobus. *AJO,* Vol.77, (1974), pp.393-9

Karseras, AG. , & Ruben, M. (1976). Aetiology of keratoconus. *Br J Ophthalmol,* Vol. 60, (1976), pp. 522-5

Kennedy, RH., Bourne, WM., & Dyer JA. (1986). A 48-year clinical and epidemiology study of keratoconus. *Am J Ophthalmol,* Vol. 101, (1986), pp. 267-73

Kim, KS., Kim, MS., Kim JM., Choi, CY. (2010). Evaluation of anterior lenticonus in alport syndrome using tracy wavefront aberrometry and transmission electron microscopy. *Ophthalmic Surg Lasers Imaging,* Vol. 41, No.3 (May-Jun 2010), pp.330-6

Koller, T., Mrochen, M., & Seiler, T. (2009). Complications and failure rates after corneal crosslinking. *J Cataract Refract Surg,* Vol. 35, No. 8 (August 2009), pp. 1358-62.

Konradsen, TR., Koivula, A., Kugelberg, M., Zetterström, C. (2010). Corneal curvature, pachymetry, and endothelial cell density in Marfan syndrome. Acta Ophthalmol (September 2010)

Krachmer, JH., Feder, RS., & Belin, MW. (1984). Keratoconus and related noninflammatory corneal thinning disorders. *Surv Ophthalmol,* Vol. 28, (1984), pp. 293-322

Kymionis, GD., Bouzoukis, DI., Diakonis, VF. (2007). Diffuse lamellar keratitis after corneal crosslinking in patient with post-laser in situ keratomileusis corneal ectasia. *J Cataract Refract Surg,* Vol. 33, (2007), pp. 2135-7

Kymionis, GD., Portaliou, DM., Bouzoukis, DI.(2007). Herpetic keratitis with iritis after corneal crosslinking with riboflavin and ultraviolet A for keratoconus. *J Cataract Refract Surg,* Vol. 33, (2007), pp. 1982-4

Liesegang, TJ., Deutch, TA., & Gilbert Grand, M. (2002-2003). *Optics, Refraction, and Contact lenses, Basic and Clinical Science Course, American Academy of Ophthalmology,* United states of America, ISSN

Maguire, LJ., Klyce, SD., McDonald ME., & Kaufmann HE. (1987). Corneal topography of pellucid marginal degeneration . *Ophthalmology*, Vol. 94, (1987), pp. 519-524

Mandic, Z., Petric ,I., Bencic, G., Vatavuk, Z., & Bojic, L. (2005). Postoperative outcomes after implantation of intraocular lenses in eyes with cataract and uveitis. *Coll Antropol.* Vol .29, No. 1, (March 2005), pp. 9-12, ISSN 03506134

Marcsai, MS., Varley, GA:, & Krachmer, JH. (1990). Development of keratoconus after contact lens wear: patient characteristics. *Arch Ophthalmol*, Vol. 108, (1990), pp. 534-8

Maruyama, Y., Wang, X., & Li, Y. (2001). Involment of sp 1 elements in the promoter activity of genes affected in keratoconus. *Invest Ophthalmol Vis Sci*, Vol. 42, (2001), pp. 1980-5

Masket, S. (1991). Horizontal anchor suture closure method for small incision cataract surgery. *J Cataract Refract Surg*, Vol. 17, (1991), pp. 689-95

Masnec-Paškvalin, S., Čima, I., Iveković, R., Matejčić, A., Novak-Lauš, K., & Mandić, Z. (2007). Comparison of Preoperative and Postoperative Astigmatism after Superotemporal or Superonasal Clear Corneal Incision in Phacoemulsiphication. *Coll Antropol* , Vol. 31, No. (2007), pp. 199-202

Mazzota, C., Balestrazzi, A., Baiocchi, S. (2007). Stromal haze after combined riboflavin-UVa corneal cross-linking in keratoconus: in vivo confocal microscopic evaluation. *Clin Exper Ophthalmol*, Vol. 35, (2007), pp. 580-2

Mendivil, A. (1996). Comparative study of astigmatism through superior and lateral small incisions. *Eur J Ophthalmol*, Vol. 6, (1996), pp. 389-92

Michaels, DD. (1980). A clinical aprprouch. *Visual optics and refraction*, (2nd ed.), Mosby, St Louis

Mohindra, I., Held, R., Gwiazda, J., & Brill, S. (1978) . Astigmatism in Infants. *Science*, Vol. 202, (1978), pp. 329-31

Morlet, N., Minassian, D., & Dart, J. (2001). Astigmatism and the analysis of its surgical correction. *Br J Ophthalmol*, Vol. 85, (2001), pp. 1127-38

Nesburn, AB., Bahri, S., & Salz, J. (1995). Keratoconus detected by videokeratography in candidates for photorefractive keratectomy. *J Refractive Surg*, Vol. 11, (1995), pp. 194-201

Nichamin, LD. (2006). Astigmatism control. *Ophthalmol Clin North Am*, Vol. 19, (2006), pp. 485-493

Oshika, T., Tsuboi, S., & Yaguchi, S. (1994). Comparative study of intraocular lens implantation through 3.2 and 5.5 mm incisions. *Ophthalmology*, Vol. 101, (1994), pp. 1183-90

Oshima, Y., Tsujikawa, K., Oh, A., & Harino, S. (1997). Comparative study of intraocular lens implantation through 3.0 mm temporal clear corneal and superior scleral tunnel self-sealing incisions. *J Cataract Refract Surg*, Vol. 23, (1997), pp. 347-53

Parunovic, A. (1995). *Korekcija refrakcionih anomalija oka*, Bjeletic, ISSN 86-17-04525-6, Beograd

Perry, HD., Buxton, JN., & Fine BS. (1980). Round and oval cones in keratoconus. *Ophthalmology*, Vol. 87, (1980), pp. 905-909

Pollhammer, M., Cursiefen, C. (2009). Bacterial keratitis early after corneal crosslinking with riboflavin and ultraviolet-A. . *J Cataract Refract Surg*, Vol. 3, No.35, (2009), pp.588-9

Pouliquen, Y., Dhermy, P., & Espinasse, MA: (1985). Keratoglobus. *J Fr Ophthalmol*, Vol. 8, (1985), pp. 43-54

Pramanik, S., Musch, DC., Sutphin, JE., & Farjo, AA. (2006). Extended long term outcomes of penetrating keratoplasty for keratoconus. *Ophthalmology*, Vol. 9, No. 113 (September 2006), pp. 1633-8

Rabinowitz, YS. (1995). Videokeratographic indices to aid in screening for keratoconus. *J Refrac Surg*, Vol. 11, (1995), pp. 371-9

Rabinowitz, YS. (1998). Keratoconus. *Surv Ophthalmol*, Vol. 42,No. 4 (Januar 1998), pp. 297-319

Rahi, A., Davies, P., & Ruben, M. (1977). Kratoconus and coexisting atopic disease. *Br J Ophthalmol*, Vol. 61,(1977), pp. 761-4

Rainer, G., Menapace, R., & Vass, C. (1999). Corneal shape changes after temporal and superolateral 3.0 mm clear corneal incisions. *J Cataract Refract Surg*, Vol. 25, (1999), pp. 1121-26

Rama, P., Di Matteo, F., Matuska, S., Paganoni, G., Spinelli, A. (2009). Acanthamoeba keratitis with perforation after corneal crosslinking and bandage contact lens use. . *J Cataract Refract Surg*, Vol. 35, No. 4, (2009), pp. 788-91

Ricchi, B., Lepore, D., & Iossa, M. (1991). Ocular anomalies in Alagille s syndrome, *J Fr Ophthalmol*, Vol 14 (1991), pp. 481-485

Roman, SJ., Auclin, FX., Chong-Sit, DA., & Ullern, MM. (1998). Surgically induced astigmatism with superior and temporal incisions in cases of with-the-rule preoperative astigmatism. *J Cataract Refract Surg*, Vol. 24, (1998), pp. 1636-41

Royce ,PM., Steinmann, B., & Vogel, A. (1990). Brittle cornea syndroma: an haritable connective tissue disorder distinct from Ehlers-Danlos syndrome type VI and fragilitas oculi, with spontaneous perforation of the eye, blue sclerae, red hair, and normal collagen lysyl hydroxylation. *Eur J Pediatr,* Vol. 149, (1990), pp. 465-9

Rumelt, S., & Rehany, U. (1998). Surgically induced keratoglobus in pellucid marginal degeneration. *Eye*, Vol.12, (1998), pp.156-158

Sawagamuchi, S., Yue ,BYT., Sugar J, Giljoy, JE. (1989). Lysosomal abnormalities in keratoconus. *Arch Ophthalmol*, Vol 108, (1989), pp. 1507-10

Sawagamuchi, S., Twinning, SS., & Yue, BYT. (1994). Alpha 2 macroglobulin levels in normal human and keratoconus corneas. *Invest Ophthalmol Vis Sci*, Vol. 35, (1994), pp. 4008-4014

Sharif, KW., Casey, TA., & Colart, J. (1992). Prevalence of mitral valve prolapse in keratoconus patients. *J R Soc Med,* Vol. 85, (1992), pp. 446-448

Seiler, T., Huhle, S., Spoerl, E., & Kunath, H. (2000). Manifest diabetes and keratoconus : a retrospective case control study. *Graefes Arch Clin Exp Ophthalmol*, Vol. 10, No. 238 (Oct ober 2000), pp. 822-5

Seiler, T., & Hafezi, F. (2006). Corneal cross- linking-induced stromal demarcation line. *Cornea*, Vol. 25, (2006), pp. 1057-9

Sii, F., Lee, GA., Sanfilippo, P., Stephensen, DC. (2004). Pellucid marginal degeneration and scleroderma. *Clin Exp Optom*, Vol 87, (2004), pp. 180-4

Simsek, S., Yasar, T., & Demirok, A. (1998). Effect of superior and temporal clear corneal incisions on astigmatism after sutureless phacoemulsification. *J Cataract Refract Surg*, Vol. 24, (1998), pp. 515-18

Smiddy, WE., Hamburg, TR., Kracher, GP & Stark WJ. (1988). Keratoconus. Contact lens or keratoplasty?. *Ophthalmology*, Vol. 95, (1988), pp. 487-92

Smolin, G. (1987). Dystrophies and degenerations, *The Cornea*, (2nd ed), Little, Brown, Boston

Spörl, E., Huhle, M., Kasper, M., & Seiler, T. (1997). Erhöhung der Festigkeit der Hornhaut durch Vernetzung. *Ophthalmologe*, Vol. 94, No. 12 (December 1997), pp. 902-6

Spörl, E., Huhle, M., & Seiler, T. (1998). Induction of cross-links in corneal tissue. *Exp Eye Res*. Vol. 66, No. 1 (Januar 1998), pp. 97-103

Spoerl, E., Wollensak, G., & Seiler, T. (2004). Increased resistance of crosslinked cornea against enzymatic digestion. *Curr Eye Res*, Vol. 29 (December 2004), pp. 35-40

Spoerl, E., Mrochen, M., & Sliney, D. (2007). Safety of UVA-riboflavin cross-linking of the cornea. *Cornea*, Vol. 26, (2007), pp. 385-9

Thornton, SP. (1994). *Radial and Astigmatic Keratotomy: The American System of Precise, Predictable Refractive Surgery*, Thorofare, Slack Incorporated, NJ

Tomkins, O., & Garzozi, HJ. (2008). Collagen cross-linking: Strengthening the unstable cornea. *Clin Ophthalmol*, Vol. 4,No. 2 (December 2008), pp. 863-7

Tuft, SJ., Moodaley, LC., & Gregory, WM. (1994). Prognostic factors of progression to keratoconus. *Ophthalmology*, Vol. 101, (1994), pp. 439-447

Waller, SG., Steinert, RE., & Wagoner, MD. (1995). Long term results of epikeratoplasty for keratoconus. *Cornea*, Vol. 14, (1995), pp. 84-8

Wang, L., Misra, M., Koch, DD. (2003). Peripheral corneal relaxing incisions combined with cataract surgery. *J Cataract Refract Surg*, Vol. 29, (2003), pp. 712-722

Wilson, SE., Guang, HE., & Weng, J. (1996). Epithelial injury induces keratocyte apoptosis: hypothesized reole of the interleukin-1 system in the modulation of corneal tissue organisation and wound healing. *Exp Eye Res*, Vol. 62, (1996), pp. 325-7

Wirbelauer, C., Anders, N., Pham, DT., & Wollensak, J. (1997). Effect of incision location on preoperative oblique astigmatism after scleral tunnel incision. *Cataract Refract Surg*, Vol. 23, (1997), pp. 365-71

Wollensak, G., Spoerl, E., & Seiler, T. (2003). Riboflavin /ultraviolet-a-induced collagen crosslinking for the treatment of keratoconus. *Am J Ophthalmol*, Vol. 135 (December 2003), pp. 620-7

Wollensak, G., & Iomdina, E. (2008). Long- term biomechanical properties after collagen crosslinking of sclera using glyceraldehyde. *Acta Ophthalmol*, Vol.86 ,No. 8, (December 2008), pp. 887-93

Wollensak, G., & Iomdina, E. (2009). Long term biomechanical properties of rabbit cornea after photodynamic collagen crosslinking. *Acta Ophthalmol*, Vol. 87, No.1, (Februar 2009), pp. 48-51

Yanoff, M., Duker, JS. (2004). *Ophthalmology*, (2nd ed.), Mosby, ISSN 0-323-01634-0, Philadelphia

Yeung, KK., Weissman, BA. (1997). Contact lens correction of patients with Marfan syndrome. *J Am Optom Assoc*, Vol. 68, No. 6, (Jun 1997), pp.367-72

Zamora, KV., Males, JJ. (2009). Polymicrobial keratitis after a collagen cross-linking
procedure with postoperative use of a contact lens: a case report. *Cornea*, Vol. 28,
No.4, (May 2009), pp. 474-6

16

Wavefront Aberrations

Mirko Resan, Miroslav Vukosavljević and Milorad Milivojević
Eye Clinic, Military Medical Academy, Belgrade,
Serbia

1. Introduction

The eye is an optical system having several optical elements that focus light rays representing images onto the retina. Imperfections in the components and materials in the eye may cause light rays to deviate from the desired path. These deviations, referred to as optical or wavefront aberrations, result in blurred images and decreased visual performance (1).

Wavefront aberrations are optical imperfections of the eye that prevent light from focusing perfectly on the retina, resulting in defects in the visual image. There are two kinds of aberrations:

1. Lower order aberrations (0, 1st and 2nd order)
2. Higher order aberrations (3rd, 4th, … order)

Lower order aberrations are another way to describe refractive errors: myopia, hyperopia and astigmatism, correctible with glasses, contact lenses or refractive surgery. Lower order aberrations is a term used in wavefront technology to describe second-order Zernike polynomials. Second-order Zernike terms represent the conventional aberrations defocus (myopia, hyperopia and astigmatism). Lower order aberrations make up about 85 per cent of all aberrations in the eye.

Higher order aberrations are optical imperfections which cannot be corrected by any reliable means of present technology. All eyes have at least some degree of higher order aberrations. These aberrations are now more recognized because technology has been developed to diagnose them properly. Wavefront aberrometer is actually used to diagnose and measure higher order aberrations. Higher order aberrations is a term used to describe Zernike aberrations above second-order. Third-order Zernike terms are coma and trefoil. Fourth-order Zernike terms include spherical aberration, and so on. Higher order aberrations make up about 15 percent of the overall number of aberrations in an eye.

2. Myopia

Myopia (nearsightedness, shortsightedness) is a refractive error where parallel light rays coming from a distance after refraction through the cornea and lens focus before the retina in the vitreous body and mature behind the focus in the state of divergence generate on retina wasteful circles (Fig. 1 and 3). Because of this, the image that one sees is out of focus when looking at a distant object but comes into focus when looking at a close object. Therefore, shortsighted people cannot see clearly at a distance (2).

Myopia can be classified by cause, degree, clinical features and age of onset. By cause myopia can be: *axial myopia*, attributed to an increase in eyes axial length (more than 24 mm), and *refractive myopia*, attributed to the condition of refractive elements of the eye, like curvature myopia (increased curvature of cornea) or index myopia (variation in the index of refraction of one or more ocular media, like in nuclear cataract). By degree myopia can be: *low myopia* (−3.0 diopters or less), *medium myopia* (between −3.0 and −6.0 diopters), and *high myopia* (−6.0 diopters or more). By clinical features myopia can be: *simple myopia*, characterized by the eye being too long for its optical power or optically too powerful for its axial length, and *degenerative (malignant, pathological, progressive) myopia* characterized by expressed fundus changes (conus myopicus, staphyloma posticum, degeneratio chorioretinae peripherica, maculopathia) and associated with a high refractive error and subnormal visual acuity after correction. This form of myopia worsen progressively over time and can become complicated with retinal tear and retinal detachment. By age of onset myopia can be: *congenital myopia*, present at birth and persisting through infancy, *youth-onset myopia* (*school myopia*) with onset between around 5 years of age and physical maturity, *early adult-onset myopia* with onset after physical maturity and up to about 40 years of age, and *late adult-onset myopia* with onset after around 55 years of age due to changes in the nucleus of the crystalline lens (2,3,4,5,6).

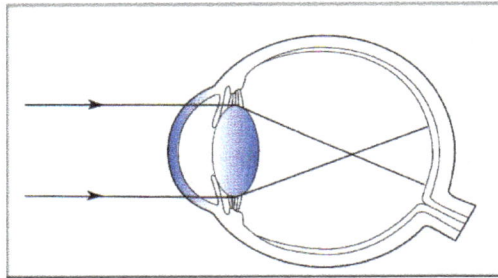

Fig. 1. Myopia with accommodation relaxed. Parallel light rays from infinity focus to a point anterior to the retina, forming a blurred image on the retina (6).

3. Hyperopia

Hyperopia (farsightedness, longsightedness) is a refractive error where parallel light rays coming from a distance after refraction through the cornea and lens focus behind the retina without participation of accommodation (Figs. 2 and 3). Causes of hyperopia are typically genetic and involve an eye that is too short or a cornea that is too flat, so that images focus at a point behind the retina (2).

Hyperopia can be classified by: cause, clinical features and accommodative status. By cause hyperopia can be: *axial hyperopia*, attributed to a decrease in eyes axial length (less than 24 mm), and *refractive hyperopia*, attributed to the condition of refractive elements of the eye like decreased curvature of cornea (cornea plana). By clinical features hyperopia can be: *simple, pathological* (resulting in amblyopia or strabismus), and *functional*. By accommodative status hyperopia can be: *total, latent*, and *manifest*. Total hyperopia occurs in state of full paralysis of accommodation (after application of cycloplegics) and represents the amount of entire refractive error. Latent hyperopia is that part of the refractive error being corrected with accommodation. Manifest hyperopia is the accommodation uncorrected part of hyperopia and becoming closer to the total one with age (2,3,4,5,6).

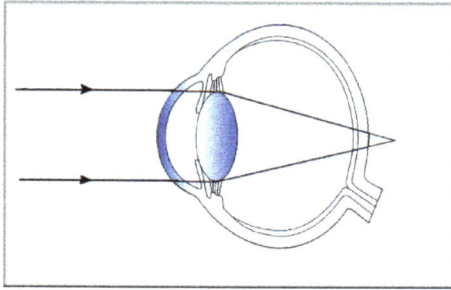

Fig. 2. Hyperopia with accommodation relaxed. Parallel light rays from infinity focus to a point posterior to the retina, forming a blurred image on the retina (6).

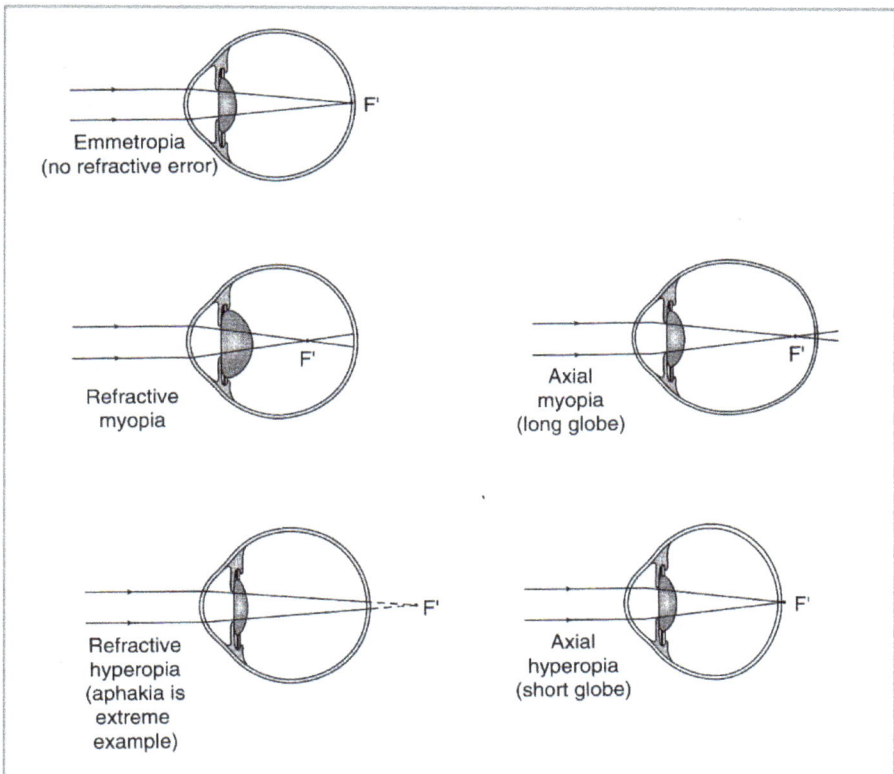

Fig. 3. Refractive errors (myopia and hyperopia) defined by the position of the secondary focal point with respect to the retina, with accommodation fully relaxed. The secondary focal point of a myopic eye is the front of the retina inside the vitreous, whereas the focal point of a hyperopic eye is behind the retina (7).

4. Astigmatism

Astigmatism is a refractive condition in which the eye optical system is incapable of forming a point image for a point object. This is because the refracting power of the optical system varies from one meridian to another. There are complex optical relationships in astigmatism: no focus (as in myopia and hyperopia), but the two focal lines corresponding to main meridians. The meridians of greatest and least refraction are defined as main (principal) meridians. Astigmatism is caused by the cornea or the crystalline lens. Clinically, most astigmatisms are corneal in origin and mainly related to the change in curvature of the cornea (3,4).

There are different types of astigmatism, according to the method of classification (2,3,4,5,6).

Astigmatism is *regular* when two main meridians are 90° to each other; it is correctable with cylindrical or spherocylindrical lenses. Otherwise, the astigmatism is *irregular*. Regular astigmatism is *with-the-rule (direct)* when the steepest corneal meridian is close to 90° (±20°) and *against-the-rule (indirect)* when the steepest meridian is close to 180° (±20°). When the astigmatism is regular but the main meridians do not lie close to 90° or 180°, it is *oblique*.

Astigmatic errors are also described by the location of secondary focal lines relative to the retina (with accommodation relaxed). *Compound myopic* astigmatism occurs when both of the main meridians are myopic, pulling the focal lines off the retina into the vitreous. In *simple myopic* astigmatism, one meridian is emmetropic and the other is myopic, one focal line is on the retina and the other is pulled into the vitreous. *Compound hyperopic* astigmatism occurs when both of the main meridians are hyperopic, pulling the focal lines behind the retina. In *simple hyperopic* astigmatism, one meridian is emmetropic and the other is hyperopic, one focal line is on the retina and the other is pulled behind the retina. *Mixed* astigmatism occurs when one meridian is hyperopic and the other is myopic (Fig. 4).

Astigmatism can be natural or surgically induced. *Natural* astigmatism is common, that is, around 15% of adult population have astigmatism > 1D and 2% have astigmatism > D. Special group of astigmatisms are those surgically induced, *postoperative* astigmatisms. Any surgical intervention in the fibrous mantle of the eye (cornea, sclera) may result in major or minor postoperatively acquired astigmatisms. Classic and most common postoperative astigmatism occurs after cataract surgery, especially after extra- and intracapsular cataract extraction. It is very minimal after phacoemulsification (2).

As noted, the cornea is usually the source of clinically significant amounts of astigmatism. The amount of *corneal* astigmatism, along with the location of meridians of least and greatest refraction, can be easily determined with a keratometer. The vast majority of corneas have with-the-rule astigmatism; a small minority of corneas have against-the-rule or oblique astigmatism, and a small minority have no astigmatism. As compared to corneal astigmatism, *internal* astigmatism is relatively small in amount, tending to slightly vary from one person to another, and is almost always against-the-rule. Main causes of internal astigmatism are the toricity of the back surface of the cornea and the tilting of the crystalline lens. There is no clinical method of measuring internal astigmatism. *Refractive (total)* astigmatism includes both corneal and internal astigmatism and can be determined with refractometry (total determination of refraction) (3).

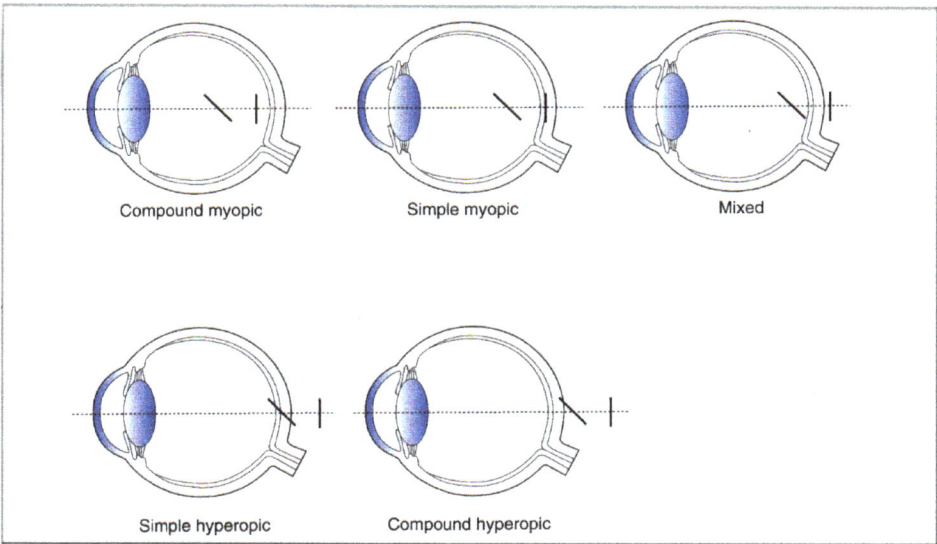

Fig. 4. The locations of focal lines with respect to the retina define the type of astigmatism (6).

5. Higher order aberrations (HOAs)

Within the past decade, rapid improvement in wavefront-related technologies, including the development of sensors for measuring optical properties of the eye in a clinical environment, allowed the ophthalmic community to move the wavefront theory of light transmission from an academic concept to one being central for better understanding of the effect of aberrations on visual performance and the corresponding image-forming properties of the eye. Imperfections in the optics of the eye are now measured and expressed as wave aberration errors. The wave aberration defines how the phase of light is affected as it passes through the eye's optical system, and is usually defined mathematically by a series of Zernike polynomials. Zernike polynomials are used to classify and represent optical aberrations because they consist of terms of same form as the types of aberrations observed when describing the optical properties of the eye, and can be used reciprocally with no misunderstanding. Moreover, the advantage of describing ocular aberrations using the normalized Zernike expansion, generally depicted as a pyramid (Figs. 5 and 6), is that the value of each mode represents the root mean square (RMS) wavefront error attributable to that mode. Coefficients with a higher value identify the modes (aberrations) that have the greatest impact on the overall RMS wavefront error in the eye and thus in reducing the optical performance of the eye (8).

The two most important HOAs are coma and spherical aberration. Coma is the distortion in image formation occurring when a bundle of light rays enters an optical system not parallel to the optic axis. Coma results in off-axis point sources such as stars appearing distorted, with a comet-like tail. Spherical aberration is the blurring of an image, occurring when light from the margin of a lens or mirror with spherical surface comes to a focus shorter than light from the central portion. The changing focal length is caused by deviations in lens or mirror surface from a true sphere.

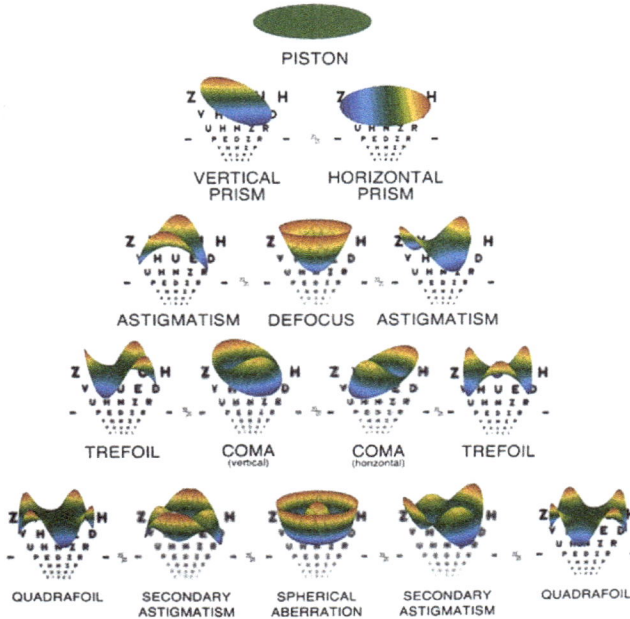

Fig. 5. This chart reveals more common shapes of aberrations created when a wavefront of light passes through eyes with imperfect vision. A theoretically perfect eye (top) is represented by an aberration-free flat plane known, for reference, as piston. (Image: Alcon Inc.)

HOAs are vision errors more complex than lower-order aberrations. HOAs have relatively unfamiliar names such as coma, spherical aberration and trefoil. These types of aberrations can produce vision errors such as difficulty seeing at night, glare, halos, blurring, starburst patterns or double vision (diplopia). No eye is perfect, which means that all eyes have at least some degree of HOAs. These aberrations are now more recognized because technology has been developed to diagnose them properly.

HOAs are measured by aberrometer (wavefront sensor). Aberrometers measure the distortion of a light wave as it is altered by passing through the optics of the eye. A plane wave of monochromatic light will be distorted by optical imperfections. Wavefront sensors do not measure light scatter (from stromal haze or corneal scars), chromatic aberrations or diffraction phenomena. Their effects on vision should be assessed by other means. A useful way to think of distortions in a wavefront is to think of the path length of parallel rays entering the pupil and projecting toward the retina. As light enters the eye from the air, its speed is retarded according to the refractive index of the material along its path to the retina. Arrival time is also influenced by the traveling distance. These two factors, refractive index and linear path variations, are measured with a wavefront sensor. A map can be made to show relevant retardation that a plane wave undergoes as it traverses the optics of the eye. Clinicians are now used to see this information displayed as Zernike polynomial expansion. In order to parcel the wavefront error into individual building blocks, a set of normalized Zernike polynomials is best fit to the measured wavefront error. The coefficient of each Zernike term reveals that term's relative contribution to the total root mean square (RMS) error (Fig. 7) (9).

radial order, *n*

↓

Lower orders

_____

Higher orders

← angular frequency, *m* →

sine phase | cosine phase

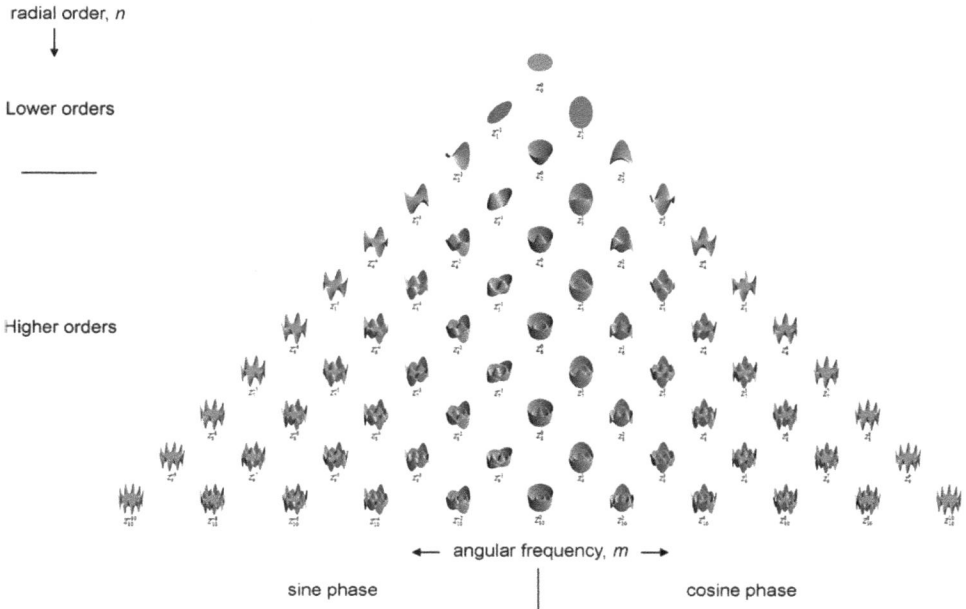

Fig. 6. The Zernike pyramid showing polynomials up to the 10th orders. The 0- to 2nd-order terms represent low optical aberrations in the eye, with 2nd-order terms (i.e. defocus and astigmatism) having the highest contribution to the overall wavefront aberration in the eye. Terms of the 3rd order and higher represent the HOAs. The 3rd- and 4th-order terms are the most prevalent HOA in the human eye (8).

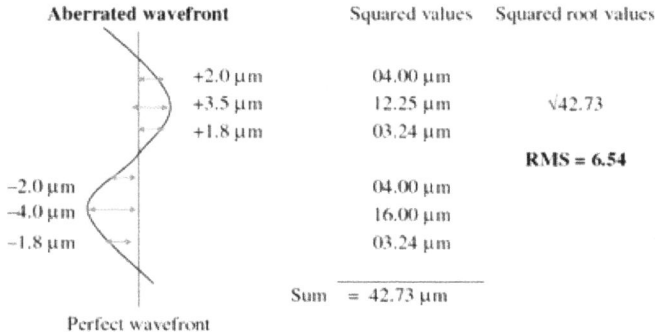

Aberrated wavefront   Squared values   Squared root values

+2.0 μm   04.00 μm

+3.5 μm   12.25 μm   √42.73

+1.8 μm   03.24 μm

                                RMS = 6.54

−2.0 μm   04.00 μm

−4.0 μm   16.00 μm

−1.8 μm   03.24 μm

Sum = 42.73 μm

Perfect wavefront

Fig. 7. Graphical representation of root mean squared wavefront error (9).

In the ametropic eye, defocus (i.e. myopia or hyperopia) is by far the largest aberration, followed by astigmatism. These are low order terms. The Zernike pyramid is useful (Table 1). As we follow down the rows from the top, we go from low order to high order. Low order encompasses the top three rows' piston, tilt, tip, and sphere and astigmatism. Row three (i.e. sphere and astigmatism) is what we normally measure and prescribe in spectacles. The fourth row is called third order aberrations, and it continues from there. Anything beyond lower order is lumped under the term of higher order aberrations (HOAs). As observed from the diagram, they have individual names such as coma, and spherical aberration. When interpreting data, we need to know whether the wavefront refers to total aberrations (9).

Plot index	Term	Binomial representation	Polynomial (ρ, θ)
1	Tip	(1,1)	$2\rho\sin(\theta)$
2	Tilt	(1,1)	$2\rho\cos(\theta)$
3	Defocus	(2,0)	$\sqrt{3}\,(2\rho^2 \angle 1)$
4	Astigmatism	(2,2)	$\sqrt{6}\,\rho^2\sin(2\theta)$
5	Astigmatism	(2,2)	$\sqrt{6}\,\rho^2\cos(2\theta)$
6	Vertical coma	(3,1)	$\sqrt{8}\,(3\rho^3 \angle 2\rho)\sin(\theta)$
7	Horizontal coma	(3,1)	$\sqrt{8}\,(3\rho^3 \angle 2\rho)\cos(\theta)$
8	Trefoil	(3,3)	$\sqrt{8}\,\rho^3\sin(3\theta)$
9	Trefoil	(3,3)	$\sqrt{8}\,\rho^3\cos(3\theta)$
10	Spherical aberration	(4,0)	$\sqrt{5}(6\rho^4 \angle 6\rho^2 + 1)$
11	Secondary astigmatism	(4,2)	$\sqrt{10}\,(4\rho^4 \angle 3\rho^2)\sin(2\theta)$
12	Secondary astigmatism	(4,2)	$\sqrt{10}\,(4\rho^4 \angle 3\rho^2)\cos(2\theta)$
13	Tetrafoil	(4,4)	$\sqrt{10}\,\rho^4\sin(4\theta)$
14	Tetrafoil	(4,4)	$\sqrt{10}\,\rho^4\cos(4\theta)$

Table 1. Zernicke pyramid (9).

In the normal ametropic eye, HOAs are a relatively small component, comprising about 10% of eye's overall aberrations. This varies between individuals. Figure 8a shows a 2-D wavefront of a normal ametropic eye with a low amount of HOAs (0.14µm), and Figure 8b shows a subtle form fruste keratoconic eye with a larger amount (0.42µm) of HOAs. Both images are for data at a 6 mm pupil size. It is important to know what the pupil size was when aberrometry was performed, and at what pupil size data was presented, as HOAs increase with increased pupil size (9).

Three different wavefront measuring principles are available to measure aberrations: (1) Hartmann-Shack, (2) Tscherning or ray tracing, and (3) automated retinoscopy. A Hartmann-Shack aberrometer is an outgoing wavefront aberrometer. It measures the shape of the wavefront that is reflected out of the eye from a point source on the fovea. An array of microlenslets is used to subdivide the outgoing wavefront into multiple beams which produce spot images on a video sensor. The displacement of each spot from the corresponding nonaberrated reference position is used to determine the shape of the wavefront. A Tscherning, or ray-tracing, aberrometer is an ingoing instrument. It projects a thin laser beam into the eye, parallel to the visual axis, and determines the location of the beam on the retina by using a photodetector. Once the position of the first light spot on the retina is determined, the laser beam is moved to a new position, and the location of the second light spot on the retina is determined. Aberrations in the optical system cause a shift in the location of the light spot on the retina. The third type, automated retinoscopy, is based on dynamic skiascopy. The retina is scanned with a slit-shaped light beam, and the reflected light is captured by an array of rotating photodetectors over a 360° area. The time difference of the reflected light is used to determine the aberrations. Visser et al. compared total ocular aberrations and corneal aberrations identified with four different aberrometers and determined the repeatability and interobserver variability. In this prospective comparative study, 23 healthy subjects underwent bilateral examination with four aberrometers: the Irx3 (Hartmann-Shack; Imagine Eyes, Orsay, France), Keratron (Hartmann-Shack; Optikon, Rome, Italy), iTrace (raytracing; Tracey Technologies, Houston, TX), and OPD-Scan (Automated Retinoscopy; Nidek, Gamagori, Japan). Six images per eye were obtained. Second-, third- and fourth-order spherical aberrations were exported for 5.0-mm pupils. Results demonstrate that significant differences in measurements were found for several total ocular aberrations (defocus [2,0], astigmatism [2,2], trefoil [3,-3], trefoil [3,3], and spherical aberration [4,0]) and corneal aberrations (defocus [2,0] and astigmatism [2,2]).

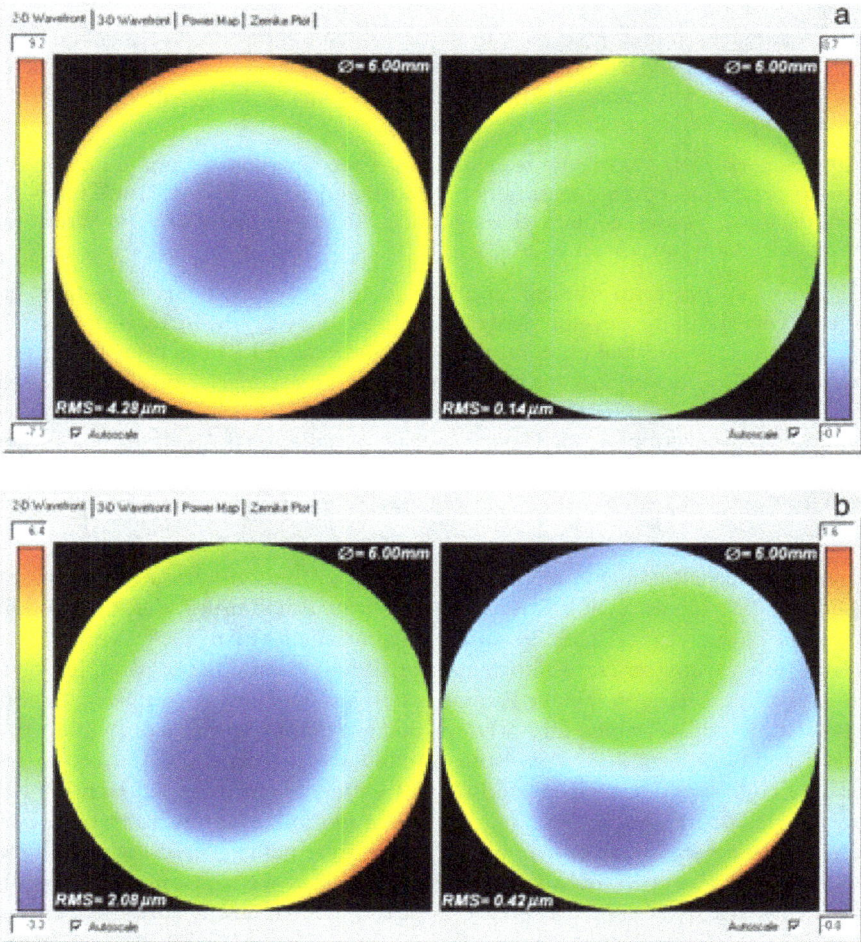

Fig. 8. HOAs represented by 2-D image: (a) eye with low degree, and (b) eye with high degree of HOAs (HOAs measured by Alcon LADARWave) (9).

The Irx3 showed the highest repeatability in measuring total ocular aberrations, followed by the Keratron, OPD-Scan, and iTrace. The repeatability of corneal aberration measurements was highest for the iTrace, followed by the Keratron and OPD-Scan. The OPD-Scan showed a lower interobserver variability, compared with the Irx3, Keratron, and iTrace. In conclusion, total ocular and corneal aberrations are not comparable when measured with different aberrometers. Hartmann-Shack aberrometers showed the best repeatability for total ocular aberrations, and iTrace for corneal aberrations (10).

In our clinic we use WaveLight Analyzer (WaveLight Germany) as aberrometer. Working in the same visible spectrum as the human eye, the WaveLight Analyzer is designed for wavefront measurements on the basis of the Tscherning principle. In order to perform measurements according to the Tscherning principle, an image of regular measurement spots is projected onto the retina and captured by a lightsensitive camera. The distortion of the light spots on the retina in relation to the reference light bundle is calculated and the wavefront error is displayed. Figure 9 shows HOAs in a male aged 32 with myopia on his left eye. Wavefront refraction: -6.54/-1.14 ax 72°, coma: 0.16μm, spherical aberration: 0.02 μm, and pupil diameter: 6.59 mm.

Can HOAs be corrected? Wavefront technology has been advanced enough only in the last few years to produce accurate measurements and diagnoses of HOAs. Some types of new wavefront designed glasses, contact lenses, intraocular lens implants and wavefront-guided laser vision correction can correct HOAs.

One of the most powerful clinical applications of aberrometry is wavefront-guided refractive surgery. With the development of wavefront analyses, the increase of the HOAs of the eye following conventional photorefractive keratectomy (PRK) has been confirmed (11). Wavefront-guided refractive surgery is a technique using excimer or other lasers to correct not only spherical and cylindrical refractive errors but also HOAs. Seiler et al. reported the first application of wavefront-guided laser *in situ* keratomileusis (LASIK) using a Tscherning aberrometer to measure the HOAs (12). McDonald performed almost simultaneously the first wavefront-guided LASIK using data obtained from the Hartmann–Shack wavefront sensor (13).

Several excimer laser platforms are available today. Although various terminology has been used to label, identify, and differentiate treatment modalities, the most commonly used include conventional laser in situ keratomileusis (LASIK); wavefront-guided treatments, which customize ablation patterns based on higher- and lower-order aberration profiles unique to the eye being treated; and wavefront-optimized treatments, which take some eye variables into account but use pre-programmed ablation profiles based on population analysis. Wavefront-guided treatments are intended to reduce preoperative HOAs, and wavefront-optimized treatments are intended to minimize the induction of postoperative HOAs; both modalities minimize significantly postoperative HOA changes compared with conventional LASIK treatments. There are some reported differences in the outcomes of wavefront-guided and wavefront-optimized platforms; however, few studies have directly compared the outcomes of these different technologies. The results in these studies are inconsistent, some indicating an advantage for wavefront-guided treatments and others finding no significant differences between the 2 treatment algorithms for patients without significant preoperative HOAs (14).

Examination

General Data		Refraction Data				Ocular Data	
		Clinical	Autoref.	Cyclopl.			
Eye:	left	Sphere D:	+0.00	...	...	K1-read. D:	...
OP State:	preOP	Cylinder D:	+0.00	...	...	@ Axis °:	0
OP Index:	01	Axis °:	...	...	...	K2-read. D:	...
Date:	16-12-2010	VD mm:	12			@ Axis °:	90

Device Settings

Diameter mm:	6.0
Zernike order:	6
Aberroscope lens:	+0.00
Camera lens:	+0.00
Accomod.lens:	+0.00

Pupil Information

Centered

Pupil Diameter mm:	+6.59
X-Offset mm:	+0.02
Y-Offset mm:	+0.06
Z-Offset mm:	+0.00

Wavefront Refraction

Sphere D:	-6.54
Cylinder D:	-1.14
Axis °:	72
Defocus:	5.33µm
Coma:	0.16µm
Astigmatism:	0.86µm
Spher.Aberration:	0.02µm

WaveLight AG

Am Wolfsmantel 5
D-91058 Erlangen - Germany
Phone: +49 9131/6186-0
info@wavelight.com
www.wavelight.com

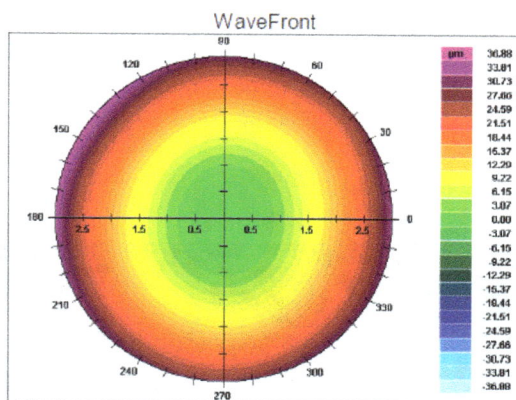

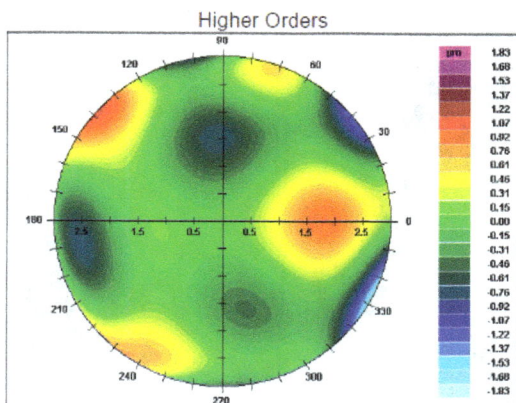

Fig. 9. Wavefront aberrations recorded on WaveLight Analyzer (WaveLight Germany).

Fares et al. compared the efficiency, predictability, safety, and induced HOAs between wavefront-guided and non-wavefront-guided ablations. Their meta-analysis showed that the increase in HOAs in patients who had wavefront-guided LASIK was lesser than in those who had non-wavefront-guided LASIK (15).

We experienced in our clinic that refractive surgical procedures (LASIK and PRK) induce HOAs and usually do not reduce visual acuity. Here is a brief overview of a case of increasing coma after successful correction of mild myopia using PRK: the patient was a male aged 27, and a PRK method was performed on his right eye with myopia. WaveLight Allegretto (400 Hz) excimer laser was used. HOAs were measured preoperatively and postoperatively on WaveLight Analyzer. Preoperative best spectacle corrected visual acuity of the right eye was with - 0.75/-0.25 ax 134° = 1.0, and postoperative uncorrected visual acuity was 1.0. Optical zone of 6.5 mm and ablated zone of 9.0 mm were used. Coma was increased from 0.02 μm preoperatively to 0.15 μm postoperatively, and sperical aberration was the same (0.08 μm) (Figs. 10 and 11).

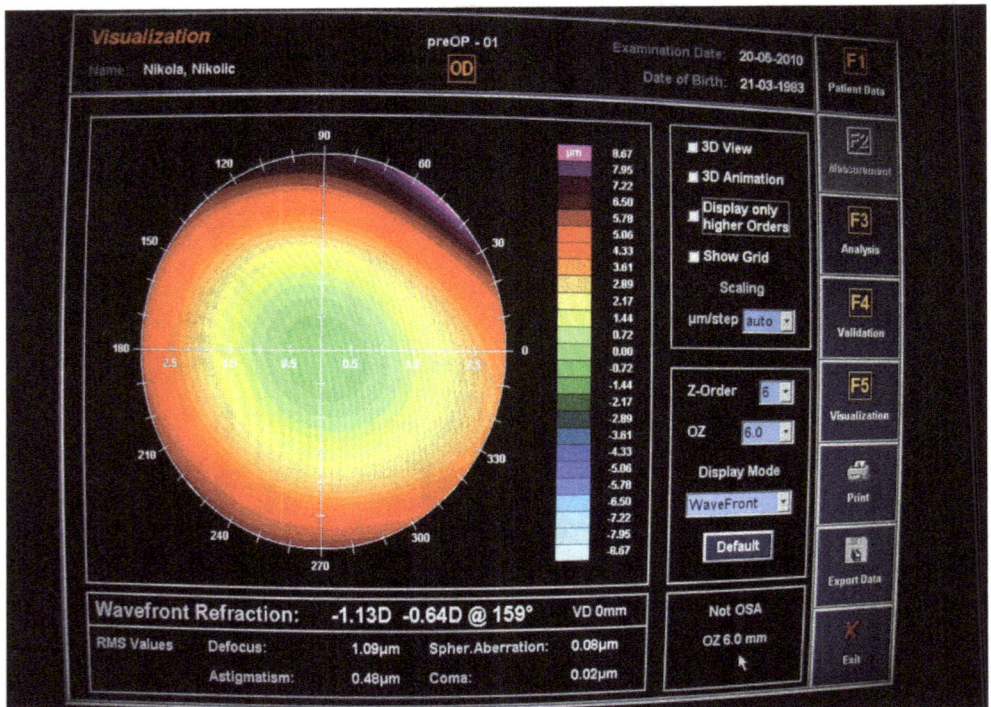

Fig. 10. Picture of wavefront aberrations preoperatively.

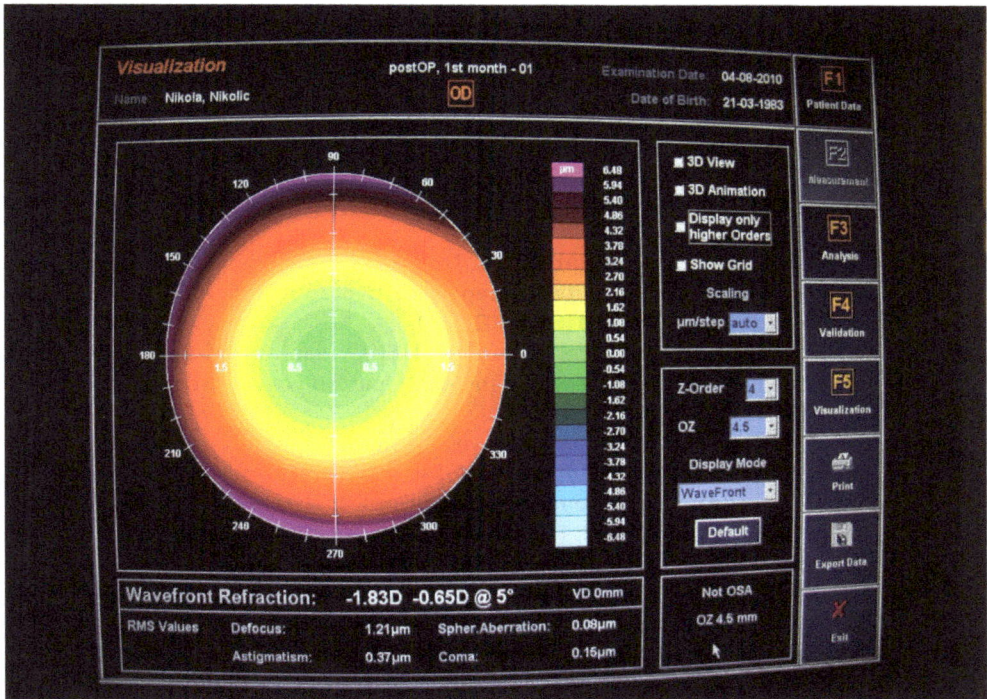

Fig. 11. Picture of wavefront aberrations postoperatively.

6. References

[1] Schwiegerling J. Theoretical limits to visual performance. Surv Ophthalmol 2000; 45:139–146.

[2] Cvetkovic D. Refraction clinic. In: Parunovic A, Cvetkovic D et al, Ed. Correction of refractive errors of the eye. Belgrade: Zavod za udzbenike i nastavna sredstva; 1995. p. 15-44.

[3] Grosvenor T. Anomalies of refraction. In: Grosvenor T, Ed. Primary care optometry. Woburn, MA: Butterworth-Heinemann; 2002. p. 3-26.

[4] Smith ME, Kincaid MC, West CE. Astigmatic lenses. In: Smith ME, Kincaid MC, West CE, Ed. Basic science, refraction, and pathology. St. Louis, Missouri: Mosby; 2002. p. 104-110.

[5] Goss DA, West RW. Optics of refractive error management. In: Goss DA, West RW, Ed. Introduction to the optics of the eye. Woburn, MA: Butterworth-Heinemann; 2002. p. 137-153.

[6] American Academy of Ophthalmology. Optics of the human eye. In: American Academy of Ophthalmology. Clinical optics. San Francisco, CA: American Academy of Ophthalmology; 2007. p. 105-123.

[7] Smith ME, Kincaid MC, West CE. The ametropias. In: Smith ME, Kincaid MC, West CE, Ed. Basic science, refraction, and pathology. St. Louis, Missouri: Mosby; 2002. p. 99-103.

[8] Lombardo M, Lombardo G. Wave aberration of human eyes and new descriptors of image optical quality and visual performance. J Cataract Refract Surg 2010; 36: 313-331.

[9] Lawless MA, Hodge C. Wavefront's role in corneal refractive surgery. Clin Experiment Ophthalmol 2005; 33: 199-209.

[10] Visser N, Berendschot TTJM, Verbakel F, Tan AN, De Brabander J, Nuijts RMMA. Evaluation of the comparability and repeatability of four wavefront aberrometers. Invest Ophthalmol Vis Sci 2011; 52:1302-1311.

[11] Seiler T, Kaemmerer M, Mierdel P, Krinke HE. Ocular optical aberrations after photorefractive keratectomy for myopia and myopic astigmatism. Arch Ophthalmol 2000; 118: 17-21.

[12] Mrochen M, Kaemmerer M, Seiler T. Wavefront-guided laser in situ keratomileusis: early results in three eyes. J Refract Surg 2000; 16: 116-121.

[13] McDonald MB. Summit-Autonomous CustomCornea laser in situ keratomileusis outcomes. J Refract Surg 2000; 16: S617-618.

[14] Perez-Straziota CE, Randleman JB, Stulting RD. Visual acuity and higher-order aberrations with wavefront-guided and wavefront-optimized laser in situ keratomileusis J Cataract Refract Surg 2010; 36: 437-441.

[15] Fares U, Suleman H, Al-Aqaba MA, Otri AM, Said DG, Dua HS. Efficacy, predictability, and safety of wavefront-guided refractive laser treatment: Metaanalysis. J Cataract Refract Surg 2011; 37:1465-1475.

Part 4

Glaucoma

17

Trabecular Surgery

Antonio Fea, Giulia Consolandi, Giulia Pignata, Davide Turco,
Paola Cannizzo, Elena Bartoli, Teresa Rolle and Federico M. Grignolo
Clinica Oculistica, Universita' degli Studi di Torino
Italy

1. Introduction

In glaucoma, the most commonly used surgical options attempt to establish communication between the anterior chamber and the subconjunctival space, either by removing part of the trabecular meshwork and thus decreasing resistance to the passage of the aqueous humour or by means of drainage tubes that conduct the aqueous humour toward extraocular subconjunctival reservoirs. Trabeculectomy is still the most widely performed glaucoma procedure worldwide. Nevertheless, it creates an artificial pathway for drainage of aqueous that is less optimal than physiologic outflow and is associated with numerous short and long-term serious complications. Surgical alternatives, such as deep sclerectomy, are more demanding, longer and seem to be surgeon-dependent. Although they achieve a high level of hypotensive effect, these forms of surgery are not exempt from potential complications and are highly dependent on the inflammatory and healing response of the patient.[1] The use of antimetabolites to regulate this healing response is also linked to a higher rate of complications.[2,3,4,5,6]

The interest in new and possibly less invasive surgical techniques to lower intraocular pressure is growing. In particular, to avoid the eventual problems linked to surgical trauma to the conjunctiva and the ensuing inflammatory response, several new *ab interno* methods that attempt to achieve intraocular pressure control have been developed. Some of these methods are aimed at obtaining flow through Schlemm's canal, whereas others point to the possibility of obtaining flow from the anterior chamber to the suprachoroidal space. Gonioscopy is used in these *ab interno* procedures in order to visualize the site of implantation.

2. Visualizing the trabecular meshwork

Trabecular bypass surgery can be performed through the same incision used for phacoemulsification in cases of combined surgery, or by means of a paracentesis, when it is performed as a sole procedure. A temporal incision is warranted because of ease of patient's head positioning. Visualization of the angle using the goniolens should be practiced in cases prior to performing surgery, in order to learn the correct techniques.

In the case of phakic patients, the instillation of a miotic is recommended to minimize the risk of lens injury. If the procedure is carried out under topical anaesthesia it is advisable to introduce lidocaine 1% into the anterior chamber, because some of the surgical manoeuvres can be uncomfortable for the patient. It is perfectly possible to carry out the surgery under topical anaesthesia with intracameral lidocaine; however, when performing the operation for the first few times, it may be advisable to use some form of locoregional anaesthetic (retrobulbar, peribulbar or sub-Tenon).

Once the incision has been made in the temporal cornea, the anterior chamber must be filled with a cohesive viscoelastic that makes it possible to enlarge the region of the angle where surgery is planned.

A perfect view of the trabecular meshwork and of the angle must be achieved. The most common error is failure to position the microscope and/or the patient adequately in order to obtain an adequate view of the trabeculum. The patient's head must be turned approximately 45° away from the surgeon. The microscope should be tilted approximately 30° towards the operating surgeon.

3. Specific devices and surgical techniques

3.1 iStent®

The iStent® trabecular micro-bypass (Glaukos Corporation, Laguna Hills, CA) is made of titanium and coated with heparin (Duraflo® powder). It is L-shaped and measures 1 mm x 0.33 mm, with a nominal snorkel bore diameter of 120 microns (fig.1). The iStent is designed to fit into Schlemm´s canal. The distal portion of the stent is bevelled and sharpened to facilitate penetration into the tissue of the trabecular meshwork. The external surface features three retention arches that impede the movement of the stent once it has been implanted. The implant weighs approximately 0.1 mg. It is delivered preloaded on an insertion device (fig.2) and it is implanted at the level of the trabecular meshwork with the aid of a Swan-Jacob type goniolens (fig.3). Two versions of the iStent are available; one for the right eye and one for the left eye. The difference lies in the orientation of the rails, designed to facilitate the penetration of the implant into the trabecular meshwork. The distal tip of the implant should point towards the patient's feet at all times.

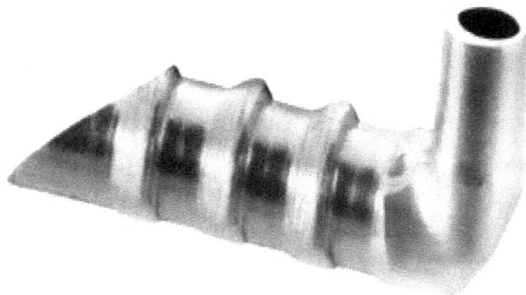

Fig. 1. iStent® trabecular bypass

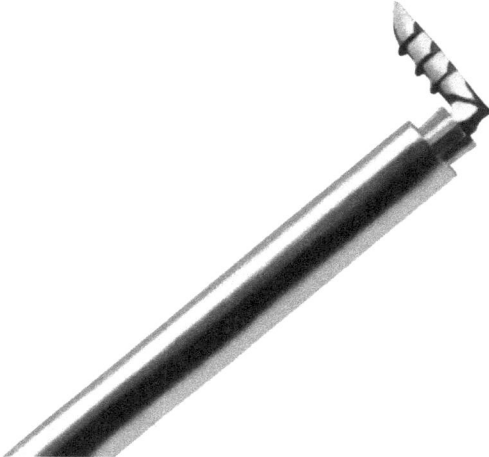

Fig. 2. iStent® trabecular bypass in iStent inserter

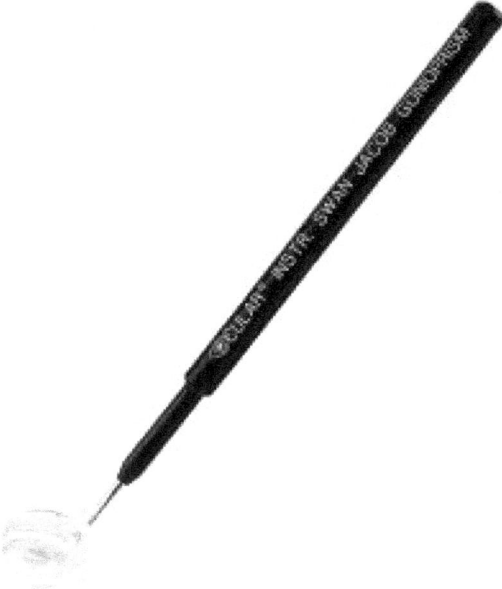

Fig. 3. Swan-Jacob goniolens

In all these techniques the patient is draped as for cataract surgery. Myosis is warranted if the surgery is not combined with phaco. Surgical steps are as follows:

1. A paracentesis is made generally using a 15 degree blade (fig.4).
2. If needed, the pupil is constricted with intracameral miotics and a cohesive viscoelastic is injected in the anterior chamber.
3. The tip of the stent, with the distal part parallel to the trabecular meshwork, should approach the trabecular meshwork at an angle of 15° to facilitate penetration of the tissue (fig.5). The stent should be placed parallel to the plane of the iris with the inner part covered by the meshwork and the lumen away from the iris. Excessive resistance indicates a path that is too perpendicular to the trabeculum or a wrong implantation site. Once the trabecular meshwork covers all of the implant, it should be released by pressing the applicator button. Only the proximal end of the stent should remain visible in the anterior chamber. The stent can be seated in its final position by gently tapping the side of the snorkel with the inserter tip. A small reflux of blood from Schlemm´s canal is common and reflects adequate positioning of the stent.
4. At the end of surgery, blood and viscoelastic are removed(Fig.6). The corneal incision can be hydrated if the paracentesis is not watertight.

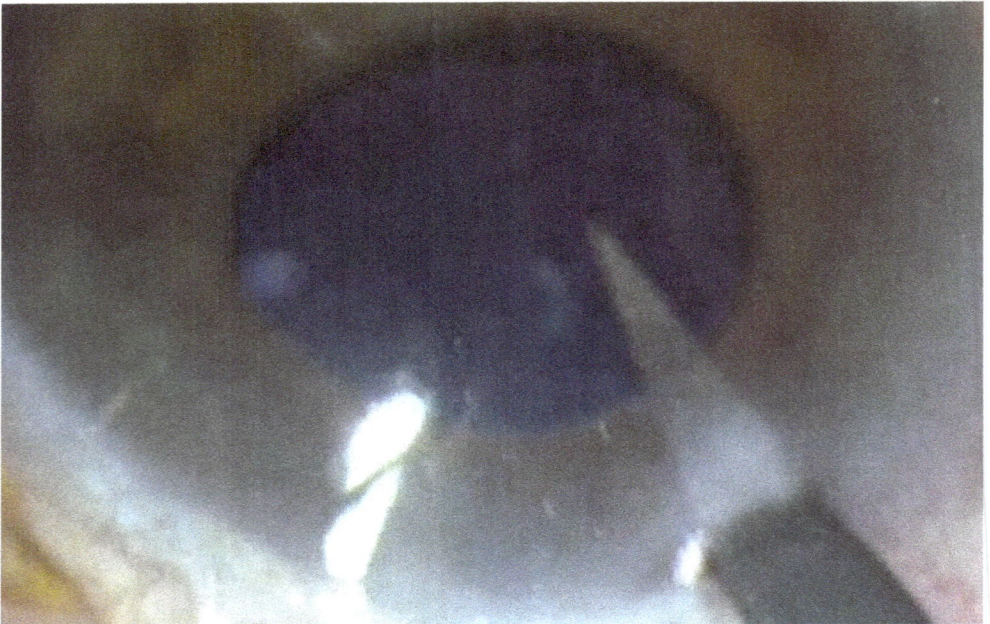

Fig. 4. A paracentesis is performed temporally.

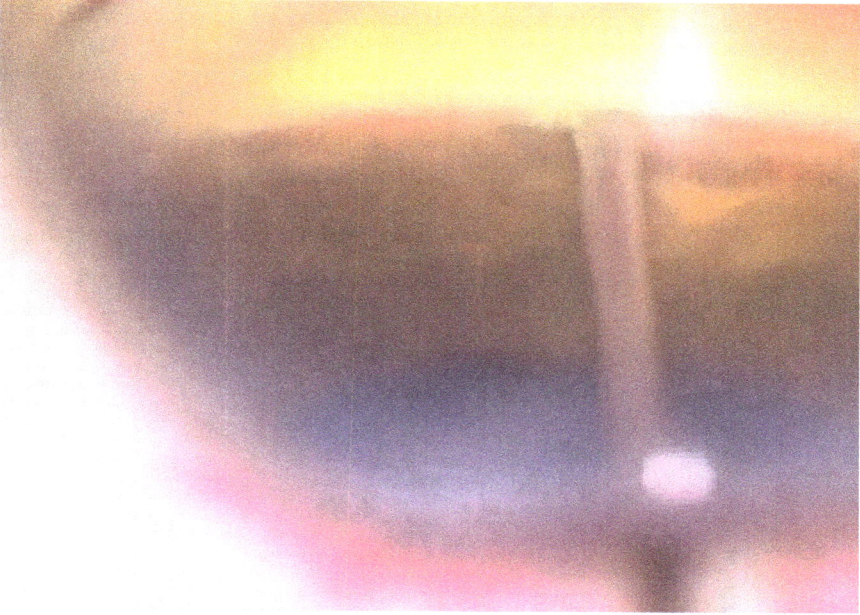

Fig. 5. The iStent is already half way within the trabecular meshwork.

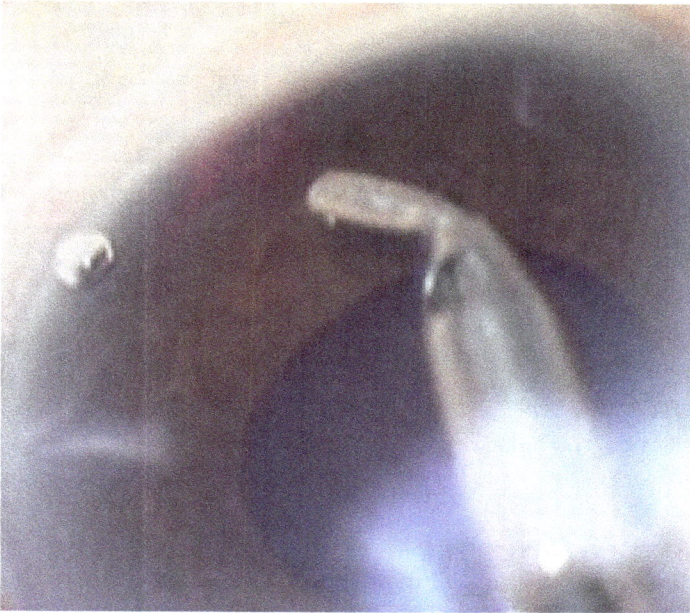

Fig. 6. Residual blood and viscoelastic are washed and aspirated by the anterior chamber with a coaxial I/A tip - the same can be done using a bimanual technique.

The post-operative suggested treatment should be similar to what is commonly used by each surgeon for an uncomplicated phacoemulsification procedure. Generally anti-glaucoma drugs are discontinued post-operatively and reintroduced if the patient does not achieve the target pressure.

iStent *inject is a* second generation trabecular bypass device that is also designed to restore conventional outflow (fig. 7). Two stents come preloaded in a sterile disposable injector that is placed on the meshwork. A stent release button on the injector is used to release the stents one at a time into the proper position (approximately 2-3 clock hours apart (fig. 8).

This new mechanism of implantation allows for implantation of two stents without exiting the inserter from the eye.

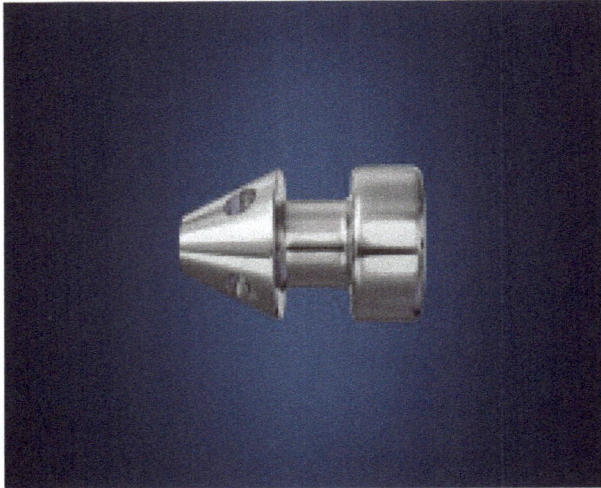

Fig. 7. iStent® inject (image provided by Glaukos)

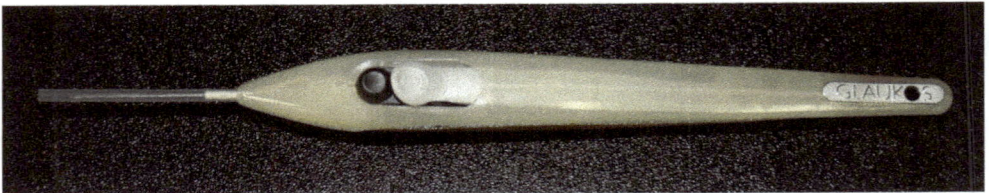

Fig. 8. iStent® inject inserter (image provided by Glaukos)

3.2 Trabectome

The Trabectome™ (NeoMedix Inc., Tustin, CA, USA) device consists of a disposable handpiece tip (19.5-gauge) that will fit through a 1.6mm corneal incision. The handpiece is connected to a console with irrigation and aspiration, and also to a simple electrocautery generator. The foot pedal controls the irrigation, aspiration and electrocautery ablation via a stepwise foot control similar to a phacoemulsification system (fig. 9).

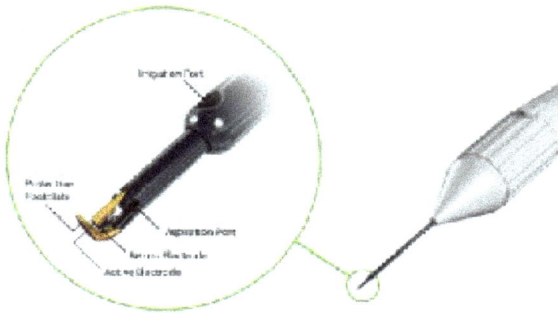

Fig. 9. Trabectome probe and tip

The tip of the handpiece is specially designed with an insulated footplate and is pointed for ease of insertion through the trabecular meshwork into Schlemm's canal. The footplate is coated with proprietary multilayered polymer, which provides thermal stability, mechanical strength, biocompatibility and chemical resistance in laboratory testing. The aspiration port is in close proximity (approximately 0.3 mm) to the cautery electrode and serves to remove debris during ablation. The irrigation is 3 mm from the surgical site and serves the dual purpose of keeping the eye pressurized and further dissipating heat energy. Although the irrigation and aspiration system role is important, the high-frequency electrocautery generator system is the pivotal point of this technology. The generator is a modified 800 EU unit from Aaron/Bovie (St. Petersburg, FL, USA) and operates at a frequency of 550 kHz with adjustable power setting in 0.1-W increment up to 10 W (recommended range 0.5–1.5 W). The target tissue is disrupted and disintegrated by applying heat energy in bursts with a high-peak power and low duty cycle. This ablation approach equates to high-energy bursts, which are bunched into small increments with comparably long time intervals in between. As a result, disruption and disintegration of tissue is achieved rather than a thermal-cooking effect such as that seen in traditional cautery of blood vessels.[7,8]

Surgical steps: steps 1 and 2 are equal to the previous procedure, although a specially designed blade is provided by the manufacturer to obtain a water-tight paracentesis. A small paracentesis is more important with this procedure because during surgery the viscoelastic material is washed out by the water flowing through the tip of the instrument. 2) The tip of the footplate is inserted through the paracentesis aiming at the trabecular meshwork and then it is inserted through the trabecular meshwork into Schlemm's canal . A foot switch activates the aspiration and electro-surgical elements that ablate and remove the strip of trabecular meshwork and Schlemm's canal as the surgeon slowly advances the instrument along the meshwork in a clockwise and then counter clockwise direction using the insertion site as a fulcrum. A strip of trabecular meshwork and Schlemm's canal spanning 80°–100° is ablated and removed under direct gonioscopic visualization. Intraoperative reflux of blood through the resulting cleft is desirable in this procedure and confirms appropriate ab interno "unroofing" of Schlemm's canal. 4) At the end of surgery any residual viscoelastic or blood present in the anterior chamber is removed. It is generally not necessary to hydrate the paracentesis.

The post-operative suggested treatment includes: antibiotics used for prophylaxis. Pilocarpine 2% qid should be used starting on the first post-operative medication and continued for a month. Lotemax is advised for three weeks and then tapered. Directly post-operative it is advised to continue the previous pre-operative anti-glaucomatous therapy, although prostaglandins should possibly be avoided. .Prof. Baerveldt recommends the eventual use of Latanoprost rather than other prostaglandins if they are absolutely necessary. Iopidine and Brimonidine can be used and are generally suggested. Anti-glaucoma medications can be reduced a month after surgery if target pressure is achieved.

3.3 Other procedures

Other approaches of gonioscopic surgery include the Ivantis method which simulates a short canaloplasty.

Two additional devices are aimed at improving flow of the aqueous humor from the anterior chamber to the suprachoroidal space. These are the Glaukos iStent *supra* and the Transcend Cypass. These devices will not be discussed, because the current data are less than one year post-operative.

4. Results

4.1 iStent

Numerous *in vitro* and *in vivo* studies support the stability, the effectiveness and the safety of the trabecular bypass iStent.

In 2004, Bahler demonstrated *in vitro* that the intraocular pressure was lowered after placement of a single stent, from 21.4 +/- 3.8 mm Hg to 12.4 +/- 4.2 mm Hg (P < .001).[9] This corresponded to an 84% increase in facility of outflow. Eyes receiving more than one stent had final IOP of 11.9 +/- 3.7 mm Hg. Nine eyes underwent sequential implantation of additional stents and seven of these had a further decrease of IOP (13.6 +/- 4.1 to 10.0 +/- 4.3; P = .02). This work suggested that bypass of the trabecular meshwork lowers IOP in cultured human anterior segments. One stent produced the greatest change in pressure. The sequential addition of more stents further lowered pressure in seven of nine eyes. Parallel to this study the founders/manufacturers of the iStent evaluated the stability of the implant on *ex vivo* eyes confirming that the L shape of the stent could not be moved even with strong traction on the stent itself.

A small clinical case series (n=6) reaffirmed the potential clinical utility of the current titanium version inserted *ab interno* and provided additional confirmation that the device stayed in place and continued to function to lower IOP with fewer medications through follow-up of one year.[10] All patients were seen day one, week one and at 1, 2, 6 and 12 months post-operatively. The mean pre-operative IOP of 20.2 ±6.3 decreased and stabilized at 14 to15 mm Hg with reduced medications out to one year. All devices remained in place and no complications were noted.

A larger prospective, 24-month, uncontrolled, multicenter, multicountry evaluation of 58 patients with uncontrolled primary open-angle glaucoma (including pseudoexfoliation and pigmentary) evaluated the effectiveness of the concurrent phacoemulsification and stent implantation.[11] Of the 48 patients in the per protocol population, 42 completed the 12 months follow-up. At baseline, mean (+/-SD) intraocular pressure (IOP) was 21.7+/-3.98 mmHg. At 12 months, mean IOP was reduced to 17.4+/-2.99 mmHg, a mean IOP reduction of 4.4+/-4.54 mmHg (p<0.001, 18.3%). At baseline, patients were taking a mean 1.6+/-0.8 medications. By 12 months, the mean number of medications was reduced to 0.4+/-0.62 (p<0.001). Half the patients achieved an IOP ≤ 18 mmHg and were able to discontinue hypotensive medication by the 12 month visit. The most commonly reported device-related adverse events were the appearance of stent lumen obstruction (seven eyes) and stent malposition (six eyes). None of the adverse events were deemed serious.

In 2010 Fea compared in a randomized study the results of phacoemulsification alone vs combined surgery (i.e. phacoemulsification and stent implantation).[12] The baseline IOP was similar in the two groups (combined group: 17.9 +/-2.6; control group: 17.3 +/-3.0 mm Hg) with a similar number of medications (2.,0 +/- 0.9 in the combined group and 1.9 +/-0.7 in the control group). Post-operative mean IOP at 15 months was 14.8 +/-1.2 and 15.7 +/- 1.1 respectively in the combined and in the control group (p=0.031). The author demonstrated that at 15 months the mean number of ocular hypotensive medications was significantly lower in the combined group (0.4 +/- 0.7 and 1.3 +/- 1.0, respectively; P = .007). Furthermore, after wash-out of ocular hypotensive medications, IOP was significantly lower in the combined group (16.6 +/- 3.1 mm Hg and 19.2 +/- 3.5 mm Hg). These results confirm the previous observation that IOP reduction could only partially be attributed to phacoemulsification and was in fact enhanced further by implantation of the iStent. The same author previously published a case report demonstrating the effectiveness of the procedure in one pseudophakic patient.[13]

More recently the effect of the iStent on flow was further elucidated by a fluorophotometic study by Fernandez-Barrientos et al.[14] Thirty-three eyes of 33 patients were randomized to either two stents and cataract surgery (n = 17, Group 1) or cataract surgery alone (n = 16, Group 2). Before surgery, flow and outflow facility were similar between Groups 1 and 2 (1.78 +/- 0.44 and 1.74 +/- 0.82 microL/min; P = 0.18; 0.12 +/- 0.03 and 0.13 +/- 0.06 microL/min/mm H; P = 0.71, respectively). At one year, outflow facility was significantly higher in the group with two stents (0.45 +/- 0.27 microL/min/mm Hg in Group 1 and 0.19 +/- 0.05 microL/min/mm Hg in Group 2; P = 0.02).

A larger prospective, randomized, open-label, controlled, multicenter clinical trial with a total of 240 eyes with mild to moderate open-angle glaucoma with intraocular pressure (IOP) ≤ 24 mmHg controlled on one to three medications compared the results of the patients who were randomized to undergo cataract surgery with iStent implantation (treatment group) or cataract surgery only (control).[15] The primary efficacy measure was unmedicated IOP ≤ 21 mmHg at one year. A secondary measure was unmedicated IOP reduction ≥ 20% at one year. Safety measures included best-corrected visual acuity (BCVA), slit-lamp observations, complications and adverse events. The study met the primary efficacy endpoint, with 72% of treatment eyes versus 50% of control eyes achieving the criterion (P<0.001). At one year, IOP in both treatment groups was statistically lower from baseline values. Sixty-six percent of treatment eyes versus 48% of control eyes achieved ≥ 20% IOP reduction without medication (P = 0.003). The overall incidence of adverse events was similar between groups with no unanticipated adverse device effects. This larger series not only further demonstrates the efficacy of the iStent in further lowering the intraocular pressure in patients undergoing cataract surgery, but also points out the safety of the procedure. A longer post-operative follow-up through two years was reported more recently.[16] Best-corrected visual acuity of 20/40 or better was reported in 93% of treatment vs. 91% of control eyes at two years. Over the two year period, post-operative adverse events occurring at a level of 5% or greater included posterior capsular opacification (6% treatment vs. 10% control), elevated IOP (4% vs. 7%, respectively), visual disturbance (3% vs. 7%, respectively) and iritis (1% vs. 5%, respectively). Furthermore, in the treatment group, stent obstruction and malposition occurred in a small percentage of eyes (4% and 3%, respectively) and resolved shortly after occurrence (with or without treatment). The authors concluded that the overall long-term safety of iStents implanted during cataract surgery was similar to that of cataract surgery alone and that the adverse event/complication rate was low through the two year post-operative period.

4.2 Trabectome

The results obtained by the Trabectome can be summarized by a single paper which reports the experience of the Trabectome group. In this retrospective case series the authors reported their experience on follow-up through one year on 143 of 1127 Trabectome surgical procedures, including 102 through one year from 738 Trabectome-only and 41 through one year from 366 Trabectome-phacoemulsification surgeries[17]. It should be pointed out that many eyes at relatively high risk for filtering surgery failure were included after prior failed trabeculectomy or other previous surgeries were included in the study. Considering glaucoma surgery only: 273 underwent SLT, 170 ALT, 20 aqueous shunt surgery, 104 trabeculectomy, five prior Trabectome and five laser iridectomy.

Considering all cases, mean pre-operative IOP of 23.8 +/- 7.7 mm Hg decreased by 39% to 16.5 +/- 4.0 mm Hg at 24 months (n = 50). Intra-operative reflux bleeding occurred in 77.6%. Medications decreased from 2.8 to 1.2 by 24 months. Sixty-five patients (5.8%) had IOP elevation > 10 mm Hg above baseline on day one. Failure led to trabeculectomy in 5.9% (n = 67) and shunt installation in 1.6% (n = 18). Kaplan-Meier failure was defined across groups with at least two weeks follow-up as IOP > 21 mm Hg with or without medications and not reduced by 20% below baseline on two consecutive visits or repeat surgery. For Trabectome-only cases, mean preoperative IOP of 25.7 +/- 7.7 mm Hg was reduced by 40% to 16.6 +/- 4.0 mm Hg at 24 months (n = 46). No prolonged hypotony, choroidal effusion, choroidal haemorrhage or infections occurred. Failure led to trabeculectomy in 8.1% (n = 60) and shunt installation in 1.9% (n = 14). Medications decreased from 2.93 to 1.2 by 24 months. For Trabectome-phacoemulsification cases, baseline IOP of 20.0 +/- 6.2 mm Hg decreased at 12 months to 15.9 +/- 3.3 mm Hg (18%) (n = 45) and medications decreased from 2.63 +/- 1.12 to 1.50 +/- 1.36. Sixteen (4.4%) of 365 had prior failed trabeculectomy and 139 of 365 (38%) had prior laser trabeculoplasty.

Although the the large number of patients who underwent surgery of the study are very impressive, there are major limitations, including the retrospective nature and the fact that a very small number of procedures reported had been followed up postoperatively. Of the 738 patients who underwent only the Trabectome procedure, only 102 had a one year follow-up and of the 366 with combined surgery only 41 were followed up to one year. Furthermore, it is not clear if the patients with a longer follow-up and with available data include those high risk patients who were originally included in the study. If this is the case it would have been very important to analyse if there was any difference in terms of efficacy in the high versus low risk patients.

Recently, Knape and Smith[18] presented the case of a patient who had intra-operative blood reflux onto peripheral iris during trabeculectomy 11 months after Trabectome surgery. After having left the eye firm after surgery, the author did not report any other episode of hyphema during the following period. He hypothesizes that the absence of overlying angle structures, including the roof of Schlemm's canal, may have allowed blood to reflux into the angle and onto peripheral iris during a sudden decrease in intraocular pressure in trabeculectomy surgery. This self-limited episode suggests that the trabeculotomy remained patent, although the patient was not compensated and points out that further studies to assess the consequences of permanent trabecular meshwork tissue removal may be warranted.

More recently, Jea[19] reported on a cohort of patients and showed that a previously failed Trabectome surgery does not seem to impact the effect of subsequent trabeculectomy.

5. Complications prevention and treatment

Bleeding: bleeding with iStent, Trabectome or other trabecular bypass procedures is generally minimal, although aspiration of the blood in phakic eyes is suggested in order to allow proper visualization.. A very rare occurrence of more significant bleeding in the anterior chamber is generally due to damage of the iris either because the surgeon did not aim at the correct site or because involuntary movements occurred during surgery. The use of air or viscoelastics can stop the haemorrhage. It is generally advisable to postpone the trabecular bypass procedure if massive bleeding occurred previously because angle visualization can be difficult and because the source of bleeding and the effect on the angle structures are easier to visualize after the hyphema has cleared.

Malposition: the iStent may at times appear malpositioned. This does not preclude the implantation of another one provided the angle can be visualized. It is advisable to move at least two or three clock hours away from the previous implant to better visualize the meshwork.

Occlusion: occlusion of the Stent by a seemingly fibrinous plug can sometimes be seen during the postoperative follow-up. This may sometimes be eliminated by a single YAG laser spot.

Endothelial damage: although possible, it has never been reported with any of the procedures described.

6. Conclusions

The idea of approaching the surgery site *ab interno* is certainly appealing. The opportunity to perform a more standardized procedure and the opportunity to preserve the conjunctiva and the sites of eventual subsequent surgery are attractive. Furthermore, creating a direct communication between Schlemm's canal and the anterior chamber is a more physiological approach to IOP reduction with a lower rate of complications and a faster surgery compared to any other available approach.

Several studies pointed out the efficacy of the iStent in the reduction of IOP, although these studies were mainly performed in conjunction with cataract surgery. Nevertheless, there is strong evidence both *in vitro* and *in vivo* that the stent insertion actually facilitates outflow independent of the concurrent phacoemulsification. The procedure is safe and complications are mainly limited to a small (and transient) blood reflux into the anterior chamber immediately upon insertion into Schlemm's canal. It should be noted, however, that all studies were performed in eyes with relatively low pre-operative IOP. At present there is no published evidence of the efficacy in patients with severe glaucoma nor what would be the impact in patients with higher baseline IOP.

Upon casual review of the number of cases reported by the papers on the Trabectome and the length of the follow-up, it may appear that the evidence of efficacy of this surgical method is more stringent. The net IOP reduction seems higher with the Trabectome compared to the iStent and patients at higher risk had been treated with this method. However, a more accurate analysis of the literature reveals that a very small number of patients have been followed for a reasonable amount of time. Futhermore, the ablation of part of the trabecular meshwork is certainly a more destructive procedure, although it seems that this fact does not impact upon the results of conventional surgery in the limited series followed for an adequate postoperative timeframe.

IOP outcomes with both approaches are usually in the mid-teens. Although mid-teens IOP might be adequate for initial and moderate patients, traditional filtering surgery with anti-fibrotic enhancement and bleb formation will probably remain the principal surgical approach to eyes with advanced glaucomatous optic neuropathy. Eventually more advanced patients may benefit from trabecular bypass surgery combined with hypotensive medications, but too little data are available at present to sustain this approach. Assuming ongoing clinical studies continue to be favourable, a strong argument can be made for use of these minimally invasive procedures which do not lead to bleb formation nor require anti-fibrotics, early in the glaucoma injury process, especially considering the difficulties of compliance with medical therapy. Neither of these procedures damages the conjunctiva superiorly, leaving surgical alternatives where necessary open. Furthermore, continued development of suprachoroidal stents (such as the iStent supra and the newer Transcend Cypass) may offer additional IOP lowering and thus serve a broader population of patients with more advanced disease.

Given that glaucoma is typically a chronic disease and that the introduction of these methods is relatively new, follow-up of the patients at the moment is limited to two years at maximum.

Trabecular surgery requires some learning curve to visualize the angle using a hand-held gonioprims and the diffuse illumination of the microscope gives a different appearance of the angle's structures as compared with slit lamp gonioscopy. Furthermore, the need for using a hand to hold the gonioprism makes any trabecular surgery strictly bimanual. During surgery, the implantation of the iStent is relatively easier compared with the Trabectome, because it does not need a continuous circumferential movement and because the chamber is well formed with viscoelastics. After the implantation of the device, the blood reflux in the anterior chamber is generally minimal with the iStent.

On the other hand, the Trabectome allows a visual feeling that the trabecular meshwork is ablated, whereas it is sometimes difficult to be sure of the correct iStent placement, especially when blood cannot be completely washed from the angle. Compared to trabeculectomy, additional costs with any device should also be considered. Furthermore at present only the Trabectome has been cleared by the FDA, although U.S. FDA approval of the iStent is expected in the near future.

7. References

[1] Janz NK, Wren PA, Lichter PR, et al. The Collaborative Initial Glaucoma Treatment Study: interim quality of life findings after initial medical or surgical treatment of glaucoma. Ophthalmology 2001;108:1954 –1965

[2] Higginbotham EJ, Stevens RK, Musch DC, et al. Bleb related endophthalmitis after trabeculectomy with mitomycin C. Ophthalmology 1996;103:650–656.

[3] Soltau JB, Rothman RF, Budenz DL, et al. Risk factors for glaucoma filtering bleb infections. Arch Ophthalmol 2000; 118:338 –342.

[4] Greenfield DS, Suner IJ, Miller MP, Kangas TA, Palmberg PF, Flynn HW. Endophthalmitis after filtering surgery with mitomycin. Arch Ophthalmol 1996;114:943–949.

[5] Fontana H, Nouri-Mahdavi K, Lumba J, Ralli M, Caprioli J. Trabeculectomy with mitomycin C: outcomes and risk factors for failure in phakic open-angle glaucoma. Ophthalmology 2006;113:930-6

[6] Anand N, Arora S, Clowes M. Mitomycin C augmented glaucoma surgery: evolution of filtering bleb avascularity, transconjunctival oozing, and leaks. Br J Ophthalmol 2006;90:175-80.

[7] Trabectome description at http://www.ncbi.nlm.nih.gov.proxy-medicina.unito.it/pubmed/16378021.

[8] Trabectome description at http://www.ncbi.nlm.nih.gov.proxy-medicina.unito.it/pubmed/18936637.

[9] Bahler C, Smedley G, Zhou J, Johnson D. Trabecular bypass stents decrease intraocular pressure in cultured human anterior segments. Am J Ophthal 2004; 138:988-994.

[10] Spiegel D, Wetzel W. Haffner DS, Hill RA. Initial clinical experience with the trabecular micro-bypass stent in patients with glaucoma. Adv Ther 2007;24:161-170.

[11] Spiegel D, Wetzel W, Neuhann T, Sturmer J, Hoh H, Garcia-Feijoo J, Martinez de la casa JM, Garcia-Sanchez J. Coexistent primary open-angle glaucoma and cataract: interim analysis of a trabecular micro-bypass stent and concurrent cataract surgery. Eur J Ophthalmol 2009; 19:393-399.

[12] Fea AM. Phacoemulsification versus phacoemulsification with micro-bypass stent implantation in primary open-angle glaucoma. J Cataract Refract Surg 2010;36:407-412.

[13] Fea A, Dogliani M, Macetta F et al. Case report: The trabecular bypass stent in a pseudophakic glaucoma patient: A 1-year follow-up. Clinical Ophthalmology 2008;2:931-934.

[14] Fernández-Barrientos Y, Garcia-Feijoó J, Martínez de la Casa JM, et al. Fluorophotometric study of the effect of the Glaukos trabecular micro-bypass stent on aqueous humor dynamics. Invest Ophthalmol Vis Sci 2010;51:3327-3332.

[15] Samuelson TW, Katz LJ, Wells JM, et al. Randomized evaluation of the trabecular micro-bypass stent with phacoemulsification in patients with glaucoma and cataract. Ophthalmology 2011;118:459-467.

[16] Craven ER. Prospective, Randomized Controlled Trial of Cataract Surgery with Trabecular Micro-Bypass Stent in Mild-Moderate Open Angle Glaucoma: Safety in Two Year Follow-up. Paper presented at 2011 American Society of Cataract and Refractive Surgeons, April, 2011; San Diego, CA.

[17] Minckler D,* Mosaed S, Dustin L, Francis B, AND the Trabectome Study Group†. Trabectome (trabeculectomy-internal approach): additional experience and extended follow-up. Trans Am Ophthalmol Soc 2008;106:149-160

[18] Knape RM and Smith MF. Anterior chamber blood reflux during trabeculectomy in an eye with previous Trabectome surgery. J Glaucoma 2010;19:499–500

[19] Jea SY, Mosaed S, Vold SD, Rhee DJ. Effect of a Failed Trabectome on Subsequent Trabeculectomy. J Glaucoma. 2011 Feb 17. [Epub ahead of print]

Permissions

The contributors of this book come from diverse backgrounds, making this book a truly international effort. This book will bring forth new frontiers with its revolutionizing research information and detailed analysis of the nascent developments around the world.

We would like to thank Shimon Rumelt, MD, MPA, for lending his expertise to make the book truly unique. He has played a crucial role in the development of this book. Without his invaluable contribution this book wouldn't have been possible. He has made vital efforts to compile up to date information on the varied aspects of this subject to make this book a valuable addition to the collection of many professionals and students.

This book was conceptualized with the vision of imparting up-to-date information and advanced data in this field. To ensure the same, a matchless editorial board was set up. Every individual on the board went through rigorous rounds of assessment to prove their worth. After which they invested a large part of their time researching and compiling the most relevant data for our readers. Conferences and sessions were held from time to time between the editorial board and the contributing authors to present the data in the most comprehensible form. The editorial team has worked tirelessly to provide valuable and valid information to help people across the globe.

Every chapter published in this book has been scrutinized by our experts. Their significance has been extensively debated. The topics covered herein carry significant findings which will fuel the growth of the discipline. They may even be implemented as practical applications or may be referred to as a beginning point for another development. Chapters in this book were first published by InTech; hereby published with permission under the Creative Commons Attribution License or equivalent.

The editorial board has been involved in producing this book since its inception. They have spent rigorous hours researching and exploring the diverse topics which have resulted in the successful publishing of this book. They have passed on their knowledge of decades through this book. To expedite this challenging task, the publisher supported the team at every step. A small team of assistant editors was also appointed to further simplify the editing procedure and attain best results for the readers.

Our editorial team has been hand-picked from every corner of the world. Their multi-ethnicity adds dynamic inputs to the discussions which result in innovative outcomes. These outcomes are then further discussed with the researchers and contributors who give their valuable feedback and opinion regarding the same. The feedback is then collaborated with the researches and they are edited in a comprehensive manner to aid the understanding of the subject.

Apart from the editorial board, the designing team has also invested a significant amount of their time in understanding the subject and creating the most relevant covers. They scrutinized every image to scout for the most suitable representation of the subject and create an appropriate cover for the book.

The publishing team has been involved in this book since its early stages. They were actively engaged in every process, be it collecting the data, connecting with the contributors or procuring relevant information. The team has been an ardent support to the editorial, designing and production team. Their endless efforts to recruit the best for this project, has resulted in the accomplishment of this book. They are a veteran in the field of academics and their pool of knowledge is as vast as their experience in printing. Their expertise and guidance has proved useful at every step. Their uncompromising quality standards have made this book an exceptional effort. Their encouragement from time to time has been an inspiration for everyone.

The publisher and the editorial board hope that this book will prove to be a valuable piece of knowledge for researchers, students, practitioners and scholars across the globe.

List of Contributors

Magdalena Zdybel, Barbara Pilawa and Anna Krzeszewska-Zaręba
Medical University of Silesia in Katowice, Poland

Zan Pan
Margaret Dyson Vision Institute, Weill Cornell Medical College, New York, NY, USA

José E. Capó-Aponte
Visual Sciences Branch, U.S. Army Aeromedical Research Laboratory, Fort Rucker, AL, USA

José E. Capó-Aponte and Peter S. Reinach
Department of Biological Science, State University of New York, College of Optometry, New York, NY, USA

Pradeep Prasad, Allen Hu, Robert Beardsley and Jean-Pierre Hubschman
Retina Division, Jules Stein Eye Institute,

Pradeep Prasad, Allen Hu, Robert Beardsley and Jean-Pierre Hubschman
Department of Ophthalmology, David Geffen School of Medicine at University of California, Los Angeles, California, USA

Yureeda Qazi, Aslihan Turhan and Pedram Hamrah
Cornea Service, Massachusetts Eye and Ear Infirmary, Department of Ophthalmology, Harvard Medical School, USA

Miroslav Vukosavljević, Milorad Milivojević and Mirko Resan
Eye Clinic, Military Medical Academy, Belgrade, Serbia

De-Quan Li and Zhijie Li
Ocular Surface Center, Cullen Eye Institute, Department of Ophthalmology, Baylor College of Medicine, Houston, TX, USA

Zuguo Liu
Xiamen Eye Institute, Xiamen University, Xiamen, China

Zhijie Li
Key Laboratory for Regenerative Medicine of Ministry of Education and Department of Ophthalmology, Jinan University, Guangzhou, China

Zhichong Wang
State Key Laboratory of Ophthalmology, Zhongshan Ophthalmic Center, Sun Yat-sen University, Guangzhou, China

Hong Qi
Department of Ophthalmology, Peking University Third Hospital, Beijing, China

Dasha Nelidova and Trevor Sherwin
Department of Ophthalmology, Faculty of Medical and Health Sciences, University of Auckland, Auckland, New Zealand

Ashok Kumar Narsani, Shafi Muhammad Jatoi, and Khairuddin Shah
Department of Ophthalmology, Liaquat University Eye Hospital, Hyderabad Sindh, Pakistan

Mohan Perkash Maheshwari
Department of Pharmacology, Baqai Medical University, Karachi Sindh, Pakistan

Elina Landa, Shimon Rumelt and Elaine Wong
Department of Ophthalmology, Western Galilee – Nahariya Medical Center, Nahariya, Israel

Claudia Yahalom
Department of Ophthalmology, Hadassah University Hospital, Jerusalem, Israel

Lionel Kowal
Department of Ophthalmology, Eye and Ear Institute, The University of Melbourne, Melbourne, Australia

John R. Phillips, Simon Backhouse and Andrew V. Collins
Department of Optometry and Vision Science, The University of Auckland, New Zealand

Luciane B. Moreira
Ophthalmology Department, Federal University of Paraná, Curitiba, Brazil

Maria C. Arbelaez
Muscat Eye Laser Centre, Oman

Samuel Arba-Mosquera
Grupo de Investigación de Cirugía Refractiva y Calidad de Visión, Instituto de Oftalmobiología Aplicada, University of Valladolid, Valladolid, Spain

Samuel Arba-Mosquera
SCHWIND Eye-Tech-Solutions, Kleinostheim, Germany

Milorad Milivojević, Miroslav Vukosavljević and Mirko Resan
Eye Clinic, Military Medical Academy, Belgrade, Serbia

Luis A. Rodriguez and Anny E. Villegas
Corneal Clinic, Centro Medico Docente La Trinidad (CMDLT), Caracas, Venezuela

Sanja Masnec Olujić
Ghethaldus Ophthalmology Policlinics, Zagreb, Croatia

Mirko Resan, Miroslav Vukosavljević and Milorad Milivojević
Eye Clinic, Military Medical Academy, Belgrade, Serbia

Antonio Fea, Giulia Consolandi, Giulia Pignata, Davide Turco, Paola Cannizzo, Elena Bartoli, Teresa Rolle and Federico M. Grignolo
Clinica Oculistica, Universita' degli Studi di Torino, Italy